1,000,000 Books

are available to read at

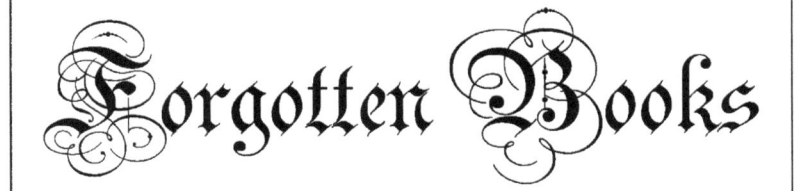

Forgotten Books

www.ForgottenBooks.com

Read online
Download PDF
Purchase in print

ISBN 978-1-334-36421-1
PIBN 10568187

This book is a reproduction of an important historical work. Forgotten Books uses state-of-the-art technology to digitally reconstruct the work, preserving the original format whilst repairing imperfections present in the aged copy. In rare cases, an imperfection in the original, such as a blemish or missing page, may be replicated in our edition. We do, however, repair the vast majority of imperfections successfully; any imperfections that remain are intentionally left to preserve the state of such historical works.

Forgotten Books is a registered trademark of FB &c Ltd.
Copyright © 2018 FB &c Ltd.
FB &c Ltd, Dalton House, 60 Windsor Avenue, London, SW19 2RR.
Company number 08720141. Registered in England and Wales.

For support please visit www.forgottenbooks.com

1 MONTH OF FREE READING

at

www.ForgottenBooks.com

By purchasing this book you are eligible for one month membership to ForgottenBooks.com, giving you unlimited access to our entire collection of over 1,000,000 titles via our web site and mobile apps.

To claim your free month visit:

www.forgottenbooks.com/free568187

* Offer is valid for 45 days from date of purchase. Terms and conditions apply.

English
Français
Deutsche
Italiano
Español
Português

www.forgottenbooks.com

Mythology Photography **Fiction** Fishing Christianity **Art** Cooking Essays Buddhism Freemasonry Medicine **Biology** Music **Ancient Egypt** Evolution Carpentry Physics Dance Geology **Mathematics** Fitness Shakespeare **Folklore** Yoga Marketing **Confidence** Immortality Biographies Poetry **Psychology** Witchcraft Electronics Chemistry History **Law** Accounting **Philosophy** Anthropology Alchemy Drama Quantum Mechanics Atheism Sexual Health **Ancient History Entrepreneurship** Languages Sport Paleontology Needlework Islam **Metaphysics** Investment Archaeology Parenting Statistics Criminology **Motivational**

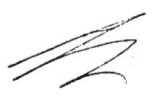

STUDIES IN THE PALAEOPATHOLOGY
OF EGYPT

THE UNIVERSITY OF CHICAGO PRESS
CHICAGO, ILLINOIS

THE BAKER & TAYLOR COMPANY
NEW YORK

THE CAMBRIDGE UNIVERSITY PRESS
LONDON

THE MARUZEN-KABUSHIKI-KAISHA
TOKYO, OSAKA, KYOTO, FUKUOKA, SENDAI

THE MISSION BOOK COMPANY

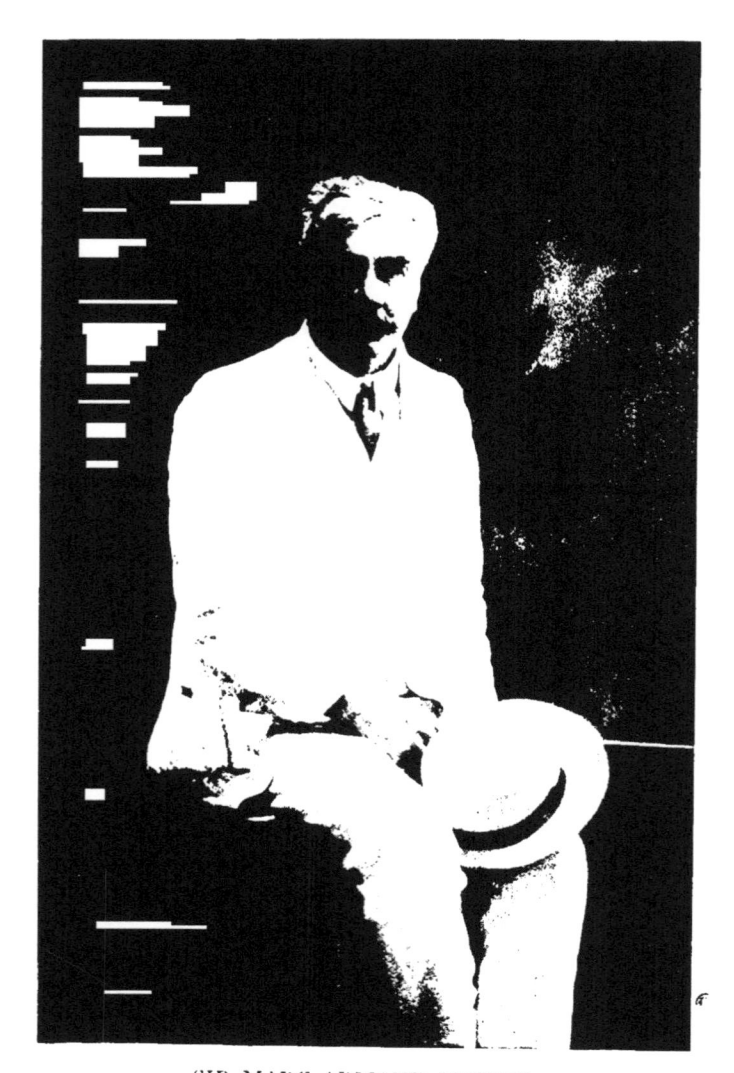

SIR MARC ARMAND RUFFER

STUDIES IN THE PALAEOPATHOLOGY OF EGYPT

By

SIR MARC ARMAND RUFFER, Kt., C.M.G., M.D.

Late President of the Quarantine Council of Egypt; formerly Director of the British Institute of Preventive Medicine; Professor of Bacteriology in the Cairo Medical School; Member of the Indian Plague Commission, etc.

Edited by

ROY L. MOODIE, Ph.D.

Associate Professor of Anatomy in the University of Illinois

THE UNIVERSITY OF CHICAGO PRESS
CHICAGO, ILLINOIS

Copyright 1921 By
The University of Chicago Press

All Rights Reserved

Published October 1921

Composed and Printed By
The University of Chicago Press
Chicago, Illinois, U.S.A.

PREFACE

Sir Marc Armand Ruffer, whose *Studies in Palaeopathology* constitute this volume, had intended to retire from active duty in 1919 and devote his attention to the preparation of a work dealing with his antiquarian studies of ancient Egypt. The present collection of papers issued under the direction of his wife, Lady Ruffer, is intended to replace that proposed undertaking. While the details of his plan are uncertain, since he left no notes on the project, it has been deemed best to select only those studies which deal with the evidences of disease in ancient Egypt. These by no means represent his life's work, but are rather the result of one of his keenest interests during the twenty years of his residence in Egypt.

When Sir Armand Ruffer left in December, 1916, on his mission to Salonika, where he had gone to reorganize the sanitary service of the Greek Provisional Government, he left with Lady Ruffer the titles and notes of several unpublished papers which he intended to finish on his return. Since his death at sea in the spring of 1917, as he was returning from Salonika, Lady Ruffer has issued five of these studies. Two of them, "Some Recent Researches on Prehistoric Trephining" and "Arthritis Deformans and Spondylitis in Ancient Egypt," appeared in 1918 in the *Journal of Pathology and Bacteriology* under the title "Studies in Palaeopathology." A third was printed by the Geological Survey of Egypt, with the title "Studies in Palaeopathology, A Pathological Specimen Dating from the Lower Miocene Period," describing spondylitis in an early crocodile.

His *Food in Egypt* has been printed in quarto by the Institut d'Egypt, and his "Consanguineous Marriages among Egyptian Kings" in the History of Medicine section of the *Proceedings* of the Royal Society of Medicine in London. One study, that on diseases of the teeth in ancient Egypt, is published in a recent number of the *American Journal of Physical Anthropology*. Another study, with the title "Alcohol and Alcoholism in Ancient Egypt," is regarded by Lady Ruffer and her advisers as too incomplete for publication.

PREFACE

The present work is the first separate volume to be devoted entirely to a discussion of palaeopathology, although there are several large memoirs which have devoted considerable space to an account of ancient pathology. Such, for instance, are the works of G. Elliot Smith and F. Wood Jones in the *Report of the Archaeological Survey of Nubia* and that of Lortet and Gaillard on the mummified fauna of Egypt. Sir Armand Ruffer made the first move toward establishing the science of palaeopathology as a distinct subject, and he gave the first definition of the science in medical literature; although there had been a prior definition of the subject by American palaeontologists. Palaeopathology has an especial appeal to students of medical literature and particularly to those who find an interest and a delight in the history of medicine. The subject is of importance also to Egyptologists in showing them something of the intimate life of the makers of the pyramids.

Acknowledgment is gladly made the publishers and editors of the *Annals of Medical History*, the *Journal of Pathology and Bacteriology*, the *British Medical Journal*, the *Cairo Scientific Journal*, the *Mémoires présentés à l'Institut d'Égypte*, the *Bulletin de la Société Archéologique d'Alexandrie*, the *American Journal of Physical Anthropology*, and Professor Karl Sudhoff, of Leipzig, for their kind permission to reprint the studies in the present volume. Professor James Ritchie, of Edinburgh, has granted the use of twenty-nine engravings from the *Journal of Pathology and Bacteriology*. It is a pleasure to express to Professor James H. Breasted our gratitude for the use of his "Chronological Summary" of Egyptian history, which, on his advice, has been taken from his *History of the Ancient Egyptians*.

My own connection with the volume began when Lady Ruffer requested me to find an American publisher for the book. Following a request of mine for permission to dedicate my monograph on the palaeontological evidences of disease, now in preparation, to Sir Armand Ruffer, which Lady Ruffer has kindly granted, there has grown up between us a most delightful friendship. My first acquaintance with Sir Armand Ruffer's studies in palaeopathology was in 1912 when I saw his "Histological Studies on Egyptian Mummies" in the library at the University of Kansas. Since my work on evidences of disease among fossil vertebrates and ancient men has a close connection with his work on ancient Egyptians, it is especially pleasant to be intrusted by Lady Ruffer with such an important undertaking as the issuing of her husband's *Studies in the Palaeopathology of Egypt.*

ROY L. MOODIE

DEPARTMENT OF ANATOMY
COLLEGE OF MEDICINE
UNIVERSITY OF ILLINOIS
CHICAGO, ILLINOIS

CONTENTS

	PAGE
LIST OF ILLUSTRATIONS	xi
BIOGRAPHICAL SKETCH	xiii
BIBLIOGRAPHY OF THE WRITINGS OF SIR MARC ARMAND RUFFER, 1888–1920	xvii
NOTE ON THE HISTOLOGY OF EGYPTIAN MUMMIES	1
POTT'SCHE KRANKHEIT AN EINER ÄGYPTISCHEN MUMIE AUS DER ZEIT DER 21. DYNASTIE (UM 1000 V. CHR.)	3
REMARKS ON THE HISTOLOGY AND PATHOLOGICAL ANATOMY OF EGYPTIAN MUMMIES	11
NOTE ON THE PRESENCE OF "BILHARZIA HAEMATOBIA" IN EGYPTIAN MUMMIES OF THE TWENTIETH DYNASTY (1250–1000 B.C.)	18
ON ARTERIAL LESIONS FOUND IN EGYPTIAN MUMMIES (1580 B.C.–525 A.D.)	20
AN ERUPTION RESEMBLING THAT OF VARIOLA IN THE SKIN OF A MUMMY OF THE TWENTIETH DYNASTY (1200–1100 B.C.)	32
ON DWARFS AND OTHER DEFORMED PERSONS IN ANCIENT EGYPT	35
HISTOLOGICAL STUDIES ON EGYPTIAN MUMMIES	49
ON OSSEOUS LESIONS IN ANCIENT EGYPTIANS	93
NOTES ON TWO EGYPTIAN MUMMIES DATING FROM THE PERSIAN OCCUPATION OF EGYPT (525–332 B.C.)	127
ON PATHOLOGICAL LESIONS FOUND IN COPTIC BODIES (400–500 A.D.)	139
ON THE DISEASES OF THE SUDAN AND NUBIA IN ANCIENT TIMES	156
PATHOLOGICAL NOTES ON THE ROYAL MUMMIES OF THE CAIRO MUSEUM	166
A TUMOUR OF THE PELVIS DATING FROM ROMAN TIMES (250 A.D.) AND FOUND IN EGYPT	179
A PATHOLOGICAL SPECIMEN DATING FROM THE LOWER MIOCENE PERIOD	184
SOME RECENT RESEARCHES ON PREHISTORIC TREPHINING	194
ARTHRITIS DEFORMANS AND SPONDYLITIS IN ANCIENT EGYPT	212
A STUDY OF ABNORMALITIES AND PATHOLOGY OF ANCIENT EGYPTIAN TEETH	268
ON THE PHYSICAL EFFECTS OF CONSANGUINEOUS MARRIAGES IN THE ROYAL FAMILIES OF ANCIENT EGYPT	322
APPENDIX	358
INDEX	367

LIST OF ILLUSTRATIONS

	FACING PAGE
Sir Marc Armand Ruffer . . . . Frontispiece	
A Trephined Skull . . . . Text figure, page 200	
Plate I. A Mummy of a Priest of Ammon with Pott's Disease . .	10
Plate II. Muscle Fibers and Fungus from the Abscess	10
Plate III–V. Arterial Lesions from Egyptian Mummies	30
Plate VI. Lesions of Variola in the Skin of a Mummy	34
Plate VII. The Dwarf Chnoum-Hotep	48
Plate VIII. Achondroplastic Dwarfs Depicted on Walls of Tombs	48
Plate IX. Other Achondroplastic Dwarfs	48
Plate X–XI. Deformed Persons in Ancient Egypt	48
Plate XII. Embalmed Liver with Image	92
Plate XIII. Embalmed Stomach and Intestines	92
Plate XIV. Embalmed Lung and Heart	92
Plate XV–XXII. Histology of Various Organs from Egyptian Mummies	92
Plate XXIII–XXXI. Osseous Lesions of Ancient Egyptians . .	126
Plate XXXII–XXXVIII. Egyptian Mummies Dating from the Persian Occupation	138
Plate XXXIX–XLIV. Osseous Lesions Found in Coptic Bodies	154
Plate XLV–XLVI. An Osteosarcoma of the Pelvis	182
Plate XLVII–XLVIII. Spondylitis Deformans in a Miocene Crocodile	192
Plate XLIX–LIV. Arthritis Deformans and Spondylitis in Ancient Egyptians	266
Plate LV–LXII. Lesions of the Teeth and Jaws of Ancient Egyptians	320
Plate LXIII–LXXI. Ancient Royal Egyptians as Seen in Their Mummies, Statues, Tombs, and Coins	356

BIOGRAPHICAL SKETCH[1]

Original investigation in medical history of late years has been furthered in remarkable ways by archaeologists, anthropologists, numismatists, antiquarians, collectors of engravings, sinologists, Egyptologists, and particularly by travelers and explorers. Indeed, the journey method of Sudhoff goes to show that he who enjoys the advantages of travel is much more likely to turn up new facts than the stationary investigator. One of the most prominent exponents of this new tendency was Sir Marc Armand Ruffer, late president of the Sanitary Council of Egypt, who lost his life at sea during the spring of 1917 on his return from Salonika, where he had gone to reorganize the sanitary service of the Greek Provisional Government. He made his mark in the medical history of ancient Egypt by his contributions to its palaeopathology, in particular the palaeohistology of the pathological lesions found in mummies of the XVIIIth–XXVIIth Dynasties.

He was born at Lyons, France, in 1859, the son of the late Baron Alphonse Jacques de Ruffer. His mother was a German. He was educated at Brasenose College, Oxford, where he took his B.A. degree in 1883, and at University College, London, becoming Bachelor of Medicine and Surgery in 1887 and Doctor of Medicine in 1889. He then became a pupil of Pasteur and Metchnikoff at the Pasteur Institute, devoting special study to the then novel subject of phagocytosis. In his papers of 1890, he gave an early and timely exposition of Metchnikoff's concept of inflammation as a protective mechanism against infection, particularly in the intestinal canal. He described the diphtheritic membrane as "a battlefield," in which pathogenic bacteria and amoeboid leucocytes contend for mastery. In 1891, Ruffer became the first director of the British Institute of Preventive Medicine, his assistant being his wife, Alice Mary Ruffer, who prepared many colored drawings. At Metchnikoff's instance, Ruffer and Plimmer took up the study

[1] Slightly modified from a memorial notice by F. H. Garrison, *Annals of Medical History*, I (1919), 218.

of cancer and established the provisional status of the quasi-parasitic formations in cancer cells. While testing the new diphtheritic serum at the Institute, Ruffer fell a victim to the disease, and he was so severely smitten with the paralytic sequelae that he felt compelled to resign his directorship. He then went to Egypt for recuperation and subsequently took up his permanent residence at the Villa Ménival, Ramleh.

Ruffer was one of the ablest organizers of medical administration in recent times. He did much to make the present Lister Institute what it is today, became professor of bacteriology in the Cairo Medical School (1896), which he reorganized, and was the president of the Sanitary, Maritime, and Quarantine Council of Egypt (1901–17), in which office he was instrumental in ridding Egypt of cholera by rigorous hygienic policing of the routes of pilgrimage at the Tor Station and elsewhere. In this work he enjoyed the confidence and support of both Lord Cromer and Lord Kitchener. He served on the Indian Plague Commission, was Egyptian delegate to sanitary conferences of 1903, 1907, and 1911, and from the outbreak of the war was highly efficient as head of the Red Cross in Egypt. He was the recipient of many honors and decorations, and was knighted in 1916. A man of the world in the widest sense, he was a remarkable linguist, a talented violoncellist, and an expert at his favorite game of billiards.

In December, 1908, in connection with the excavations made in Nubia by Reisner, Elliot Smith, Wood Jones, and Derry prior to the flooding of the country by the raising of the Assuan dam (1907), Ruffer began to exhibit microscopic sections of pathological lesions in mummies at the Cairo Scientific Society. In this field Fouquet was the pioneer (1889), but Ruffer made it his own by his expert skill in microtomic technique and staining methods. To overcome the hard, brittle, and friable character of the tissues, before cutting them with a Minot microtome, he softened them in a solution of alcohol and sodium bicarbonate, with subsequent hardening in alcohol. For this new branch of pathological histology he devised the term "palaeopathology." His "preliminary note" of 1909 (*British Medical Journal*, I [1909], 1005) was followed by a striking series of papers on the presence of Bilharzia haematobia in Egyptian mummies of the XXth Dynasty, 1250–1000 B.C. (*ibid.*, I [1910], 16), on a varioloid eruption in the skin of a mummy of the same period (*Journal of Pathology and Bacteriology*, Cambridge, XV [1910–11], 1–3, 1 pl.), on arterial lesions in mummies of 1580 B.C.—525 A.D. (*ibid.*, 453–62, 3 pls.), on the osseous lesions in Egyptian skeletons, ranging from 2980 B.C. to the Greek period (*ibid.*, XVI [1911–12], 439–65, 9 pls.), on dental, osseous, and articular lesions in Coptic bodies of 400–500 A.D. (*ibid*, XVIII [1913–14], 149–62, 6 pls.), on a tumor of the pelvis from the catacombs of Kom el Shougafa, 250 A.D. (*ibid.*, 480–84, 2 pls.), and a monograph on "Histological Studies on Egyptian Mummies" (Cairo, 1911). In 1910, Elliot Smith and Ruffer described a case of Pott's disease in a mummy of the XXIst Dynasty, *ca.* 1000 B.C. (Giessen, 1910), perhaps the earliest landmark we have in the history of tuberculosis. In these studies Ruffer showed the presence of calcified Bilharzia eggs in the kidneys of two mummies, a common cause of prehistoric haematuria, as shown in the hieroglyphs and medical papyri; also the common occurrence of arthritis, spondylitis deformans, dental caries, rarefying periodontitis, pyorrhea alveolaris, Bouchard's nodes, malarial enlargement of the spleen, biliary calculi, and particularly arteriosclerosis (atheroma) which was found even in the aorta of Ramses II, and was as frequent three thousand years ago as it is today. Its causation Ruffer leaves an open question, since, in his view, alcohol, tobacco, meat diet, strenuous exercise, and "wear and tear" could, none of them, have availed to produce it. His final studies of dental and osseous lesions in specimens dug up at Faras (100 B.C.—300 A.D.) and at Merawi (750–500 B.C.) in the Sudan (*Sudhoff's Mitth.*, XIII [1914], 453) led him to the conclusion that these people were short lived, dying before fifty. The war interrupted his work, which was cut short forever by his untimely death, but he had already planned a volume of studies which is represented by the present collection of papers.

Ruffer's large-hearted, sympathetic personality made him well loved by every class and nationality in the cosmopolitan city of Alexandria. Some native pashas on the Municipal Council, of which Ruffer was for some years vice-president, remarked to Lady Ruffer after her husband's death that no one had ever been so mourned and regretted by them as he even after three years. A young medical officer remarked, during the war: "Sir Ruffer always treats us as if we were his equals; he listens sympathetically to all that interests us, and never talks down to us."

Ruffer's love for the game of billiards has already been mentioned by Dr. Garrison, and it is interesting to learn also of his great love for music; being an accomplished celloist and possessed of a rich baritone voice, he and Lady Ruffer spent many delightful evenings at the piano.

Among other brilliant traits was his unusual pentecostal gift, a real gift of tongues, unusual even for a versatile European. This gift was a very real aid to him in his work on the Quarantine Council, where he had to come in contact with representatives of so many nationalities, often being able to converse with them in their native tongue. This ability, added to his tact and discretion in handling the difficult affairs of the Council which often involved as many as eighteen nations, brought his efforts to establish quarantine stations on the boarder lands to a success. His greatest monument of all, perhaps, is the quarantine station at El Tor, established for the return of Mecca pilgrims in the Peninsula of Sinai, where he encouraged research work on plague, cholera, and dysentery, and from which station several of his own studies were issued.

Ruffer's friend and co-worker for many years, Harry G. Plimmer, says in his obituary notice in *Nature*, May 10, 1917: "As a colleague Ruffer was ideal, ever ready to help and advise, and never thinking of himself; and he was one who had the truest, kindliest, and most appreciative affection for his many friends."

The loss of such a man is truly a great one, and this volume of his studies will go far to keep alive his memory among men with whom he so loved to work and live.

BIBLIOGRAPHY OF THE WRITINGS OF SIR MARC ARMAND RUFFER 1888-1920

1. "Sur l'élimination par les urines des matières solubles vaccinantes fabriquées par les microbes en dehors de l'organisme." *Comptes rendus des séances de l'Academie des Sciences*, 1888, pp. 1-3.
2. The same (cont'd). *Comptes rendus des séances de la Société de Biologie*, XL (October 20, 1888), 696-97. (With M. Charrin.)
3. "Mécanisme de la fièvre dans la maladie pyocyanique." *Comptes rendus des séances de la Société de Biologie*, XLI (March 9, 1889), 208-10. (With M. Charrin.)
4. "Les matières solubles vaccinantes dans le sang des animaux." 1889. 2 pp.
5. "Influence du système nerveux sur l'infection." 1889. 2 pp.
6. "Rabies and Its Preventive Treatment." Lecture given at the Society of Arts, December 6, 1889. 9 pp.

    (The above were written while working at the Pasteur Institute, Paris.)

7. "Nature of the Disease Produced by Inoculation of the Bacillus Pyocyaenus." 1889. Paper read before University College Medical Society, March 7, 1889. 33 pp.
8. "Remarks on the Prevention of Hydrophobia by M. Pasteur's Treatment." *Brit. Med. Jour.*, London, II (1889), 637-43.
9. "On the Phagocytes of the Alimentary Canal." *Quart. Jour. Micros. Sci.*, XXX (February, 1890), 481-505. 1 pl.
10. "On the Destruction of Micro-Organisms by Amoeboid Cells." Paper read before British Medical Association, August 30, 1890. *Brit. Med. Jour.*, London, II (1890), 491-93.
11. "Chronic Hydrocephalus," Part I. Reprinted from *Brain*, XIII (1890), 117-44. Abstract from thesis written to obtain the degree of Doctor of Medicine at the University of Oxford, June, 1888.
12. "Chronic Hydrocephalus," Part II. *Brain*, XIII (1890), 240-69.
13. "On the Destruction of Micro-Organisms during the Process of Inflammation." *Brit. Med. Jour.*, London, I (1890), 1177-83. 2 pls. of pencil drawings by Lady Ruffer.
14. "Preliminary Note on Processes Taking Place in the Diphtheritic Membrane." *Brit. Med. Jour.*, London, II (July 26, 1890), 202-3.
15. "Recherches sur la déstruction des microbes dans les cellules améboïdes dans l'inflammation." 1890. 21 pp. (This paper is a continuation and enlargement of the subject of Paper 13.)
16. "Recent Advances in Bacteriology." *Medical Annual*, 1892. 14 pp. and 2 pls. of water-color drawings by Lady Ruffer.

17. "Immunity against Microbes," Part I. *Quart. Jour. Micros. Sci.*, XXXII (1891), 99-109.
18. "Immunity against Microbes," Part II. *Quart. Jour. Micros. Sci.*, XXXII (1891), 417-50. 2 double-page pls. of water-color drawings by Lady Ruffer.
19. "Remarks Made at the Discussion on Phagocytosis and Immunity at the Pathological Society of London, March 15, 1892." *Brit. Med. Jour.*, London, I (1892), 591-96.
20. "The New Science—Preventive Medicine." *The Nineteenth Century*, December, 1891. 19 pp.
21. "Further Investigations on the Destruction of Micro-Organisms by Amoeboid Cells." *Lancet*, II (December 26, 1891), 377.
22. "Preliminary Note on Some Parasitic Protozoa Found in Cancerous Tumours." *Brit. Med. Jour.*, London, II (July 16, 1892), 113. (With J. H. Walker.)
23. "Second Note on Parasitic Protozoa in Cancerous Tumours." *Brit. Med. Jour.*, London, II (November 5, 1892), 993. (With J. H. Walker.)
24. "On Some Parasitic Protozoa Found in Cancerous Tumours." *Jour. Path. and Bacteriol.*, I (1892), 198-215. 3 pls. of water-color drawings by Lady Ruffer. (With J. H. Walker.)
25. "Do the Interests of Mankind Require Experiments on Living Animals, and If So, Up to What Point Are They Justifiable?" Remarks made at the Church Congress of 1892. 5 pp.
26. "The Morality of Vivisection." *The Nineteenth Century*, November, 1892. 6 pp.
27. "Should Experiments on Animals Be Prohibited by Law?" *Lit. Rev.*, 1892. 8 pp.
28. "The British Institute of Preventive Medicine." Paper read to further its objects at Birmingham, 1892.
29. "On Protozoa and Cancer." *Trans. Path. Soc. Lond.*, XLIV (1893), 209-16. 1 pl. of drawings by Lady Ruffer.
30. "Further Researches on Parasitic Protozoa Found in Cancerous Tumours." *Jour. Path. and Bacteriol*, II (October, 1893), 3-25. 4 pls. colored. (With H. G. Plimmer.)
31. "A Visit to the Institut Pasteur, by an Old Student." *Brit. Med. Jour.*, London, I, January 7, 1893.
32. "The Celebration of Louis Pasteur's Seventieth Birthday: Its Signification." *Med. Mag.*, February, 1893. 10 pp.
33. "Sur les parasites des tumeurs épithéliales malignes." Extrait du *Traité de pathologie générale*, Tome II (décembre, 1895). 12 pp. and 1 pl. woodcut reproduction of water-color illustrations by Lady Ruffer.
34. "Discussion on Diphtheria . . . . and Its Treatment by Serum." *Glasgow Med. Jour.*, July, 1895. 7 pp.
35. "Measures Taken at Tor and Suez against Ships Coming from the Red Sea and the Far East." *Lancet*, London, II (December 30, 1899), 1801-8.

36. "A Contribution to the Study of the Presence and Formation of Agglutinins in the Blood." 14 pp. (With M. Crendiropoulo.)
37. "On the Toxic Properties of Bile and on Antihaemolytic (Haemosozic) Serum." *Jour. Path. and Bacteriol.*, Edinburgh and London, IX (1903-4), 278-310. (With M. Crendiropoulo.)
38. "Note on Haemosozic Sera. 3 pp. (With M. Crendiropoulo.)
39. "On Haemolytic and Haemosozic Serums." *Brit. Med. Jour.*, London, II (1904), 581.
40. "On Substances Favouring and Inhibiting the Action of the Haemolysins of Bile and Serum." 9 pp. (With M. Crendiropoulo.)
41. "Sur le pouvoir hémosozique du chlorine du sodium et son mode d'action." 1½ pp. (With M. Crendiropoulo.)
42. "On a Hitherto Undescribed Change in the Urine of Patients Suffering from Nephritis." *Brit. Med. Jour.*, London, II (1905), 544. (With G. Calvocoressi.)
43. "On the Lesions Produced by Oxyuris Vermicularis." *Brit. Med. Jour.*, London, I (1901), 208-9.
44. "Contribution to the Technique of Bacteriology." *Brit. Med. Jour.*, London, II (1900), 1305-6. 1 fig. (With M. Crendiropoulo.)
45. "Note on the Dialysis of Toxins through Collodion Walls. 1½ pp. (With M. Crendiropoulo.)
46. "On Some Results Obtained by Disinfection and Isolation against Cholera." 3½ pp. (With Zackariades Bey.)
47. "On the Lysogenic and Haemosozic Properties of Urine." 23 pp. (With M. Crendiropoulo and G. Calvocoressi.)
48. "Researches on the Bacteriological Diagnosis of Cholera by the Medical Officers at the Quarantine Council of Egypt, under the Direction of Sir Armand Ruffer." *Brit. Med. Jour.*, London, I (1907), 735-42.
49. "Perpetual Sanitary Supervision of Ports: Permanent Measures to Be Taken in Harbours." *Bericht über den XIV. Intern. Kongress für Hygiene und Demographie*, Berlin, 1907. 9½ pp.
50. "On the Etiology of Dysentery." *Brit. Med. Jour.*, London, II (September 25, 1909), 862-66. (With J. G. Willmore.)
51. "The Serum Treatment of Dysentery." *Brit. Med. Jour.*, November 12, 1910, pp. 1-12. (With J. G. Willmore.)
52. "Sur la guérison du tétanos expérimentale chez le cobaye." 1913. *Comptes rendus des séances de la Société de Biologie*, Paris, LXXIV (1913), 1277-79. (With M. Crendiropoulo.)
53. "Sur la guérison du tétanos expérimentale des cobayes. *Presse Médicale*, November 8, 1913. 19 pp. (With M. Crendiropoulo.)
54. "Note on the Anti-Haemolytic (Haemosozic) Properties of Normal Urine." *Brit. Med. Jour.*, London, I (1904), 1418.
55. "Note on the Presence of 'Bilharzia Haematobia' in Egyptian Mummies of the XXth Dynasty." *Brit. Med. Jour.*, London, I (January 1, 1910), 16.

56. "Remarks on the Histology and Pathological Anatomy of Egyptian Mummies." *Cairo Sci. Jour.*, IV (January, 1910), 1–5.
57. "Note on an Eruption Resembling That of Variola in the Skin of a Mummy of the XXth Dynasty." *Jour. Path. and Bacteriol.*, XV (1910), 1–3. (With A. R. Ferguson.)
58. "Potts'che Krankheit an einer ägyptischen Mumie aus der Zeit der 21. Dynastie." *Zur historischen Biologie der Krankheitserreger*, 3. Heft, Giessen, 1910. 2 pls., 1 colored, by Lady Ruffer. (With Elliot Smith.)
59. "On Arterial Lesions Found in Egyptian Mummies." *Jour. Path. and Bacteriol.*, XV (1911), 453–62. 3 pls.
60. "On Dwarfs and Other Deformed Persons." *Bull. de la Soc. Archéol. d'Alexandrie*, No. 13 (1911), 1–17. 3 pls. of photographs, 2 pls. of drawings from the tombs, by Lady Ruffer.
61. "Histological Studies on Egyptian Mummies." *Mémoires presentés à l'Institut Égyptien*, Tome VI, Fasc. iii, 39 pp., 11 pls., roy. 4to (mars, 1911).
62. "On Osseous Lesions in Ancient Egyptians." *Jour. Path. and Bacteriol.*, XVI (1912), 439–65. 9 pls. of photographs. (With A. Rietti.)
63. "Notes on Two Egyptian Mummies Dating from the Persian Occupation of Egypt." *Bull. de la Soc. Archéol. d'Alexandrie*, No. 14 (1912), 1–18. 7 pls. of photographs. (With A. Rietti.)
64. "Pathological Notes on the Royal Mummies of the Cairo Museum." *Mittheil. z. Gesch. der Med. und der Naturwissensch.*, No. 56, XIII (1914), 239–68.
65. "Note on the Diseases of the Sudan and Nubia in Ancient Times." *Mittheil. z. Gesch. der Med. und der Naturwissensch.* No. 58, XIII (1914), No. 6, 453–60.
66. "On Pathological Lesions Found in Coptic Bodies." *Jour. Path. and Bacteriol.*, XVIII (1913), 149–62. 2 pls.
67. "On a Tumour of the Pelvis Dating from the Roman Times and Found in Egypt." *Jour. Path. and Bacteriol.*, XVIII (1914), 480–84. 2 pls. (With J. G. Willmore.)
68. "A Pathological Specimen Dating from the Lower Miocene Period." (Extrait de *Contributions à l'Étude des Vertébrés miocènes de l'Égypte*.) Cairo: Survey Dept., 1917. 2 pls. 7 pp.
69. "The Use of Natron and Salt by the Ancient Egyptians." *Cairo Sci. Jour.*, IX (1917), 34–53.
70. "Some Recent Researches on Prehistoric Trephining." *Jour. Path. and Bacteriol.*, XXII (1918), 90–104. 1 fig.
71. "Arthritis Deformans and Spondylitis in Ancient Egypt." *Jour. Path. and Bacteriol.*, XXII (1918), 152–96. 6 pls. of photographs.
72. "Food in Egypt." *Mémoires présentés à l'Institut Égyptien*, I (1919), 1–88.
73. "On the Physical Effects of Consanguineous Marriages in the Royal Families of Ancient Egypt." *Proc. Royal Soc. of Med., Sect. of Hist. of Med.*, London, XII (1919), 1–46. 27 figs.
74. "Abnormalities and Pathology of Ancient Egyptian Teeth." *Amer. Jour. Phys. Anthrop.*, III (1920), No. 3, 335–82. 8 pls.

NOTE ON THE HISTOLOGY OF EGYPTIAN MUMMIES

(*British Medical Journal*, I [London, 1909], 1005)

Some time ago my friend Professor Elliot Smith, F.R.S., gave me some fragments of mummies of the XXIst Dynasty (dating from 1250–1000 B.C.), and I endeavored to examine these fragments by histological methods. As far as I knew, then, this was practically the first attempt to study microscopically the minute structure of tissues mummified for about three thousand years; at any rate, I found nothing bearing on this subject in the literature at my disposal, but I was informed that Professor Looss of Cairo had shown the striation of mummified muscular fibres to his colleagues. I demonstrated some of my sections at the Sheffield meeting of the British Medical Association and at the December meeting (1908) of the Cairo Scientific Club. Quite lately my friend Mr. Shattock has read a paper on a similar subject before the Royal Society of Medicine.

METHOD

It was found impossible to obtain good microscopical sections without first restoring, to some extent at any rate, their flexibility to the tissues, as their brittleness and hardness broke the edge of the microtome knives; even when a fair section was obtained, this invariably crumbled up when transferred to the slide. I need not describe the various methods tried and rejected, but it will be sufficient to note that, by combining an alkaline salt such as carbonate of soda with a hardening reagent such as alcohol or formol, the mummified tissue placed in the mixture gradually swells up and resumes its former shape.

The solution which has given me the best results is composed of alcohol, 100 parts, 5 per cent carbonate of soda solution, 60 parts. In many cases, however, such a solution softens the tissues too much, and more alcohol must then be added.

After a period of time, the length of which depends on the bulk and nature of the tissue, the solution is replaced by 30 per cent alcohol, and more alcohol is added day by day. After two or three days the softened tissue is transferred to absolute alcohol, then chloroform, paraffin, and cut secundum artem. During these manipulations the tissue remains pliable, though it shrinks a good deal. Very thin sections do not present any particular advantages, and I generally use three divisions of Minot's microtome. Such preparations, after maceration in 1 in 10,000 caustic potash, give excellent pictures.

RESULTS

I have prepared sections of muscle (voluntary, cardiac, and involuntary), blood vessels, skin, intestine, stomach, liver, kidney, bone, mammary glands, and testicles, and the main characters of all these organs and tissues can be readily recognized. The striation of muscular fibres, for instance, the muscular coats, the submucous tissue, and occasionally even the glands of the intestines and the convoluted tubules, the straight tubules and glomeruli of the kidneys, the various layers of the skin can be identified with certainty. I have no doubt that coarse pathological changes, such as inflammation, cirrhosis, tubercle, or cancer could be demonstrated by this method.

POTT'SCHE KRANKHEIT AN EINER ÄGYPTISCHEN MUMIE AUS DER ZEIT DER 21. DYNASTIE (UM 1000 V. CHR.)[1]

(Sudhoff und Sticker, *Zur historischen Biologie der Krankheitserreger* [Giessen, 1910], 3. Heft)

Es ist nichts Neues, die Entdeckung eines Falles von Pott'scher Krankheit in Überresten aus Altägypten anzukündigen. Wir glauben jedoch, dass unser Fall das erste echte Beispiel jener Krankheit ist, das an ägyptischen Mumien gefunden wurde, dessen Wichtigkeit durch die Tatsache wächst, dass uns ihr typisches Bild ermutigt hat, mehrere später ausgegrabene Fälle als tuberkulös zu identifizieren.

Die Wirbelsäulen archaischer Ägypter, welche von Dr. Fouquet als Beispiele Pott'scher Krankheit beschrieben wurden (siehe J. de Morgan, *Recherches sur les origines de l'Égypte*, Paris, 1897, Appendice par le Dr. Fouquet), sind für uns typische Beispiele von Osteoarthritis, so wie sie Dr. Wood Jones unter dem Namen "Spondylitis deformans" beschrieben und abgebildet hat. (*The Archaeological Survey of Nubia, Bulletin No. 2*, Cairo, 1908, Plate LIV.)

Diese Erkrankung war in Ober-Ägypten so verbreitet,—besonders wahrscheinlich in prädynastischer Zeit—, dass gelegentlich einer von uns (G. E. S.) Beweise davon an jedem ausgewachsenen Skelett in einem grossen allgemeinen Begräbnisplatze fand. Sie war auch zur Zeit der persischen Dynastien, zirka 525–332 v. Chr., verbreitet, und in Unter-Ägypten zeigen selbst die Skelette von makedonischen Soldaten und deren Familien (seit zirka 332 v. Chr.) —kürzlich von Dr. Breccia ausgegraben—oft unverkennbare Merkmale dieser Krankheit. (M. A. R.)

Professor Poncet stellt auch die Diagnose tuberkulöser Erkrankung an der Wirbelsäule eines Affen, den Professor Lortet in einem alten thebanischen Begräbnisplatz gefunden (Lortet et Gaillard, *La faune momifiée de l'ancienne Égypte*, Lyon, 1905, pp. 228–31,

[1] This paper was written with Grafton Elliot Smith as senior author.

Fig. 95), und sagt Seite 231: "Ich will als Beweis hierfür nur die Ähnlichkeit dieser Wirbelankylosen mit denjenigen anführen, die wir oftmals beim Menschen konstatierten und deren tuberkulösen Ursprung wir dargewiesen haben. . . . . Diese Diagnose wird noch bekräftigt durch die Tatsache, dass die Tuberkulose beim Affen sehr häufig vorkommt."[1]

Wir können der Diagnose von Professor Poncet nicht beipflichten, da wir mit der Mehrzahl der Pathologen behaupten, dass— was auch immer die Ursache von Spondylitis deformans sein mag— der Tuberkelbazillus nicht als Faktor in deren Ätiologie nachgewiesen worden ist, und dass eine scharfe Unterscheidungslinie zwischen ihr und der Rückenwirbeltuberkulose (Pott'scher Krankheit) gezogen werden muss.

Einer von uns (G. E. S.) fand vor ungefähr fünf Jahren—bei der Prüfung menschlicher Überreste, die Dr. Reisner in einem Begräbnisplatz des alten Kaiserreiches (Ausgrabungen der Hearst-Expedition) in Gizeh entdeckt hat—das Skelett eines kleinen Kindes (vielleicht aus der Zeit um 2700 v. Chr.), an welchem die typische krankhafte Veränderung von vorgerücktem Hüftleiden zu sehen war. Obgleich dasselbe höchstwahrscheinlich durch Tuberkulose entstanden war, konnte man keinen positiven Beweis dafür erbringen.

Im ersten *Bulletin* des Archaeological Survey of Nubia (p. 38) beschreibt Dr. Wood Jones eine Mumie mit ausgesprochener pathologischer Veränderung des Hüftgelenks (linkes Iliosakral-Gelenk) und der letzten beiden Lendenwirbel. Auch das linke Ellbogengelenk war stark verändert; von diesem liefen Fistelgänge aus, die sich auf der Hautoberfläche öffneten.

Damals wurde die Diagnose einer tuberkulösen Erkrankung gestellt, aber Professor A. R. Ferguson von der medizinischen Schule in Kairo setzte dem entgegen, dass die Natur der Knochenneubildung nicht auf eine tuberkulöse Veränderung hindeute. Auch Dr. Charles Todd vom Public Health Department suchte vergeblich nach Tuberkelbazillen in den Lungen.

[1] "Je n'en veux pour preuve que la similitude de cettes ankyloses vertebrales avec celles que nous avons maintes fois constatées chez l'homme et dont nous avons démontré l'origine tuberculeuse. ... Ce diagnostic est encore corroboré par ce fait que la tuberculose est très commune chez le singe."

Seit jener Zeit hat Dr. Derry (im Verlaufe seiner anthropologischen Arbeiten im Zusammenhang mit dem Archaeological Survey of Nubia) eine Reihe von kranken Wirbelsäulen—aus der Zeit von 2000 bis 3000 v. Chr. und sogar noch früher—gefunden, die eine so vollkommne Ähnlichkeit mit den Fällen besitzen, die hier beschrieben werden sollen, dass—wenn letztere für tuberkulös erklärt werden dürfen, dieselbe Diagnose bei der Untersuchung der früher gefundenen Wirbelsäulen gestellt werden muss (siehe *Archaeological Survey of Nubia, Bulletin No. 3*, p. *32, No. 4*, pp. *20*, *26* und *No. 5*, pp. *21* und *22*).

Die Mumie, mit der wir in diesem Bericht zu tun haben, war die irdische Hülle eines Priesters des Ammon aus der 21. Dynastie (zirka 1000 v. Chr.) und befand sich unter der grossen Sammlung menschlicher Körper der Seconde trouvaille de Deir el Bahari, die 1891 von M. Grébaut vom Service des Antiquités in der Gegend der grossen thebanischen Hauptstadt aufgefunden wurden.

1904 überantwortete Sir Gaston Maspéro (Generaldirektor des Service des Antiquités) vierundvierzig dieser Mumien (seit 1891 im Museum der Altertümer von Kairo aufbewahrt) an das anatomische Museum der medizinischen Schule von Kairo. Unter diesen fand einer von uns beiden (G. E. S.) die Mumie dieses typischen Buckeligen; leider trug sie aber keinen Zettel, der bezeichnet hätte, aus welchem Sarg sie genommen war, und auch auf den diesen Leichnam umhüllenden Leinwandbandagen keine Angabe, um uns die Identifizierung oder die Festsetzung ihrer genauen chronologischen Stellung zu ermöglichen.

Die besonders gut erkennbare Technik des Einbalsamierungsvorgangs, wie solche in den Tagen der 21. Dynastie angewandt wurde, ist ausführlich anderswo beschrieben (G. E. S., " A Contribution to the Study of Mummification in Egypt," *Memoires présentés à l'Institut Égyptien*, Vol. V, Fasc. 1, 1906), lässt uns jedoch mit Sicherheit feststellen, dass diese Mumie in der genannten Zeit einbalsamiert worden war.

Das allgemeine Aussehen der Überreste dieser Mumie eines jungen erwachsenen Mannes wurde in der von Mrs. Cecil Firth freundlichst verfertigten Skizze (Tafel I, Figur 1) ausgezeichnet porträtiert. Tafel I, Figur 2, ist eine unretouchierte Photographie, die die Ansicht des Körpers von vorne darstellt, nachdem die vordere Körperwand entfernt war.

Augenscheinlich hatte hier eine ausgedehnte Zerstörung der Mitte des 1. Lendenwirbels und der unteren drei oder vier Rückenwirbel stattgefunden; das Rückgrat hatte in der unteren Rückengegend nachgegeben, und es war eine ausgesprochene unregelmässige Einknickung entstanden. Die Rückengegend der Wirbelsäule bildet einen Winkel, dessen Spitze in der Verschmelzungsstelle des 8. und 9. Rückenwirbels liegt. Der erste Lendenwirbelkörper hat vorne und oben einen Ansatz zu einer starken neuen Knochenbildung genommen (wie Tafel I, Figur 2, gut zeigt); soweit durch Prüfung mit dem Messer gefunden werden konnte, war die Konsolidierung der Wirbelkörper eine vollständige und keine andere Knochenneubildung zu entdecken.

Von der rechten Seite des 1. Lendenwirbelkörpers sieht man eine breite abgeplattete Anschwellung ausgehen, die sich nach unten längs eines Stranges hinzieht, demjenigen entsprechend, welchen an der linken Seite der Lendenmuskel (Musculus psoas) bildet, bis in die rechte Darmbeingrube (Fossa iliaca), in welcher sie sich verliert. Keine Spur von einer Öffnung in der Haut war am Oberschenkel oder am Bein oder in der Lendengegend zu finden, wo Abszesse von Krankheiten der Wirbelsäule sich bei einigen Fällen zu öffnen pflegten, die einer von uns im Sektionsraum zu Kairo zu untersuchen Gelegenheit hatte.

MIKROSKOPISCHE UNTERSUCHUNG

Bruchstücke von Trachea, Larynx und Bronchialdrüsen wurden mikroskopisch nach einer Methode untersucht, die einer von uns (M. A. R.) schon besprochen hat. Man erweichte die Gewebe in einer Lösung, die wie folgt zusammengesetzt war:

```
Alkohol............................30 cc
Wasser.............................50 cc
5% kohlensaure Natronlösung..........20 cc
```

legte sie dann in immer konzentrierteren Alkohol, in absoluten Alkohol, in Chloroform, und bettete sie schliesslich in Paraffin ein. Schnitte solcher Gewebe wurden mit Hämatoxylin oder speziell für

Tuberkelbazillen gefärbt, etwas Abnormes konnte jedoch nicht daran entdeckt werden.

Mit einer kleinen Trepankrone von ungefähr 15 mm Durchmesser entfernten wir sodann von dem vermutlichen Psoasabszess einen Gewebszylinder. Es zeigte sich, dass eine deutliche Höhlung, gross genug, um einen kleinen Finger durchzulassen, die obere Schicht vom Knochen trennte, und durch diese Höhlung konnte mit Leichtigkeit eine Sonde nach dem Oberschenkel geschoben werden. Deutliche muskulöse Fasern konnten mit blossem Auge nicht gesehen werden.

Behufs Kontrolle dieser Beobachtung wurde mit derselben Trepankrone ein Probestück an der entsprechenden Stelle in der linken Fossa iliaca entnommen. Nur eine dünne Gewebeschicht trennte den Knochen hier von der Oberfläche, und dies war unzweifelhaft quergestreifte Muskelsubstanz. So ergab sich also der positive Beweis für eine krankhafte Veränderung in der Gegend des rechten Lendenmuskels (Musc. psoas).

LINKE ODER GESUNDE SEITE

Das angebohrte Stück bestand aus gelblich-weissem, fleckigem Material von Aussehen und Konsistenz normaler einbalsamierter Muskelfaser (siehe Tafel II, B). Es fühlte sich hart an, wenn auch nicht körnig, und kleine biegsame Muskelfaserstreifen konnten leicht abgetrennt werden (siehe Tafel II, C). Wegen der sehr tief gelb gefärbten Materie, die die Struktur einbalsamierter Gewebe immer verdunkelt, vermochte man nach einfachem Zupfen durch histologische Untersuchung sehr wenig zu finden. Nach der Erweichung kleiner Stückchen durch 12–24 Std. in $1/10000$ Ätzkalilösung war aber die Muskelfaser leicht zu erkennen. Die Querstreifung war unverkennbar und an einigen Stellen war das Sarkolemma nachweisbar, doch waren, wie es meist bei einbalsamierten Muskeln der Fall ist, keine Zellkerne zu unterscheiden.

Schnitte hiervon wurden auch nach der oben beschriebenen Methode präpariert, und die Präparate zeigten, dass der Muskel sehr gut erhalten und kein Leichen-Packungsmaterial zwischen die Fasern gedrungen war. Die Querstreifung, obgleich gut erkennbar, war vielleicht nicht so vollkommen erhalten wie an Muskeln anderer

Mumien. Dieser Punkt ist nicht so sehr wichtig, da es beträchtliche Unterschiede im Erhaltungszustand ägyptischer Mumien gibt, selbst bei denjenigen der nämlichen Dynastie.

RECHTE ODER KRANKE SEITE

Der Stand der Dinge auf dieser Seite war makroskopisch und mikroskopisch ein durchaus anderer. Erstens musste man von der Oberfläche des herausgebohrten Stückes eine verhältnismässig grosse Menge pulverigen schwarzen Stoffes, hauptsächlich aus Holzkohle bestehend, entfernen.—Zweitens sah das durch das Ausbohren erhaltene Stück ganz anders aus wie dasjenige von der linken Seite. Es zeigte eine schmutziggelbe Farbe, war aber stellenweise glänzendweiss und hie und da mit pechschwarzen Flecken getupft (siehe Tafel II, A). Seine Konsistenz war hart, aber kleine Partien zerkrümelten rasch unter dem Finger, was allein schon genügte, um den Unterschied zwischen der Muskelstruktur rechts und links zu veranschaulichen. In den inneren Partien des ausgebohrten Stückes zeigte der leicht zerkrümelnde Stoff ein schmutziggelbes Aussehen und ein ganz wenig Beimischung des oben beschriebenen schwarzen Pulvers.

In Deckglaspräparaten konnte man erkennen, dass die schwarzen Bestandteile des ausgebohrten Stückes fast gänzlich aus kleinsten Teilchen von Holzkohle und Pflanzenüberresten bestanden, die augenscheinlich als Verpackungs- oder Ausstopfungsmaterial gedient hatten. Ausserdem fand man eine gewisse Menge eines gelben glänzenden Stoffes (Harz?).—Die Bemühungen, aus dieser schwarzen Substanz Schnittpräparate zu machen, waren von keinem Erfolge gekrönt, da dieser Stoff in der ihn erweichenden Lösung nicht aufquoll, sondern hart und zerbrechlich blieb.

Der gelbliche Stoff veränderte sich nicht merklich in der erweichenden Lösung, nichtsdestoweniger wurden aber ziemlich gute Erfolge erzielt. Die Präparate zeigten: (a) muskulöse Fasern, obgleich nicht zahlreich, so doch genügend gut erhalten, um die Querstreifung und des Sarkolemma zu zeigen.

Die Muskelfasern waren (b) in einen körnigen Stoff, bestehend aus unregelmässigen rundlichen Körpern, eingebettet, von keiner besonderen Struktur, aber mit Hämatoxylin und Eosin (siehe Tafel

II, F) gut sich färbend. Man war versucht, diese Körper für Leukozyten anzusehen; obgleich aber diese Diagnose nicht unwahrscheinlich ist, konnte doch kein typisches weisses Blutkörperchen nachgewiesen werden. Vermischt mit diesen Körperchen war (c) eine gewisse Menge Holzkohle (siehe Tafel II, E und F) und eines gelblich-krystallartigen Stoffes (siehe Tafel II, F), welche augenscheinlich Packungsmaterial waren.

Man konnte auch (d) eine grosse Anzahl von eiförmigen Körperchen (siehe Tafel II, G) sehen, welche sich mit Hämatoxylin schwach und gleichmässig färben liessen, und deren äussere Enden etwas verdickt waren und tiefer sich färbten (siehe Tafel II, G). Ihre Konturen waren scharf, und bei manchen war eine deutliche Membran zu erkennen. Sie lagen vereinzelt, öfter auch in Gruppen von 6 bis 12, manchmal sogar von 30 bis 40 zusammengeballt. In manchen Fällen hatten sie alle gleichmässige Struktur (siehe Tafel II, G), aber manchmal waren sie mehr oder weniger deformiert (siehe Tafel II, J). Nach ihrer Form und Struktur zu urteilen, sehen wir sie als Schimmel-Sporen an; denn sich verästelnde Myzelien waren deutlich an vielen Präparaten zu sehen (siehe Tafel II, H). Mikrokokken oder Bazillen konnten durch keine Methode nachgewiesen werden.

Um es kurz zusammenzufassen: Der linke Psoas bestand aus normalen Muskelfasern; dagegen war die Oberfläche des rechten Psoas mit einer grossen Menge schwarzen staubigen Stoffes, bestehend aus Holzkohle, Pflanzenfaser, Harz (?) etc., als Packungs- und Ausstopfungsmaterial gebraucht, bedeckt. Die tiefen, mehr gelben Teile bestanden aus Muskelfasern, welche in einer grossen Menge körnigen Stoffes (Leukozyten?) eingebettet lagen, vermischt mit einer gewissen Menge von Holzkohle etc. (Packungsmaterial) und Schimmel.

SCHLUSSFOLGERUNG

Der mikroskopische Befund des rechten Psoas unterstützt die Diagnose, zu der man nach einer Prüfung mit blossem Auge gelangte, nämlich das Vorhandensein eines Psoasabszesses auf der rechten Seite.

Es wurde zwar kein Eiter gefunden, der mit Sicherheit erkannt werden konnte, aber man muss sich vergegenwärtigen, dass während des Einbalsamierungsprozesses der meiste Eiter mechanisch weggewaschen oder aufgelöst oder zur Unkenntlichkeit verändert wurde durch das sogenannte "Natronbad." Dass der rechte Psoas in einem weicheren, halb flüssigen Zustand sich befand, als der Korper aus der konservierenden Lösung genommen wurde, wird bewiesen durch die Tatsache, dass das Ausstopfungsmaterial (Holzkohle etc.) tief zwischen die Muskelfasern gedrungen ist.

Eine andere wichtige Tatsache, die zugunsten dieser Ansicht spricht, ist, dass sich eine Höhlung zwischen Muskel und Knochen der rechten Seite befand, wogegen sich an der linken Seite keine derartige Höhlung auffinden liess. Der rechte Muskel muss deshalb durch irgend einen pathologischen Prozess schon bei Lebzeiten mehr oder weniger von dem Knochen losgelöst gewesen sein.

DESCRIPTION OF PLATES I-II

PLATE I

Fig. 1.—A drawing, by Mrs. Cecil M. Firth, of the mummy of a priest of Ammon of the XXIst Dynasty (1000 B.C.), showing in lateral view the protrusion of the spine so commonly seen in Pott's disease.

Fig 2.—An untouched photograph of the anterior aspect of the mummy, showing the huge psoas abscess into which the pus from the tuberculous lesion in the lumbar vertebrae had drained. The mass was soft at the time of embalming.

PLATE II

(Drawings by Alice M. Ruffer)

A.—Portion of the external surface of the right psoas muscle (diseased side) removed by a trephine.

B.—Portion of the external surface of the left psoas muscle (normal side) removed by a trephine.

C.—Small, isolated fragment of A.

D.—Small, isolated fragment of B.

E.—Cover-glass preparation of the yellow substance of A. (Leitz, Oc. 1, Obj. 4.)

F.—A small portion of E greatly enlarged. (Leitz, Oc. 1, Obj. 1/12.)

G.—Spores of mold. The same diameter.

H.—A branched fragment of fungus. The same magnification.

I.—Fungus and spores more or less degenerated. The same magnification.

REMARKS ON THE HISTOLOGY AND PATHOLOGICAL ANATOMY OF EGYPTIAN MUMMIES

(Cairo Scientific Journal, Vol. IV [January, 1910], No. 40)

At the meeting of the British Medical Association in Sheffield (July, 1908) and at a meeting of the Cairo Scientific Society (December, 1908), I gave a demonstration of the microscopic structure of mummified tissues. The organs examined came from mummies of the priests of the twentieth dynasty, and had been given me by Professor Elliot Smith. On the same occasion, and in a note published in the *British Medical Journal* (January, 1909), I described the method which I then used for the preparation of such specimens. My intention now is to give a short account of the results obtained by this and similar methods during the last year, but before doing so, I wish to thank Sir Gaston Maspero, Professors Flinders Petrie, Elliot Smith, and Keatinge, for providing me with the necessary material.

Urinary calculi.—Professor Flinders Petrie gave me three stones found by him in a predynastic skeleton, and which he had correctly diagnosed as urinary calculi.

The largest of these stones weighs 30 grammes, and measures 4.5 centimetres in its greatest length, and 3 centimetres in its greatest thickness. It is roughly pear-shaped, with a whitish smooth surface streaked here and there with yellow (incrustations of fine sand?).

The second calculus weighs 24 grammes, and measures 4 centimetres in its greatest length, and 2.5 centimetres in its greatest thickness. It is roughly triangular in shape, and its surface resembles that of the first.

The third stone weighed 11.7 grammes only, and resembled the second in shape. Professor Aders Plimmer, of the Physiological

Laboratory, University College, London, kindly analysed it for me, and found its composition to be as follows:

	Per Cent
Water	6.5
Organic Matter	34.8
P_2O_5	37.6
MgO	19.7
CaO	0.8
Total	99.4*

*The insoluble residue gave a strong murexide reaction.

The centre of this calculus is yellow, the periphery irregularly laminated, and by the usual methods crystals of uric acid are easily obtained. Microscopically, the insoluble residue consists of organic débris, staining with haematoxylin (leucocytes and epithelial cells possibly). Anatomical elements or eggs of parasites[1] were not recognisable. The third calculus, therefore (and probably the others also), is a mixed phosphatic and uric acid calculus, which are common enough in Egypt at the present time.

Liver of Ranefer.—I received from Professor Flinders Petrie a fragment of an organ found in the tomb of Ranefer.

It looked like some internal organ, or part of such an organ, imbedded in a large quantity of mud. The mud was removed and then the typical arrangement of liver cells was easily recognised; the blood vessels, biliary tubes and connective tissue had disappeared.

Tissues of predynastic mummies.—The fragment of tissue just described was about five thousand years old and the remarkable results obtained encouraged me to study microscopically the prehistoric bodies of the Hearst collection, which are now in the museum of the School of Medicine at Cairo, and which, I am informed, date from eight thousand years ago at least. The method used so far is fatal to these tissues, as they first crumble to pieces and then dissolve almost completely. By using a macerating fluid with a slightly different composition, however, good sections are easily prepared, and these I intend to describe fully on some future

---

[1] Nearly all the specimens described in this paper are now deposited in the Museum of the Government School of Medicine, Cairo.

occasion. It is extraordinary that the striation of the voluntary muscular fibres and the nuclei of some cells should be perfectly plainly visible eight thousand years after death.

Diseases of arteries in mummies of the eighteenth to twentieth dynasties.—In order to dissect the arteries, the following method was adopted after many failures.

The whole mummy or the limbs to be examined are immersed in a solution having the following composition:

	Per Cent
Carbonate of soda	2
Formol	0.5
Tap water	97

The skin becomes soft after twenty-four hours or longer and is then stripped off. The parts are replaced in the macerating fluid until this has penetrated to the bones, when the large arteries are easily dissected out. The muscles are separated from one another by simply running the finger along the intermuscular septa, and nerves, ligaments of joints, cartilages, etc., are readily seen. The arteries are still remarkably elastic; whereas the muscles, though soft, do not return to their former size after stretching.

a) The first aorta examined consists of a piece $4\frac{1}{2}$ inches long, covered, throughout its whole length almost, by a hard calcareous plate. Small pieces of this plate were decalcified in the following solution:

	Per Cent
Absolute alcohol	98
HNO_3	2

washed several times in 30 per cent alcohol, hardened and cut secundum artem. Microscopical preparations show the main alterations of calcareous degeneration.

b) Another aorta was taken from one of the mummies (eighteenth to twentieth dynasties) given me by Professor Flinders Petrie. Its arch had been hacked away by the embalmer, who had also cut right through all the coats just above the bifurcation of the vessel. The thoracic aorta from a point just above the origin of the left subclavian artery, and the whole of the abdominal artery, were intact and easily removed. The internal coat is studded with small calcareous patches and the two largest, each the size of a shilling, are situated just above the bifurcation. The left subclavian artery, at a point just above its origin, is almost blocked by a raised, ragged calcareous excrescence, as large as a threepenny bit (calcified atheromatous ulcer). Small atheromatous patches, not calcified, are scattered through the whole length of the aorta, and these, owing to the dark coloration of the tissues, are more easily felt than seen.

The common carotid arteries show small patches of atheroma, but the most marked changes are found in the pelvic arteries and in those of the lower limbs.

The common iliac arteries are studded with small patches of atheroma and calcareous degeneration. The other arteries of the pelvis are converted by calcification into rigid, "bony" tubes, down to their minute ramifications. So stiff and brittle are they that it was impossible to dissect them out entire, as in spite of every possible care they were invariably broken. The minute intra-muscular arteries were easily felt on triturating the muscles under the fingers.

Both arms and the legs (about 6 inches below Poupart's ligament) had been lost, but on the right side the common femoral and the profunda were dissected out. Both are converted into rigid calcareous tubes.

It is to be noted that as far as could be made out from the examination of the cartilages of the ribs the mummy was not that of a very old person.

c) A Greek mummy given me by Sir Gaston Maspero also shows atheromatous patches in the aorta and brachial arteries. From the examination of the cartilages, etc., I concluded at the time that the man was not above fifty years old at the time of death.

d) I had an opportunity also of examining the legs of an old woman of the twentieth dynasty. The body has been very carefully embalmed, and all the muscles and most of the arteries removed, sand and linen filling their places. The posterior tibial artery, however, was dissected out and found ossified from end to end.

Arterial disease, therefore, was of frequent occurrence among Egyptians of old, and indeed temporal arteries of mummies in various museums are as tortuous as they are at the present day, even in people who died when comparatively young.

I may add that very interesting microscopical preparations were obtained from all arteries which had been isolated.

Lesions of lungs.—Owing to the shrivelled state of the lungs, naked-eye evidence of pulmonary disease is not easily obtainable. With the microscope, however, pathological changes were detected in the lungs of several mummies.

a) The lungs of one mummy (twentieth dynasty) present all the signs of diffuse anthracosis, the alveoli and the alveolar interspaces containing an enormous quantity of jet-black or dark yellow material (soot). Some of the alveoli are so full of this black stuff that at first I thought that an emulsion of finely divided charcoal had been poured down the trachea into the bronchi. I realized my mistake when I found that the material had penetrated into the depths of the tissues and that there were evident signs of inflammation in the alveoli. This condition of things is frequently found at the present time, among miners, cooks, and persons living in a smoky atmosphere, and I have no doubt that this person was engaged in some work necessitating his presence in smoke-laden air.

b) The two lungs (twentieth dynasty) to be described now present nothing abnormal to the naked eye, but nevertheless I expected to find pathological change in them, as small pieces had been left behind and were sticking to the pleura. I suspected that pathological adhesions had probably existed during life.

Under the microscope, all the alveoli are seen to be crammed with cells, some of the characteristics of which, e.g., nuclei, can be recognized still.

No micro-organisms are visible except in one place where numerous micrococci are packed in an alveolus. Although they still stain by Gram's method, I am unable to say to what species of micrococci they belong. In spite of the almost total absence of micro-organisms and judging from the pathological appearances only, I do not hesitate in making the diagnosis of pneumonia, which had advanced to the stage of hepatisation.

c) This lung came from a mummy dating from the Greek period. There is nothing abnormal in the apex and upper half of this organ, which became flexible after softening in the usual manner, and floats in 60 per cent of alcohol. On the contrary, the lower part immediately sinks in that fluid. Moreover, on section, the upper portion of the organ is spongy looking, the lower part shows a dense, almost solid section, much resembling muscle. Consolidation of the lower lobe, therefore, had evidently taken place.

Microscopic examination of the upper part of the lung shows here and there patches of inflammation, and a few short bacilli, with rounded edges, scattered in groups through the tissue.

The alveoli of the lower part of the lung are full of exudation in which very few anatomical elements are plainly recognisable, and an enormous number of the bacilli just mentioned.

The liver of the same mummy was also examined. The interlobular connective tissue is much denser than usual, and strands of the tissue run between the liver cells. The interesting point, however, is the large number of the same bacilli in the tissues and in blood vessels.

These bacilli stain well with haematoxylin,[1] methylene blue, fuchsin, but not with Gram's method. They are ovoid in form about the size of plague bacilli, though plumper, and, except in a few cases, without a clear interspace between their extremities. A careful examination of numerous preparations left me with the impression that they had certainly been present during life and that they were pathogenic. Indeed, had a bubo been found I should have diagnosed the case as one of plague. At present, with the very scanty knowledge of the changes undergone by micro-organisms in mummified tissue, it will be best not to make any definite diagnosis.

It is clear, however, that micro-organisms retain their characters unaltered in mummified tissue. I have found in organs that had evidently undergone putrefaction Gram-positive and Gram-negative micro-organisms, and others the spores of which gave all the typical staining reactions. Considering that the nuclei of some mummified or simply dried tissue stain characteristically, this result was not unexpected.

[1] I use Böhmer's haematoxylin, not less than one year old. I do not know why this simple and excellent stain is not used more extensively for micro-organisms.

Renal lesions.—(*a*) The kidneys of one mummy given me by Professor Flinders Petrie had not been removed by the embalmers. The right kidney presents nothing abnormal, but the left measures only 4.5 centimetres in length, 3.5 centimetres in breadth, and weighs 3 grammes.

Microscopically, there are no signs of inflammation except for some slight thickening of the capsule and of the connective tissue in some parts of the medulla. I am not satisfied that where the connective tissue looks denser, this appearance is due to a pathological change, and not to an unequal expansion of the organ in the softening fluid. Any cirrhosis would be easy of detection, for the connective tissue stains well, the epithelium is remarkably well preserved, and there is no desquamation whatever. The atrophy was congenital, therefore, a condition not infrequently found at the present day.

b) The kidneys of another mummy of the eighteenth to twentieth dynasties (1580–1050 B.C.) contained multiple abscesses with well-staining bacilli, and other lesions, which so far I have not yet diagnosed. The bacilli are found in the abscesses and their immediate neighbourhood, but nowhere else. They are short, straight bacilli, which take haematoxylin and basic aniline dyes readily, but not Gram's stain. They greatly resemble the bacillus coli, as seen at the present day.

c) In the kidneys of two mummies of the twentieth dynasty[1] I have demonstrated a large number of calcified eggs of Bilharzia haematobia situated for the most part among the straight tubules. These kidneys had other lesions as well, which, owing to the shrunken state of the organs, I am unable to define as yet.

Renal disease, therefore, was not infrequent among Egyptians living over three thousand years ago.

Conclusion.—The only object of this paper has been to draw attention to the possibilities opened up by this method of study, with the hope of encouraging others to take up the same subject. I have purposely avoided giving histological details, as I hope to publish these and other results fully at some not very distant date.

[1] See also *British Medical Journal*, January, 1910, p. 16.

NOTE ON THE PRESENCE OF "BILHARZIA HAEMATOBIA" IN EGYPTIAN MUMMIES OF THE TWENTIETH DYNASTY (1250–1000 B.C.)

(British Medical Journal, January 1, 1910)

In a previous note published in this *Journal*, I described a process by which mummified tissues could be prepared for histological examination. I ventured to predict that it was highly probable that, by this method, one would be able to recognize pathological changes, such as cirrhosis, cancer, etc.

Thanks to the kindness of Professor Elliot Smith, Professor Flinders Petrie, and Professor Keatinge, I have obtained several organs from mummies of the eighteenth to the twentieth dynasty, and I may state at once that such diseases as atheroma, pneumonia, renal abscesses, and cirrhosis of the liver are plainly recognizable. In the renal abscesses and in other lesions I have stained microorganisms with methylene blue, fuchsin, haematoxylin, and even by Gram's method.

At the present time there is perhaps no disease more important to Egypt than that caused by the Bilharzia haematobia. So far no evidence has been produced to show how long it has existed in this country, although medical papyri contain prescriptions against one of its most prominent symptoms—namely, haematuria. The lesions of this disease are best seen in the bladder and rectum, but unfortunately these are just the two mummified organs which I have not been able to obtain so far. Nevertheless, in the kidneys of two mummies of the twentieth dynasty, I have demonstrated in microscopic sections a large number of calcified eggs of Bilharzia haematobia, situated, for the most part, among the straight tubules. Although calcified, these eggs are easily recognizable and cannot be mistaken for anything else. I may add that I showed some of my sections to Professors Looss and Ferguson, whose paramount authority on such a subject cannot be disputed, and both confirmed my diagnosis.

I have examined microscopically the kidneys of six mummies. The kidneys of two were apparently healthy; the left kidney of another was congenitally atrophied; those of the fourth contained multiple abscesses with well-staining bacteria and other lesions, which so far I have not diagnosed; those of the fifth and sixth showed Bilharzia eggs, and the latter had other lesions as well, which, owing to the shrunken state of the organ, I am unable to define accurately as yet.

ON ARTERIAL LESIONS FOUND IN EGYPTIAN MUMMIES (1580 B.C.—525 A.D.)

(*Journal of Pathology and Bacteriology*, Vol. XV [1911])

The mummies examined came from the XVIIIth–XXVIIth Dynasties (1580 B.C.–525 A.D.), and from the time of the Persian conquest (500 B.C.). I also dissected a Greek[1] and a Coptic mummy, the latter dating from the fifth or sixth century after Christ.

The investigations therefore range over a period of two thousand years—namely, from 1580 B.C. to 525 A.D.

I take this opportunity of thanking Sir Gaston Maspero, Professor Flinders Petrie, Professor Elliot Smith, Dr. Derry, and Dr. Keatinge for help. To the last gentleman my thanks are specially due for giving me a number of arms and legs from broken-up mummies of the XXIst Dynasty (1090–945 B.C.). These limbs were of no possible use as museum specimens, and I had no hesitation, therefore, in dissecting them. Most of the preparations came from them.[2]

DIFFICULTIES OF THE INQUIRY

The chief difficulty consisted in the extensive mutilations made during the process of embalming. Dr. Elliot Smith has shown that at the time of the XXIst Dynasty, the embalmers removed the whole of the viscera, the aorta, and most of the muscles of the body. The body cavity and the holes left in the limbs after removal of the muscles are found filled with mud, sand or rags, or all three.

The sole of the foot is packed with sawdust mixed with some "resinous" material. The muscles and big blood vessels of the

[1] This mummy was given me as coming from the Greek period. Judging from the way it was embalmed, I am of opinion that it really dated from the XXIst and certainly not later than the XXIId Dynasty.

[2] The only papers I know on the subject are: (*a*) Shattock, "Microscopic Sections of the Aorta of King Merneptah," *Lancet*, London, January 30, 1909; and (*b*) Armand Ruffer, "Remarks on the Histology and Pathological Anatomy of Egyptian Mummies," *Cairo Scientific Journal*, Vol. IV, January, 1910. Some of my pathological sections were shown at a meeting of the Cairo Scientific Society in December, 1908.

neck are also gone, the larynx is either pushed upwards or has been removed, and the neck is filled with mud or rags. The cheeks are filled out with a fatty material mixed with sand and sawdust, and the brain removed. It is only by accident, therefore, that the whole or a portion of the aorta, or one of the large arteries is left behind. Fortunately for our purpose, one artery, namely the posterior peroneal, owing to its deep situation, often escaped the embalmer's knife. In a few cases also, when the embalmers had evidently scamped their work, the arm or leg was untouched.

After the removal of the foreign material, and when the limb is plunged in the softening solution, the walls of the cavity thus left are often found lined with a hard black material, not easily removed by water or a weakly alkaline solution. It must be taken away mechanically, and this often proves a very tedious process. When left standing in the hot and damp summer atmosphere of our laboratory, a brown gummy sticky fluid exudes out of this material. The same gummy substance is also found in bandages kept under similar conditions. I hope shortly to have some chemical evidence as to its nature.

The limbs of such mummies of the XXVIIth Dynasty as I examined were intact, but the body cavity had been almost cleaned out. The thoracic cavity contained an enormous quantity of jet black material showing a glistening surface, which I should certainly never have suspected of containing any tissue. In one case, however, a lump of this substance, which to the naked eye appeared to contain no tissue whatever, was placed in running hot water. The black substance slowly dissolved out, and then a small piece of aorta appeared, which, after long washing, showed exquisite calcareous patches. Mr. Lucas, who has chemically examined some of the material found in the mummies, will doubtless, later on, give the result of his researches. Suffice it to say that the black shiny material is not bitumen. Indeed, it is a striking fact that up to the present I have never found bitumen in any mummy, even in those of the Ptolemaic period.

The Coptic mummy had apparently been simply dried, and there was no evidence of its having been embalmed in any way.

METHOD OF ISOLATING THE ARTERIES

The mud, sand, bandages, and gummy material are first picked out with forceps, or slowly scraped away; a most unpleasant task, as the dust floating in thick clouds about the room is most irritating to the lungs. The "packing" does not appear to contain pathogenic microbes, as, in spite of numerous cuts and scratches, no inflammation followed.

The limbs or trunk are thoroughly washed, and deep incisions are made into the skin wherever necessary. The parts to be examined are then placed in a solution containing carbonate of soda 1 per cent and formol 0.5 to 1 per cent, and soaked for twenty-four to forty-eight hours, when the skin can be taken off as a rule. After a few days of this treatment, the remaining muscles, fasciae, etc., are soft enough to allow the arteries to be dissected out. Unfortunately, the condition of the tissues is very variable, part of one limb, for instance, softening quickly, the remainder more slowly, In some cases, without any apparent reason, the muscles remain as hard as stone.

The arteries, especially the larger ones, such as the aorta, femoral, brachial, etc., are completely flattened out, looking as if they had been well ironed, and are therefore often difficult to find. If they have undergone marked fibroid or calcareous changes, the lumen may be patent and the vessel easily seen.

The arteries are dissected out and placed in a fresh solution of the aforementioned fluid for twenty-four hours. All adhering connective tissue is now removed, and the vessels are plunged into glycerine to which a few drops of formol have been added. This solution must be changed two or three times in the course of the next few weeks, as some coloring matter invariably dissolves out.

For microscopic examination small pieces of a calcified artery are placed in alcohol containing nitric acid, or better into Marchi's solution.[1] After twenty-four hours or longer the decalcified piece is washed in water for some hours, hardened, embedded in paraffin, and cut in the usual manner.

[1] I have given up alcohol and nitric acid, as Marchi's solution gives much better results.

Fibrous pieces were hardened in alcohol in the usual way. It is very difficult to know, however, whether a given artery does or does not contain small calcareous patches, so that for practical purposes it is always better to decalcify first. Marchi's solution does no harm, and by adopting this process much time will be saved.

DESCRIPTION OF ARTERIES EXAMINED

1. *Aorta (XXIst Dynasty)* consists of a piece 4½ inches long, covered almost throughout its whole length by a hard calcareous plate.

2. *Aorta (XVIIIth–XXth Dynasties).*—The arch had been hacked away by the embalmer, who had also cut right through all the coats just above the bifurcation of the vessel. The thoracic aorta from a point just above the origin of the left subclavian artery and the whole of the abdominal aorta were intact and easily removed. The internal coat is studded with small calcareous patches, and the two largest, each nearly the size of a shilling, are situated just above the bifurcation. The left subclavian artery at a point just above its origin is almost blocked by a raised, ragged, calcareous excrescence, as large as a threepenny-bit (calcified atheromatous ulcer). Small atheromatous patches, not calcified, are scattered through the whole length of the aorta, and these, owing to the dark coloration of the tissues, are more easily felt than seen.

The common carotid arteries show small patches of atheroma, but the most marked changes are found in the pelvic arteries and in those of the lower limbs.

The common iliac arteries are studded with small patches of atheroma and calcareous degeneration. The other arteries of the pelvis are converted by calcification into rigid "bony" tubes, down to their minute ramifications. So stiff and brittle are they that it was impossible to dissect them out entire, and in spite of every possible care they were invariably broken. The minute intramuscular arteries were easily felt on triturating the muscles under the fingers.

Both arms and the legs (about 6 inches below Poupart's ligament) had been lost, but on the right side the common femoral and profunda were dissected out. Both were converted into rigid calcareous tubes.

It is to be noted that, as far as could be made out from the examination of the cartilages of the ribs, the mummy was not that of a very old person.

3. *Atheromatous patches in the aorta and brachial arteries in a Greek mummy.*—From the examination of the cartilages, etc., I concluded at the time that the man was not above 50 years old at the time of death.

4. *Piece of thoracic aorta (XXVIIth Dynasty)*, altogether 4½ inches long. It contains seven calcareous patches, two of which are figured in Plate III, Fig. 3. No other lesion.

5. *Aorta from a Coptic mummy.*—Small hard calcareous patches scattered throughout its length. The two largest are just above the bifurcation and are almost the size of a sixpenny-piece.

6. and 7. *Pieces of two aortae, thoracic (XXIst Dynasty).*—No lesions.

8. *Posterior tibial artery.*—From a woman of the XXIst Dynasty, calcified from end to end.

9. *Posterior peroneal artery.*—A piece about 4 inches long. Artery stiff, lumen patent; evidently calcareous in places. After soaking, artery still very stiff; calcareous patches visible from outside. On opening, internal and middle coats almost completely calcified in places. In other places, vessel studded with minute calcareous nodules projecting into the lumen of the tube, hardly any healthy tissue being left between nodules.

10. *Anterior tibial artery.*—Apparently healthy, though lumen patent. On careful examination with lens, small points about the size of a pin's head, of a darkish brown color. Microscopically these points were found to be foci of disease.

11. *Posterior tibial artery.*—One piece about 6 inches long. This is completely calcified, the whole being converted into a rigid calcareous tube.

12. *Posterior peroneal.*—Apparently quite normal. The contrast between this smooth, highly flexible artery and the diseased vessels is most striking.

13. *Posterior peroneal artery.*—Quite soft and flexible, but here and there small highly colored brown patches project into the lumen.

14. *A small piece of anterior tibial artery and dorsalis pedis.*—Walls not markedly thickened, but distinctly nodular, with dark brown small nodules projecting into lumen.

15. *Femoral, profunda, and branches.*—Very tortuous and almost completely calcified.

16. *Posterior tibial and branches.*—Almost completely calcified from end to end.

17. *A piece of artery found mixed with the packing of the leg.*—Apparently quite normal.

18. *Part of posterior tibial and peroneal artery.*—Stiff, but no other changes to the naked eye.

19. *Piece of ulnar artery, about 3 inches long.*—Lumen patent and artery stiff after soaking and being plunged in glycerine for weeks. It has a curiously mottled, brown and white appearance. On cutting sections, fairly extensive calcification was discovered.

20. *Several small pieces of a brachial artery.*—In glycerine it becomes beautifully transparent, light yellow in color, but in spite of several weeks' soaking the longitudinal folds do not disappear. From the outside small brownish spots are seen studding it. On opening, these spots are seen to be small nodules projecting into the lumen. Some have a whitish centre with a brown irregular margin.

21. *Ulnar artery.*—Apparently quite normal.

22. *Part of palmar arch, soft and flexible.*—Small brownish patches in first digital branch.

23. *Ulnar artery.*—Apparently normal.

24. *Brachial, ulnar, and two inches of radial arteries.*—Ulnar and radial almost completely ossified. Brachial studded throughout its length with brownish prominent patches projecting into lumen of the tube. These are mostly quite soft, but the centre of some is undoubtedly calcified. The whole artery is markedly thicker than it should be.

N.B.—When not otherwise stated the mummies belonged to the XXIst Dynasty.

The results noted may be summed up as follows:

1. *Complete or incomplete calcification.*—There is no difficulty in recognising completely or partially calcified arteries. Even before they are placed in the softening solution, or at any rate shortly afterwards, their hard, "osseous" structure is manifest. Arteries, such as are depicted in Plate III, Fig. 1, are as rigid as calcified arteries of the present day.

When slit up, even with the finest scissors and the greatest care, the calcareous middle and inner coats have a tendency to detach themselves from the adventitia, and to break up into small brown roughly rectangular plates (see Plate III, Fig. 2). In this picture a small artery just branching off shows well-marked calcareous change.

After decalcification in picric acid and staining, microscopical sections of such arteries are most interesting and will be best understood by examining Plate IV, Fig. 9 This shows, under a low power, a decalcified posterior peroneal artery, stained by Van Gieson's method, from a mummy of the XXIst Dynasty. The section is perhaps not quite satisfactory, in so far that, nearly the whole of the artery being diseased, it is difficult to find points of comparison between healthy and calcareous tissue. Only shreds of endothelium and fenestrated membrane, for instance, are left at a, a_1, and a_2.

The point of interest is that the muscular coat has been changed almost wholly by calcification, following on degeneration of the muscle fibre, into a magma of no particular structure. The disease clearly did not begin in one spot, but in several foci which coalesced, as at *b*, for example. When the section is stained with haematoxylin alone the calcified parts are coloured so black that hardly any structure is recognisable. Plate IV, Fig. 10, represents part of a calcified ulnar artery under a high power (same stain as previously). In this section the muscular fibres at *a* have been completely destroyed by calcification, so that no structure is recognisable. At *b*, on the other hand, the annular fibres are still indicated, though somewhat vaguely, whereas at *c* they are plainly visible. To the naked eye this artery appeared to be completely calcified.

Partial calcification was best seen in the aorta, and is well illustrated by Figs. 3 and 4 in Plate III. Here we see calcareous patches in two aortae. Fig. 3 represents part of the abdominal aorta of a mummy of the XXVIIth Dynasty, and Fig. 4 a piece of a thoracic aorta dating from the same dynasty. The flattened vessel did not open out again, in spite of long soaking in glycerine, but remained angular.

The calcareous patches are quite obvious, and it is unnecessary to describe them any further. In the aorta depicted in Plate III, Fig. 3, they projected to a considerable extent into the lumen of the tube.

Such aortae are not good objects for microscopical examination, because, however careful the decalcification, the calcified part almost invariably falls off. In the calcified part nothing can be seen except a few shreds of muscular tissue lying between oval or round masses of calcified material staining almost black with haematoxylin.

In the coats of the aorta, beneath the wholly calcified parts, one sees almost normal muscular fibres, but here and there are small round darkly staining masses such as have been already described in the posterior peroneal and radial arteries. These are manifestly patches of incipient calcareous degeneration.

An interesting point is that very often the disease seems to pick (see, for instance, Plate III, Fig. 4) just the point of origin of the smaller arteries.

On examining carefully the inner lining of such an artery, one often sees small brownish nodules. These, however, are much more evident in the smaller arteries and will be described more fully hereafter. Indeed, in the larger vessels they are much more easily felt than seen.[1]

In one subclavian artery of the XVIIIth–XXth Dynasties the lumen of the artery near its origin was almost blocked by a ragged calcareous excrescence, depicted in Plate III, Fig. 5. There can be no doubt that this person narrowly escaped embolism.

2. *Partial calcification and atheroma.*—When an artery like the femoral or brachial is partly or completely calcified, there can be no difficulty in recognising such a lesion. The case is different, however, when the lesions are slight, as they are completely obscured by the colouring matter and the opacity of the tissue.

Good results can be obtained, however, by soaking pieces in glycerine to which a few drops of formol have been added, when, after a few days, the tissues become transparent. In many cases, even before the artery is opened, one sees through the coat (Plate III, Fig. 8) small dark brown patches, which are then also felt easily. When the artery is opened these patches are seen to protrude into the lumen (Plate III, Figs. 6 and 7), and sometimes they have a hard white centre (Plate III, Fig. 6), which is manifestly calcareous to the touch.

In pieces of such an artery, hardened and stained in the usual way, these patches are found to be just under the fenestrated membrane, which is easily recognised at one or both edges of the preparation (Plate V, Figs. 11*b* and 12). The inner membrane of the artery is often intact; sometimes the lesion has evidently broken through it (Plate V, Fig. 12).

The lesion, therefore, is in the middle coat of the artery, the muscle fibres of which are transformed into dark deeply staining strands, which have evidently undergone some very marked degeneration (Plate V, Fig. 11*d, e, f,* and Fig. 12).

Very often nothing more can be seen, and there is no sign of emigration of leucocytes in or around the diseased tissue.

[1] In this connection it must not be forgotten that, for some unexplained reason, air bubbles are often present between the middle and inner coat. These cause the inner coat to bulge outwards, causing an appearance as if the aorta were studded with small atheromatous patches. A little pressure at once causes them to flatten out and disappear.

In some arteries, however, I have seen around the degenerated patch small irregular bodies, which may or may not be leucocytes (Plate V, Fig. 13a).

I do not attach much importance to this absence of leucocytes, as I know from experience that leucocytes are hardly ever found in mummies, even in such tissues and lesions where we know that they must have been present in considerable numbers during life. Why this should be the case need not be discussed here.

I have already drawn attention to the fact that some arteries, although not necessarily showing any sign of calcification or other degeneration, feel like whip-cord and are plainly thickened, though they are not atheromatous. I regret that I cannot show any satisfactory microscopical specimens illustrating this fibroid change. When we remember that the thickness of an artery in microscopical sections of the tissues from fresh bodies depends on many conditions, it will be manifest that in mummified bodies comparison and inferences are practically impossible. Moreover, at present I cannot always distinguish, with certainty, fibrous from unstriated muscular tissues in mummies. I repeat, however, that to the naked eye and to the touch some arteries are distinctly thickened and fibrous.

DISCUSSION OF RESULTS

Nature of the lesions.—There can be no doubt respecting the calcification of arteries, and that it is of exactly the same nature as we see at the present day, namely, calcification following on atheroma.

The small patches seen in the arteries are atheromatous, and though the vessels have without doubt been altered by the three thousand years or so which have elapsed since death, nevertheless the lesions are still recognisable by their position and microscopical structure.

The earliest signs of the disease are always seen in or close below the fenestrated membrane—that is, just in the position where early lesions are seen at the present time. The disease is characterised by a marked degeneration of the muscular coat and of the endothelium. These diseased patches, discrete at first, fuse together later, and finally form comparatively large areas of degenerated tissue, which may reach the surface and open out into the lumen of the tube. I need not point out how completely this description agrees with that of the same disease as seen at the present time.

I have already mentioned the absence of leucocytes and cellular infiltration, and need not therefore return to it here.

In my opinion, therefore, the old Egyptians suffered as much as we do from arterial lesions identical with those found in the present time. Moreover, when we consider that few of the arteries examined were quite healthy, it would appear that such lesions were as frequent three thousand years ago as they are to-day.

ETIOLOGY

The etiology of this disease three thousand years ago is as obscure as it is in modern people. One cause which is supposed to play a part in modern times, namely *tobacco*, can certainly be eliminated, as this drug was not used in ancient Egypt.

Syphilis also can be eliminated with considerable certainty, as no pathological specimens of this disease in ancient Egyptians have as yet been discovered.

Alcohol played a part in Egyptian social life, in so far that on festive occasions some of the old Egyptians certainly got drunk, as is shown by pictures found in Egyptian tombs. Beer was a common beverage, and wine was not only made in the country but also imported.

It is clear, however, that the Egyptians as a race are not and never have been habitual drunkards.

If I may be allowed a short digression, I would remark in this connection that my personal experience has led me to call in question the importance of alcohol as a cause of arterial disease. During the Mussulman pilgrimage, I have made over eight hundred post-mortem examinations of people who had certainly never touched alcohol in their lives, and I have found that disease of the arteries is certainly as common and occurs as early in total abstainers as in people who take alcohol regularly.

Another favourite cause invoked for the production of arterial disease is the supposed increased wear and tear of modern life.

This has always appeared to me an extraordinary theory, considering that people, even as late as the beginning of last century, worked far harder and had much greater difficulty in getting their living than in the present day. In my opinion, the theory that the wear and tear of human life has increased is a myth, the fact being that our life is easier and that we work less than did our ancestors.

There is no evidence that old Egyptians worked hard either mentally or physically. Indeed, the time-tables of workmen which have been discovered show that the Egyptian navvies of ancient times toiled practically the same hours as the Egyptians do now. They enjoyed a holiday every seven days, as do many nations at the present time.

I do not think we can accuse a very heavy meat diet. Meat is and always has been something of a luxury in Egypt, and although on the tables of offerings of old Egyptians haunches of beef, geese, and ducks are prominent, the vegetable offerings are always present in greater number. The diet then as now was mostly a vegetable one, and often very coarse, as is shown by the worn appearance of the crown of the teeth.

Nevertheless, I cannot exclude a high meat diet as a cause with certainty, as the mummies examined were mostly those of priests and priestesses of Deir el-Bahri, who, owing to their high position, undoubtedly lived well. I must add, however, that I have seen advanced arterial disease in young modern Egyptians who ate meat very occasionally. In fact, my experience in Egypt and in the East has not strengthened the theory that meat-eating is a cause of arterial disease.

Finally, strenuous muscular exercise can also be excluded as a cause, as there is no evidence that ancient Egyptians were greatly addicted to athletic sport, although we know that they liked watching professional acrobats and dancers. In the case of the priests of Deir el-Bahri, it is very improbable, indeed, that they were in the habit of doing very hard manual work or of taking much muscular exercise.

I cannot therefore at present give any reason why arterial disease should have been so prevalent in ancient Egypt. I think, however, that it is interesting to find that it was common, and that three

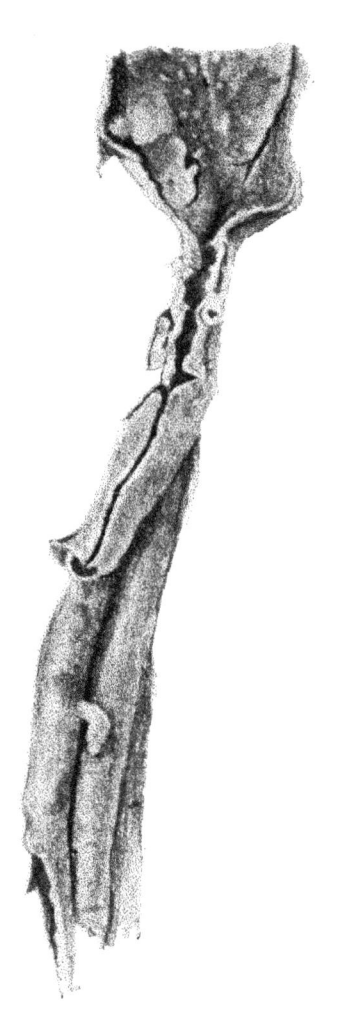

Fig. 1

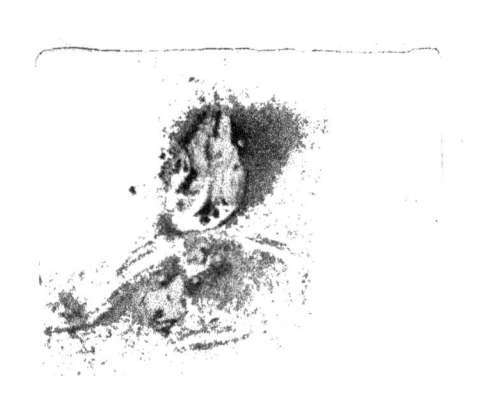

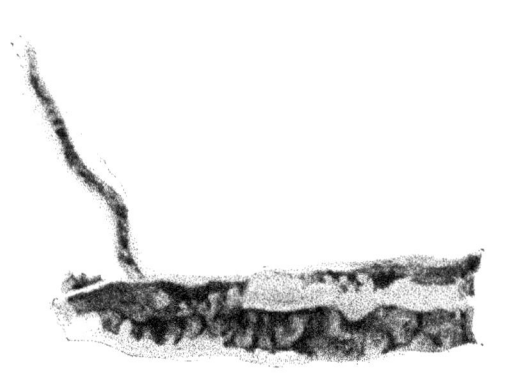

Fig. 2

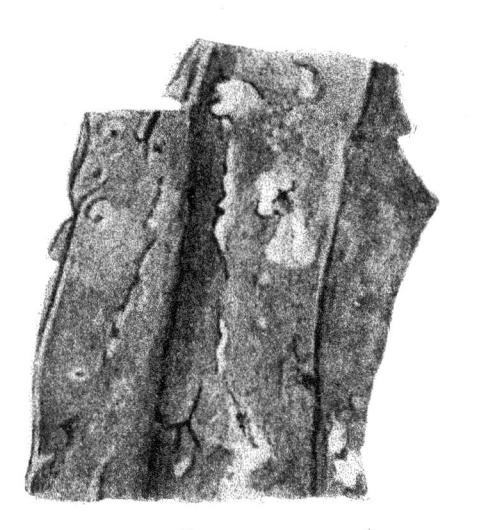

Fig. 4

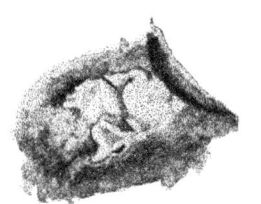

Fig. 5

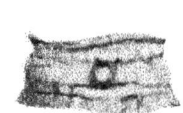

Fig. 6

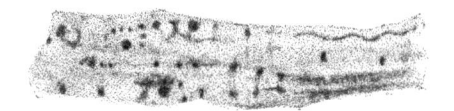

Fig. 7

PLATE IV

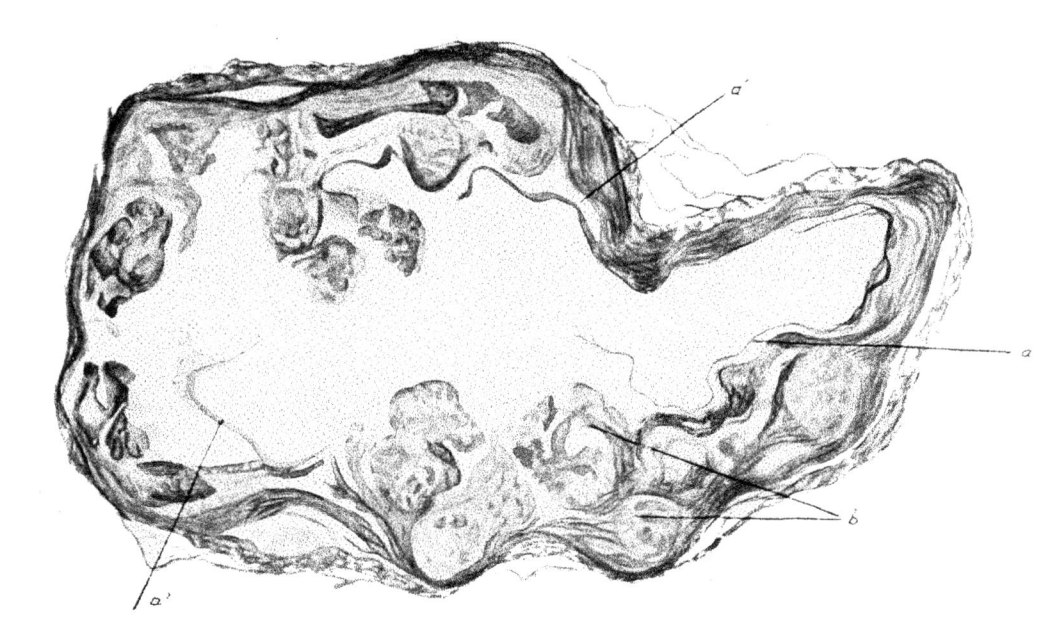

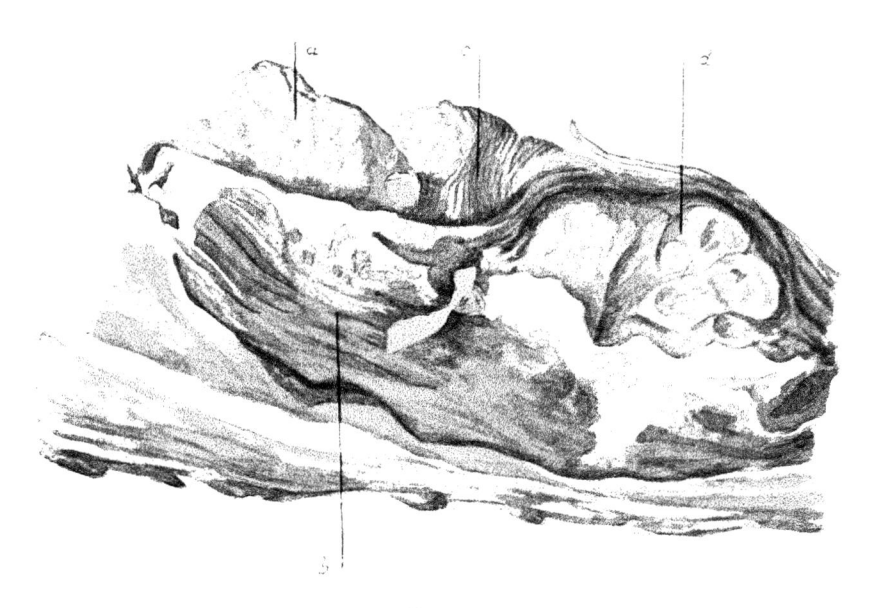

FIG. 9

FIG. 10

PLATE V

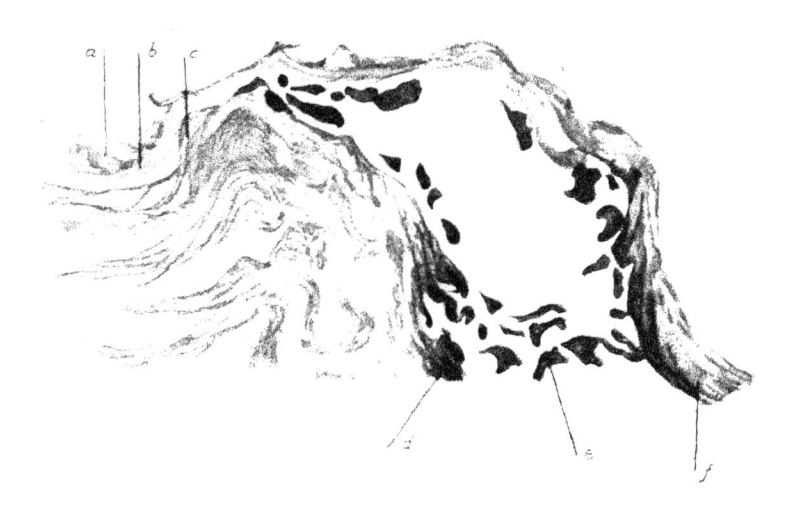

FIG. 11

FIG. 12

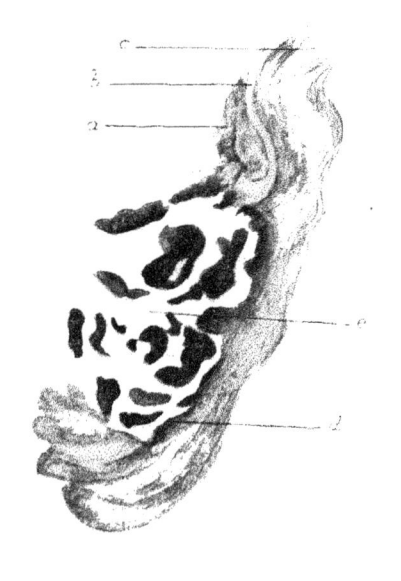

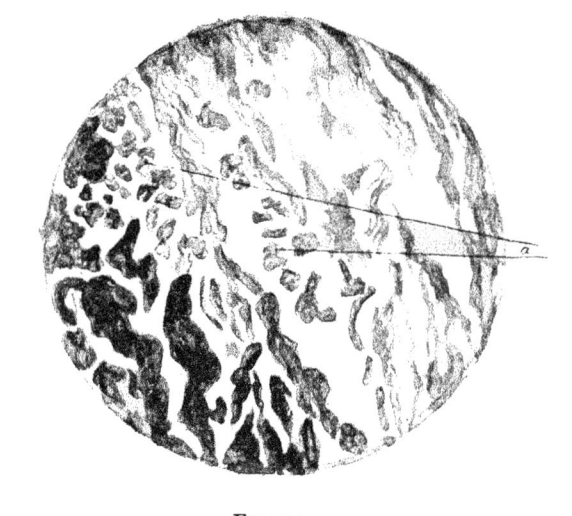

FIG. 13

thousand years ago it represented the same anatomical characters as it does now.

DESCRIPTION OF PLATES III–V

(For particulars see text)

PLATE III

Fig. 1.—Pelvic and arteries of thigh completely calcified (XVIIIth–XXth Dynasties).

Fig. 2.—Completely calcified profunda artery after soaking in glycerine (XXIst Dynasty).

Fig. 3.—Partly calcified aorta (XXVIIth Dynasty).

Fig. 4.—Calcified patches in aorta (XXVIIth Dynasty).

Fig. 5.—Calcified atheromatous ulcer of subclavian artery (XVIIIth–XXth Dynasties).

Fig. 6.—Patch of atheroma in anterior tibial artery (glycerine). The centre of the patch is calcified (XXIst Dynasty).

Fig. 7.—Atheroma of brachial artery (glycerine) (XXIst Dynasty).

Fig. 8.—Unopened ulnar artery, atheromatous patch shining through (glycerine) (XXIst Dynasty).

PLATE IV

Fig. 9.—Section through almost completely calcified posterior peroneal artery (low power). Van Gieson staining. a, a_1, a_2, remnants of endothelium and fenestrated membrane; b, calcified patches. Many more are seen.

Fig. 10.—Section through calcified patch of ulnar artery. Same stain. (Leitz, Oc. 1, $\times \frac{1}{12}$.) a, d, calcified patches; b, partially calcified muscular coat; c, annular muscular fibre.

PLATE V

Fig. 11.—Section through atheromatous patch of anterior tibial artery. Same stain. (Leitz, Oc. 1, $\times \frac{1}{12}$.) a, remains of endothelium; b, fenestrated membrane; c, muscular coat; d, f, membrane coat undergoing degeneration; e, completely degenerated remnants of muscular coat.

Fig. 12.—Section through atheromatous patch of ulnar artery. Same stain. (Leitz, Oc. 1, $\times \frac{1}{12}$.) (Reference letters the same as in Fig. 11.)

Fig. 13.—Section at edge of atheromatous patch. Haematoxylin stain. (Leitz, Oc. 1, $\times \frac{1}{12}$.) a, leucocytes (?). The atheromatous part on the left stains intensely dark with haematoxylin.

AN ERUPTION RESEMBLING THAT OF VARIOLA IN THE SKIN OF A MUMMY OF THE TWENTIETH DYNASTY (1200–1100 B.C.)[1]

(*Journal of Pathology and Bacteriology*, Vol. XV [1911])

The body from which the skin was taken was that of a tall man of middle age. It was brought to the attention of one of us by Professor G. Elliot Smith during his investigations into the process of mummification as illustrated in the royal mummies in the Cairo Museum of Antiquities. The body was the seat of a peculiar vesicular or bulbous eruption which in form and general distribution bore a striking resemblance to that of small-pox. The portion of skin we were permitted to remove, and which forms the subject of the present note, was taken from the adductor surface of the right thigh. The eruption on the inner surface of the thigh was, as the drawing shows (see Plate VI, Fig. 1), a closely set vesicular one, and it was in this situation that the general resemblance to small-pox was most noticeable.

Small portions of skin were treated by the following method:[2] (1) The tissue was softened in a solution of sodium carbonate mixed with alcohol (alcohol, 100 parts; water, 15 parts; 5 per cent solution of sodium carbonate, 60 parts); (2) this solution was replaced by 30 per cent alcohol, and the tissue gradually brought thereafter into absolute alcohol, and embedded in paraffin.

A reference to Plate VI, Fig. 2 (a low-power drawing of a microscopical section), shows that the superficial epithelial covering is very much disintegrated, all traces of Malpighian layer and its papillae having disappeared. No nuclear staining is discernible in any of the sections, a considerable number of which were stained and examined. The skin is everywhere broken up into a series of deeply staining lamellae or blocks. The dermis shows a more definite structure, and its wavy fibrillae and bundles are easily dis-

---
[1] This paper was written with A. R. Ferguson as junior author.
[2] Marc Armand Ruffer, *British Medical Journal*, I (London, 1909), 1005.

cernible. No distinct vessels, however, can be made out. On looking at the skin layer with a planatic magnifier, the presence of the dome-shaped vesicles is clearly demonstrated. They must have originated and developed in the middle of the prickle layer, i.e., in the situation in which the small-pox eruption is first seen.

In the fully matured state of the vesicles, as they are present in the skin under consideration, their bases are formed by the deepest (Malpighian) layer, whilst the elevated superficial layers of the epidermis form their roofs. In one or two of the sections examined there are traces of the vertical septa and curtains which subdivide the developing vesicle in small-pox.

The structure of the dermis has been much less interfered with, and wavy or curling hyaline fibrillae of the fibro-areolar tissue are as distinct as in many similar sections from freshly fixed tissues. There are no traces of cellular infiltration beneath the vesicles.

Sections stained by Gram's method reveal very large numbers of bacteria, the large majority of which are strongly Gram-positive. By far the largest proportion of these occur in the connective tissue of the dermis, where they are met with either in dense clusters or diffusely sprinkled throughout the tissue, following the lines of separation of the fibrillar bundles. Occasionally, however, they are seen to follow the track of what may have been a small vessel, the direction of which is more or less oblique to the surface (see Plate VI, Fig. 3). Owing to the tenacity with which the epithelial layer retains the Gram's stain, the presence of bacteria amongst the epithelial remains is impossible to establish. Careful search, however, in sections stained with methylene-blue, leaves no doubt as to their presence here also. They appear to be more numerous in the neighbourhood of the vesicles than elsewhere. The organisms present in the largest numbers are short, plump bacilli, often swollen at one end, so as in many instances to resemble one of the drum-stick bacilli. Others are distinctly beaded in form or have a torpedo shape. A cluster of bacilli with such characters bears a superficial resemblance to a group of diphtheria-like organisms. A few micrococci also occur; these are more apparent in sections stained with methylene-blue (see Plate VI, Fig. 4).

It is certainly unusual to find the sub-epithelial tissue so invaded by bacteria in small-pox as in the skin under consideration. Nor do we wish to maintain that these organisms played any part during the progress of the malady (supposing it to have been small-pox); but, after careful examination of a large number of sections, we are of opinion that these bacteria were present in the body at the time of death, although they have probably multiplied enormously after death. It may be firmly surmised that bacteria already present in the tissues might in some cases greatly multiply locally between the time of death and the mummification proper.

The specimen which we have described thus provides several points of quite exceptional interest, among which may be mentioned:

1. The probable existence of small-pox as evidenced by as characteristic an eruption as the conditions of preservation of such ancient material permits.

2. The conservation of the form of minute organisms such as bacteria after such a phenomenal period.

3. The demonstrability of bacteria in mummified tissues by modern staining methods.

DESCRIPTION OF PLATE VI

FIG. 1.—Naked-eye view of skin.

FIG. 2.—Microscopic section of skin under low power.

FIG. 3.—Section through dermis; Gram and eosin; Zeiss, *DD*, Compens. Oc. 6.

FIG 4.—Section through dermis; methylene-blue; Zeiss, *DD*, Compens. Oc. 6.

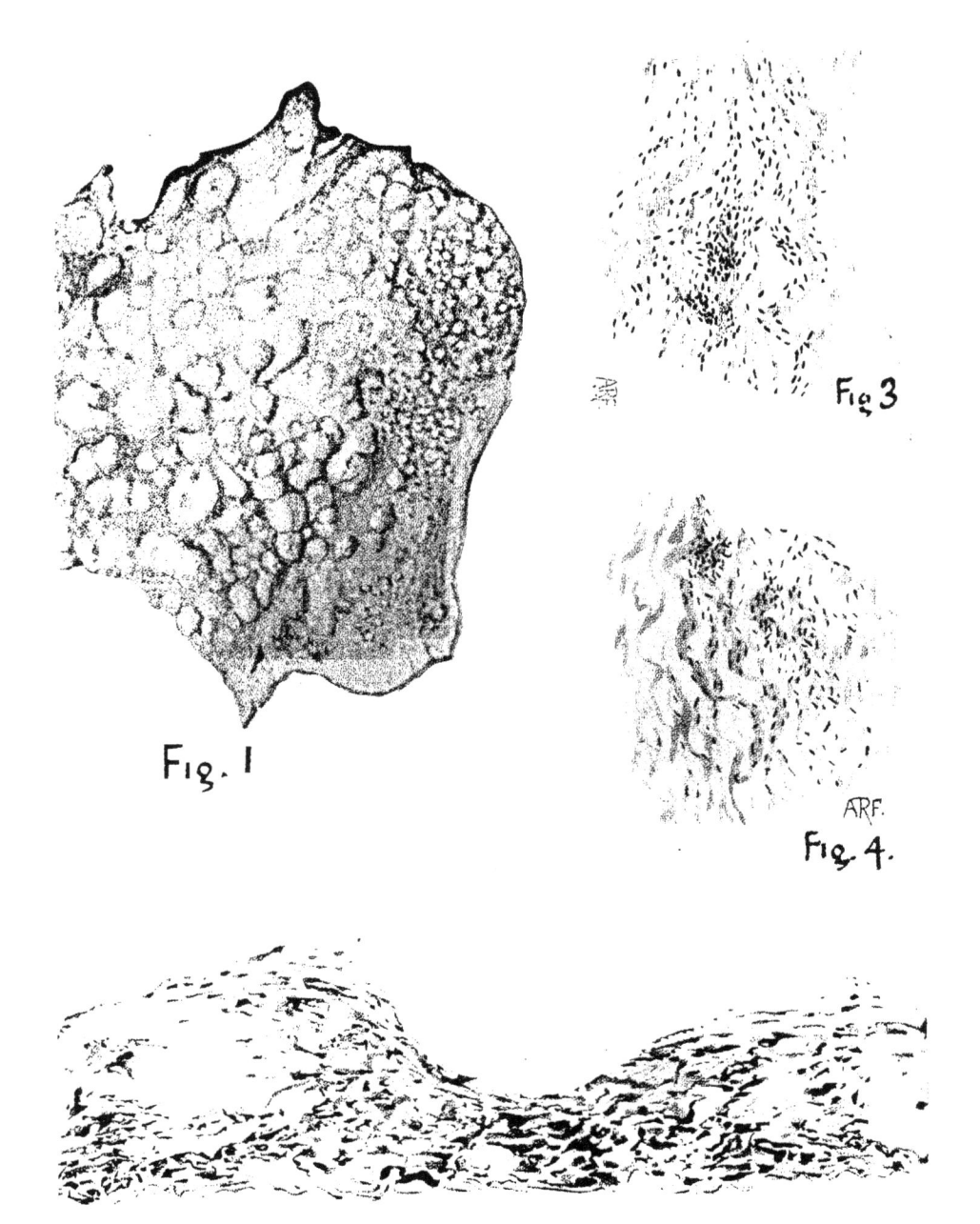

Fig. 1

Fig. 3

Fig. 4

ON DWARFS AND OTHER DEFORMED PERSONS IN ANCIENT EGYPT

(*Bulletin de la Société Archéologique d'Alexandrie*, No. 13)

It is not a little strange that certain deformed individuals should have had, from time immemorial, and should even now have a peculiar fascination for some men and women. Of these misshapen human creatures, perhaps the most popular have been dwarfs and hunchbacks. Even at the present time, dwarfs are kept in the household of several Eastern potentates, and some have a distinct influence at court.

It is altogether outside the scope of this paper to try and explain this strange taste, the reasons for which are very complicated. There is a superstition for instance, not only in the Levant but also in some parts of Europe, that to touch a hunchback's hump brings good fortune. Mythology and folklore have endowed dwarfs or gnomes with supernatural powers. Hunchbacks also enjoy an unmerited reputation as merry grigs; witness the French expression *s'amuser comme un bossu*.

Dwarfs were kept as pets in the palaces of kings, princes, and nobles during the Renaissance and Middle Ages. I would suggest, though without being able to adduce any proof, that this fashion was introduced in Europe by the Crusaders returned from the East. Painters such as Raphael, Titian, Mantegna, Veronese, Carpaccio, and others introduced dwarfs into their pictures, nor did they disdain to paint their portraits. An excellent account of this branch of art has been written by Richer.[1]

Among the Romans, *nani* were kept in rich houses for the amusement of inmates and guests.[2] The fashion may have come from Syria, but not from Greece, as dwarfs do not seem to have been a feature in households of Greece proper before the Roman conquest. In Lucian's banquet, the host introduces a dwarf to amuse his

---

[1] Dr. Paul Richer, *L'Art et la Médecine*.
[2] See Smith's *Dictionary of Archeology*.

guests, and he falling foul of the pompous philosopher present, a fierce fight ensues between the two ill-matched adversaries, the philosopher getting much the worst of it. At Rome, great ladies especially delighted in dwarfs, as Livia and Seneca's wife; and the prevalence of the fashion at Rome is marked by Suetonius, when he mentions particularly that Augustus did not care for them.

There is no clear distinction between *nanus* or *pumilio* or *pumilus*, the dwarf, and *morio*, the jester, since the jesters seem to have been selected for their absurd appearance as well as for that power, often found in the malformed, of making comical remarks for which mediaeval jesters were in demand. There seem to have been several kinds of dwarfs. One of them[1] is described as "acuto capite et auribus longis" and in another place[2] it is said "si solum spectas hominis caput, Hectora credas, si stantem videas Astyanacta putas," which indeed exactly describes the deformity due to the comparatively big head and short limbs of an achondroplastic dwarf. Some dwarfs were possibly cretins or myxoedematous dwarfs.[3] Misshapen limbs as well as small stature added to their price, and the most revolting part of the fashion was that the deformity was sometimes caused by artificial means, the children being kept in a case or frame which would stunt or distort their growth.[4] The Romans kept female as well as male dwarfs.

Amongst the extreme cases recorded on ancient authority one may notice Philetus, a contemporary of Hippocrates, who was so small that he "had to ballast himself to avoid being carried away by the wind"; the Egyptian dwarf mentioned by Nicephorus Callistus, who "at the age of 25 years did not exceed *a partridge in size*," and lastly the poet Arisastus, of whom Athenaeus records that he was so small that "no one could see him." I leave the reader to make whatever allowance he thinks fit for exaggeration.

Little is known about dwarfs among the Jews, except that they are mentioned among those who were forbidden access to the temple.

---

[1] Mart. vi. 39.   [2] Mart. xiv. 212.

[3] Mart. viii. 12.

[4] I confess to much scepticism with regard to the possibility of making dwarfs artificially.

In Egypt, dwarfs were common, and indeed, the pictures, statuettes, etc., found in this country copied nature with such fidelity that in many cases it is possible to recognise to what disease the deformity was due.

Nevertheless, many Egyptologists, instead of regarding dwarfs as pathological specimens, look upon them as having been pygmies brought into Egypt from Central Africa. In order to illustrate this view I can do no better than quote the most modern, excellent, and learned work, namely the *History of Egypt* by Breasted.

Breasted relates that:

in the young king's [Pepi II, about 2400 B.C.] second year, Harkhuf, one of the king's best officers, was for the fourth time despatched to Yam,[1] whence he returned bringing a rich pack train and a dwarf (Figs. 41, 75) from one of the pygmy tribes of Central Africa.

Breasted adds:

These uncouth, bandylegged figures were highly prized by the noble class of Egypt; they were not unlike the merry genius Bes in appearance, and they executed dances in which the Egyptians took the greatest delight. The land from which they came was connected by the Nile dwellers with the mysterious regions of the West, the sojourn of the dead, which they called "the land of the spirits" and the dwarfs from this sacred land were especially desired for the dances with which the king's leisure hours were diverted.

I have copied Fig. 41 (Plate VIII, Fig. 1), and Fig. 75 of Breasted's book is represented here by the excellent photograph of the dwarf Chnoum-hotep, given me by my friend His Excellency E. Brugsch Pasha (Plate VII). A glance at these figures shows that they do not represent pygmies, but typical achondroplastic dwarfs.

Granted that Egyptians brought pygmies back from Central Africa, it does not follow that all or even the majority of dwarfs in Ancient Egypt were pygmies. I have examined carefully hundreds of illustrations of people depicted in ancient Egyptian monuments, without finding a true pygmy among them.

On the contrary, the dwarfs figured in tombs are always typically pathological specimens. Indeed, Edward Tyson in 1699 had

[1] A country in the South, probably Central Africa.

already pointed out the mistake into which some authors had fallen by grouping together pygmies and dwarfs. He wrote:

Now by *Men Pygmies* we are by no means to understand *Dwarfs*. In all Countries, and in all Ages, there have been now and then observed such Miniature of Mankind, or under-sized Men. Cardan (de subtilitate lib. II, p. 458) tells us that he saw one carried in a Parrot's cage, that was but a Cubit high. Nicephorus tells us (Nicephor. Histor. Ecclesiast. lib. 12. cap. 37) that in *Theodosious* the Emperour's time, there was one in Aegypt that was no bigger than a Partridge; yet what was to be admired, he was very Prudent, had a sweet clear Voice, and a generous Mind; and lived Twenty Years. So likewise a King of *Portugal* sent to a Duke of *Savoy*, when he married his daughter to him, an *Aethiopian* Dwarf but three Palms high (Happelius in Relat. Curiosis. No. 85, p. 677). And *Thévenot* (Voyage de Levant lib. 2. c. 68.) tells us that the Present made by the King of the *Abyssins*, to the Grand Signor, of several *little black Slaves* out of *Nubia*, and the countries near Aethiopia, which being made Eunuchs, were to guard the Ladies of the Seraglio. And a great many such like Relations there are. But these being only Dwarfs, they must not be esteemed the Pygmies we are enquiring about, which are represented as a *Nation*, and the whole Race of them to be of the like stature.[1]

I

I will begin by the description of a dwarf who has already figured as an achondroplastic dwarf in Dr. P. Richer's book.

The name of this person was Chnoum-hotep (Plate VII), and his limestone statuette, now in the Cairo Museum, was found at Saqqarah. He lived in the Vth Dynasty (about 2700 B.C.), that is, about 4,500 years ago.

Le nain a la tête grosse, barrelée, cantonnée de deux vastes oreilles. La figure est niaise. [I do not agree with Sir Gaston here, as the face to me appears rather cunning than otherwise.] L'œil, ouvert étroitement, est retroussé vers les tempes, la bouche mal fendue. La poitrine est robuste et bien développée, mais le torse n'est pas en proportion avec le reste du corps; l'artiste a eu beau s'ingénier à en voiler la partie inférieure sous une ample jupe blanche, on sent qu'il est trop long pour les bras et pour les jambes. Le ventre se projette en pointe et les hanches se retirent pour faire contrepoids au ventre. Les cuisses n'existent guère qu'à l'état rudimentaire, et l'individu entier, campé qu'il est sur des petits pieds contrefaits, semble être hors d'aplomb et prêt à tomber face contre terre.

The description is from every point of view perfectly correct. It is obvious that the large head and bust are out of all proportion

[1] *A Pathological Essay Concerning the Pygmies of the Ancients*, by Edward Tyson, A.D. 1699, now edited, with an introduction treating of pygmy races and fairy tales, by Bertram C. A. Windle.

to the diminutive lower limbs. The knot in the girdle is well above the symphysis pubis, which, judging from the position of the umbilicus, I take to be level with or just a little below the tips of the fingers. The femur is very short, and there is same diminution in length of the bones of the legs. The feet are squat and flat. The bones of the upper limbs, as compared to the length of the trunk, are much shorter than they should be, as the tips of the fingers only reach the top of the thigh.

The arms do not hang down straight, but away from the sides, and the palms of the hands are turned forwards. There is probably some deformity of the legs also, but this is hidden by the skirt. The hands are squat. A certain amount of lordosis[1] is present also. Otherwise the little man is strongly built, and the muscular development of the arms specially well marked.

In fact, this statuette shows the chief characteristics of an achondroplastic dwarf, namely disproportion between the size of the trunk and limbs, the latter being much too short for the former, a head too large in proportion to the size of the body, and good muscular development. The description of achondroplasia in any modern textbook of medicine exactly applies to this dwarf.

The only other possible diagnosis, namely that of myxoedema, is negatived by the fact that this person held a high position at court. His tomb was one of the finest and richest at Saqqarah, and according to Maspero he was "Chief of the Perfumes" or "Head of the Wardrobe." No myxoedematous dwarf, whose mental faculties are generally impaired, could have held court functions, which, among the intrigues of the East, must have required no little tact and cleverness.

Achondroplastic dwarfs are not stupid as a rule, and are often distinctly cunning. Some have occupied important functions at court as jesters. Muscularly they are well developed and not unfrequently at the present time earn their living as dancers and acrobats.[2] As will be seen presently, they had definite duties assigned them in Egyptian households.

[1] I.e., forward curvature of the lumbar spine.

[2] Both in Paris and London achondroplastic dwarfs are appearing on the music-hall stage at the present time.

The other illustration, which Breasted gives as representing pygmies, comes from a tomb of the Old Empire and represents four dwarfs working at jewelry. The copy which is shown here (Plate VIII, Fig. 1) demonstrates that these persons were not pygmies, but achondroplastic dwarfs of the same class as Chnoum-hotep. Though the body is well developed, the arms and especially the lower limbs are stunted. The picture shows incidentally how carefully Egyptian artists followed nature sometimes, as in the extreme left of the picture a fat man has been introduced whose obesity is in sharp contrast with the spare bodies of this fellow workman.

Several other achondroplastic dwarfs have been copied by archaeologists on monuments of ancient Egypt. Perhaps the oldest is the "dwarf of Zer" (Plate VIII, Fig. 2) discovered by Flinders Petrie at Abydos, and dating from about 4715–4658 B.C.

The drawing, a mere outline on a bowl of metamorphic rock, is wonderfully spirited, as Petrie has remarked. Some of the characteristics of an achondroplastic dwarf are obvious, as for instance the great length and breadth of the trunk as compared with the lower limbs. The shortness of the thighs and the great muscular development are noticeable, but the right lower limb is so foreshortened that it is practically impossible to say where the thigh ends and the leg begins. The arms are short also. The head, however, is not characteristic, being small and the features sharp and intelligent. Nevertheless, the other characteristics justify the diagnosis of achondroplasia. It is only right to add that Petrie had recognised the dwarfish nature of this person.

Many similar dwarfs are depicted on Egyptian monuments, and a few more instances may be given.

Plate VIII, Fig. 3, shows two dwarfs from the tomb of Aba, about 2400 B.C.,[1] at work in the manufacture of necklaces. The contrast between the size of the trunk and the lower limbs is well marked, though other details are obscured.

In the same work[2] a dwarf (Plate VIII, Fig. 4), perhaps one of the four just mentioned, is seen standing under his master's chair holding a mirror in his hand. The dwarf looks exceedingly small,

[1] N. de G. Davies, *Deir el Gebrawi*, Plate XIII.
[2] Plate XVII.

but as the Egyptian artist always drew the master much larger in proportion to the other people in the picture, no opinion can be formed regarding the real size of the little man.

Two more achondroplastic dwarfs (Plate VIII, Fig. 5) are represented on the walls of a tomb at Deshasheh, dating from the middle of the Vth Dynasty (about 2700 B.C.).[1] The one on the left of the picture holds a necklace in his right hand and carries a box on his head, whereas the other is busy at the work table. In both the characteristic deformity is accurately shown.

In the same tomb a dwarf is represented (Plate VIII, Fig. 6) holding a sling (?) in his hand and standing in the prow of a boat. The contrast between the slim oarsman and the squat dwarf is very noticeable.

In the tombs of Sheikh Said, dating from the Vth Dynasty probably, a dwarf (Plate VIII, Fig. 7) holding a monkey in leash stands under his master's chair, and another (Plate VIII, Fig. 8) leads a greyhound. Although both figures are in a bad state of preservation, yet the deformities are recognisable.

The female dwarf (Plate IX, Fig. 9) discovered at Athribis[2] dates from the IVth Dynasty. It is not a very good specimen, though the squat figure shows off the slim, naked girl walking in front.

Other achondroplastic dwarfs might doubtless be found on Egyptian monuments, but in my opinion the examples copied here are sufficient to show that this disease has been in existence for the last five thousand years at least, and that it presented then the same pathological characteristics as it does now.

The occupations of these little people, in the majority of cases, appear to have been of two kinds. The first was the care of pet animals, and it is not a little odd that in comparatively modern times they should have been similarly employed. The Egyptian dwarf is seen leading his master's greyhound or holding a monkey in leash, the Italian dwarf is caressing a greyhound (see Tiepolo's picture in the Berlin Museum), and Valesquez has painted an English dwarf holding a greyhound in leash (see the picture of Don Antonio, the Englishman, by Velasquez in the Madrid Museum).

[1] Petrie, *Deshasheh*.   [2] Petrie, *Athribis*, Plate I.

Another occupation was the care and making of jewelry. An eminent Egyptologist has suggested to me that valuables were entrusted to dwarfs, because their deformities provided an easy means of identification if they ran away with their master's property. This view appears to me to be probably correct.

II

I may now pass on to the description of some other malformed persons depicted on Egyptian tombs. The first that I would draw attention to represents two young people copied by Mr. Percy Newberry, from the walls of tombs at Beni-Hassan, dating from the XIth and XIIth Dynasties (about 2000 B.C.). One of them has already been figured by Richer in the work quoted already (Plate IX, Fig. 10b and Fig. 11). The diagnosis here is easy, for the position of the feet is typical of talipes equino-varus.[1] Notice the contrast between these youths and the achondroplastic dwarfs previously described, for in the case of the club-footed people, the proportion between the length of the limbs and that of the body is almost normal.

The female dwarfs (Plate IX, Fig. 13) with well-marked talipes equino-varus are represented on the walls of the tomb at El Amarna, dating from the XVIIIth Dynasty (1375 B.C.). Next to them the artist has represented one of the king's daughters, and the contrast between the slim child and the deformed little figures is most striking.

III

Two other figures show the typical features of Pott's disease. In the first (Plate IX, Fig. 15) discovered in the tombs of Beni-Hassan (XIth–XIIth Dynasties about 2000 B.C.) the characteristic deformity occupies the upper dorsal and lower cervical region. In consequence, the head is protruded slightly forwards. The other (Plate IX, Fig. 14) was copied from a tomb at El Amarna and dates from the XVIIIth Dynasty. The hump in this case occupies the lower dorsal or lumbar region.

These are the only two examples of Pott's disease that I have found so far on old Egyptian monuments. They acquire impor-

[1] Anglice: club-foot.

tance from the fact that they date from nearly two thousand years before Christ.

Mme Constantine Sinadino of Alexandria owns a little marble statuette dating from the Greek period, which shows the characteristic deformity of Pott's disease (Plate X, Fig. 2).

Another statuette in the Alexandria Museum hollowed in the shape of a pot, and dating from the Graeco-Roman period, shows a similar deformity (Plate X, Fig. 3).

IV

There is some evidence also that rickets existed in Old Egypt. The man outlined in Plate IX, Fig. 10*b*, shows considerable enlargement of the cranium, which is evident on comparing his head with those of his companions. The smallness of the face accentuates the deformity. The squareness of the trunk suggests an adult man, the breadth being out of proportion to the length of the body. On the other hand, the trunk does not appear to be much too long for the limbs.

The lower limbs are greatly deformed and the bowed legs are typical of rickets. The foot is flat, whereas the arch of the foot in people from the same period is high.

In my opinion, we are here in presence of a case of rickets, with evident deformity of the legs, and probably some amount of hydrocephalus also. Achondroplasia and myxoedema are plainly out of the question.

A dwarf (Plate IX, Fig. 12) from another tomb at Beni-Hassan shows deformities similar to the preceding one. The head, however, does not appear to be larger than usual. The little person was pot-bellied, for the abdomen is prominent, and the curve of the waist, usually emphasised in Egyptian pictures, is absent here. The bowed legs are characteristic of rickets. The arch of the foot has almost disappeared.

V

I now proceed to describe one statuette and two bas-reliefs in which the etiology of the deformities is not quite plain.

The first (Plate X, Fig. 2) is a small statuette, now in the Ashmolean Museum at Oxford. The work is rough, and the figure in a bad state of preservation, for the left leg is broken. It is interesting to find that the British artist who repaired it was obliged to make a plaster leg bending outwards in order that it should fit the other leg. Although the lower limbs are short as compared to the trunk, yet the disproportion is not marked enough to warrant the diagnosis of achondroplasia. The deformity was probably due to rickets. The statuette dates from the Ist Dynasty and is at least five thousand years old.

A bas-relief (Plate IX, Fig. 16) of the Ist Dynasty figured by Flinders Petrie (*Royal Tombs*, II, Plate XXVIII, the tomb of Zer-Ta) shows another interesting dwarf. The work is primitive and coarse, though the figure is full of movement. The prominent pathological features are the bowed legs, the stout body, and the shortness of the arms. Owing to the want of finish in the carving, the size of the head cannot be ascertained with accuracy, though it appears somewhat too large as compared with the body.

An exact diagnosis is in my opinion impossible. Considering the absence of any marked disproportion between the size of the body and that of the legs, considering also the well marked deformity of the legs, I conclude that the disease which had produced these deformities was probably rickets.

Perhaps the most striking figure which has been assumed to be a dwarf (see Richer, *loc. cit.*) is that of the celebrated "Queen of Punt" (see Plate XI) which was carved in relief on the walls of the Temple of Deir el Bahri and is now in the Cairo Museum.

The authorities of the Cairo Museum consider this person to have been a steatopygous woman. Richer, on the other hand, thinks that the deformity was typical of achondroplasia. He expresses himself as follows:

> Derrière lui, le roi de Poun [Anglice:Punt], se trouve sa femme. Celle-ci a sa chevelure soigneusement peignée et ramassée en queue épaisse par derrière,... ...Quant à ses traits, ils sont assez réguliers, quoiqu'un peu virils, mais tout le reste de sa personne est repoussant. Ses bras, sa poitrine, ses jambes, sont comme chargés de chairs ramollies; le bassin se projette en arrière, et accuse ure déformité que l'artiste égyptien a rendue avec une naïveté surprenante.
>
> Faut-il voir là l'ensellure et la proéminence des fesses signalées par Parrot, chez certains nains, ou bien, comme le pense M. Bordier, ne s'agirait-il pas de

la représentation du type des Boschemans, avec l'ensellure et la stéatopygie charactéristiques ? Broca fait une remarque qui ruine cette dernière hypothèse. Il fait remarquer que l'humérus paraît plus court que le radius. Or, ce fait ne se rencontre dans aucune race, moins chez les Boschemans que chez aucune autre. Nous ajouterons que la disproportion des membres très courts avec le torse trop long, leur surcharge graisseuse, s'ajoutent aux signes ci-dessus relevés, pour faire de cette figure une véritable naine se rattachant à la catégorie des achondroplasiques.

The problem is rendered more difficult by the fact that the legs, abdomen, and head are drawn in profile and the chest almost full face.

My opinion agrees with Richer's in so far that I do not think that the Queen of Punt was either a steatopygous woman nor a Bushwoman. The first hypothesis is disproved by her face, which is certainly not that of a Bushwoman but is rather of a Semitic type.

The diagnosis of steatopygia can also be shown to be incorrect.

The chief characteristic of a steatopygous woman is the disproportion between the size of the buttocks and thighs. If, in the case of the Queen of Punt, a horizontal line be drawn just below the top of the thigh, it will be noticed that, as a matter of fact, the buttocks do not stand out at all prominently above that line; whereas in a steatopygous woman, a Hottentot, for instance, the prominence is very noticeable. In the Queen of Punt, the most marked characteristic is the pronounced lordosis. The lumbar spine is bent forwards, the whole abdomen has sunk, and the umbilicus is only a little above the level of a line drawn across the lower edge of the gluteal fold. Very remarkable also is the depression of the symphysis pubis. In any case, the lordosis alone is sufficient to account for the size of the buttocks.

It is true that steatopygous women look as if they had lordosis, but in them, if the deformity exists at all, it is very slight indeed.

Although, therefore, I consider the diagnosis of steatopygia as not proven, yet neither do I consider Her Majesty of Punt as an achondroplastic dwarf.

In the first place, it cannot be proven that the Queen was smaller than her companions. On the bas-relief she is just as tall as the men preceding and following her. The point is perhaps not of great importance, as it may be argued that the artist drew her the same size as her companions for the sake of symmetry. Much more important, however, is the fact that although there is undoubtedly some disproportion between the length of the trunk and that of the lower limbs, yet this is rendered very prominent by the depression of the umbilicus. Were it not for the depression of the abdomen, the umbilicus would be situated about one and a half centimetres higher than it is in the photograph, which would correspond pretty nearly to the centre of the figure.

Another important fact against the diagnosis of achondroplasia is that the arms are by no means short, and I can see no reason for supposing, as Broca did, that the humerus was shorter than the radius. The hand and fingers are shapely and very unlike the squat extremities of the achondroplastic dwarf.

One fact must not be forgotten, which appears not to have been noticed by all those who have examined this bas-relief, namely that the Queen of the Punt had a daughter. Part of the bas-relief discovered by Mariette has unfortunately been lost and the missing portion showed the daughter of the Queen. The fact is mentioned by Naville (*The Temple of Deir el Bahri*), and Sir Gaston Maspero informs me that the daughter showed the same deformities as the mother, though to a slighter degree. Although achondroplasia has been known to be hereditary, yet it appears to me that the extreme lordosis of the Queen would certainly have interfered with parturition, and that it is very probable therefore that the deformity was an acquired one.

I confess my inability to propose any definite diagnosis for the present. The lordosis is self-evident, but I cannot account for the redundant flesh on the limbs and trunk, whereas the face, hands, feet, and apparently the breasts also, have remained normal. I say flesh and not fat advisedly, for the enlargement of the thighs, etc., resembles far more the jelly-like tissues of certain cases of elephantiasis than adipose tissue.

The deformity is not due to filaria, for all the limbs and the trunk are enlarged. I have seen in Egyptian women enlargement of one limb exactly corresponding to that seen in the Queen of Punt, and neither during the day nor at night did I find parasites in their blood. This deformity may perhaps occur in several limbs? I cannot say.

VI

Among the dwarfs of Egypt, the gods Bes and Phtah have also been mentioned. The first is supposed to have been copied from a rickety dwarf and the other from an achondroplastic dwarf. I have examined a great many statuettes of the latter without arriving at any definite conclusion for the present. Some statuettes, however, show a distinct swelling in the region of the navel, most resembling an umbilical hernia. The former, in my opinion, is not a dwarf at all. As, however, the discussion of this question would entail entering into a great many archaeological problems, I must leave this subject until another occasion. For the same reason, it would also be inexpedient to describe the many dwarfish figures found in Egypt which date from the Greek and Roman times.

The old Egyptians kept not only human dwarfs, but animal dwarfs also. On the walls of the tombs of Beni-Hassan there are representations of dwarf cattle and dogs, the latter resembling somewhat the dachshund of the present day (Plate IX, Figs. 18 and 19).

A point which as far as I know has escaped everybody's attention is that giants were employed also, for in the same tombs some men are depicted who were without doubt at least a foot taller than their fellows. It may be that these men were simply Shillouk slaves, but at any rate the point requires investigation.

CONCLUSIONS

The statuettes, bas-reliefs, and paintings found in ancient Egyptian tombs show that:

1. Achondroplasia has existed for at least five thousand years.
2. Rickets has probably existed for the same period, and certainly since 2000 B.C.
3. The deformities characteristic of Pott's disease and of talipes equino-varus were put on record about four thousand years ago.
4. In addition to the deformities of the skeletons mentioned, there are a number of others to be found on Egyptian monuments in which the diagnosis remains doubtful.

48 STUDIES IN THE PALAEOPATHOLOGY OF EGYPT

DESCRIPTION OF PLATES VII-XI
(For particulars see text)

PLATE VII
The dwarf Chnoum-Hotep.

PLATE VIII
Achondroplastic dwarfs.

PLATE IX
FIG. 9.—Female achondroplastic dwarf following a young girl.
FIG. 10.—A boy with talipes equino-varus and a rickety dwarf.
FIG. 11.—A boy with talipes equino-varus.
FIG. 12.—A rickety dwarf.
FIG. 13.—Two female dwarfs with talipes equino-varus.
FIG. 14.—A hunchback.
FIG. 15.—Another hunchback.
FIG. 16.—A dwarf. (Diagnosis?)
FIG. 18.—Dwarf bull led by a man.
FIG. 19.—Dwarf dog.

PLATE X
FIG. 1.—Statuette from the Ashmolean Museum at Oxford representing a female dwarf. (Diagnosis?)

FIG. 2.—A hunchback, from Mme Constantine Sinadino's collection (Greek period).

FIG. 3.—A hunchback. Terra-cotta pots in the Alexandria Museum (Greek period).

PLATE XI
The Queen of Punt. Bas-relief from Deir el Bahri.

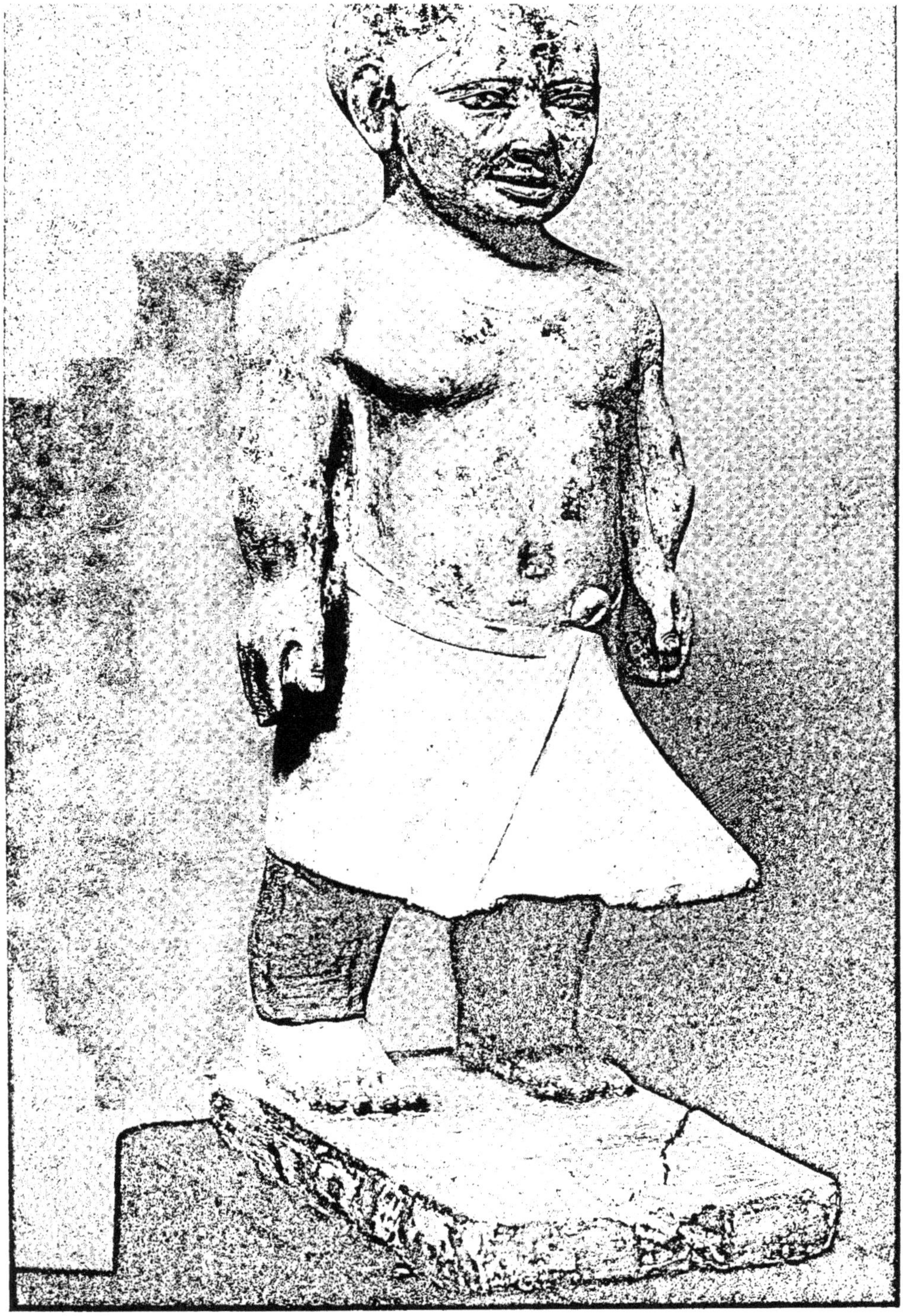

PLATE VIII

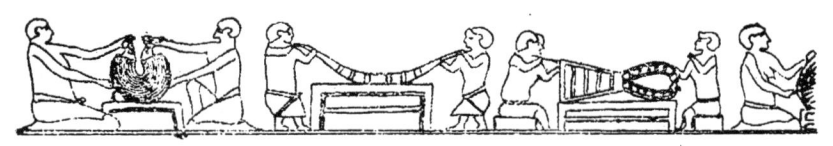

Fig. 1.

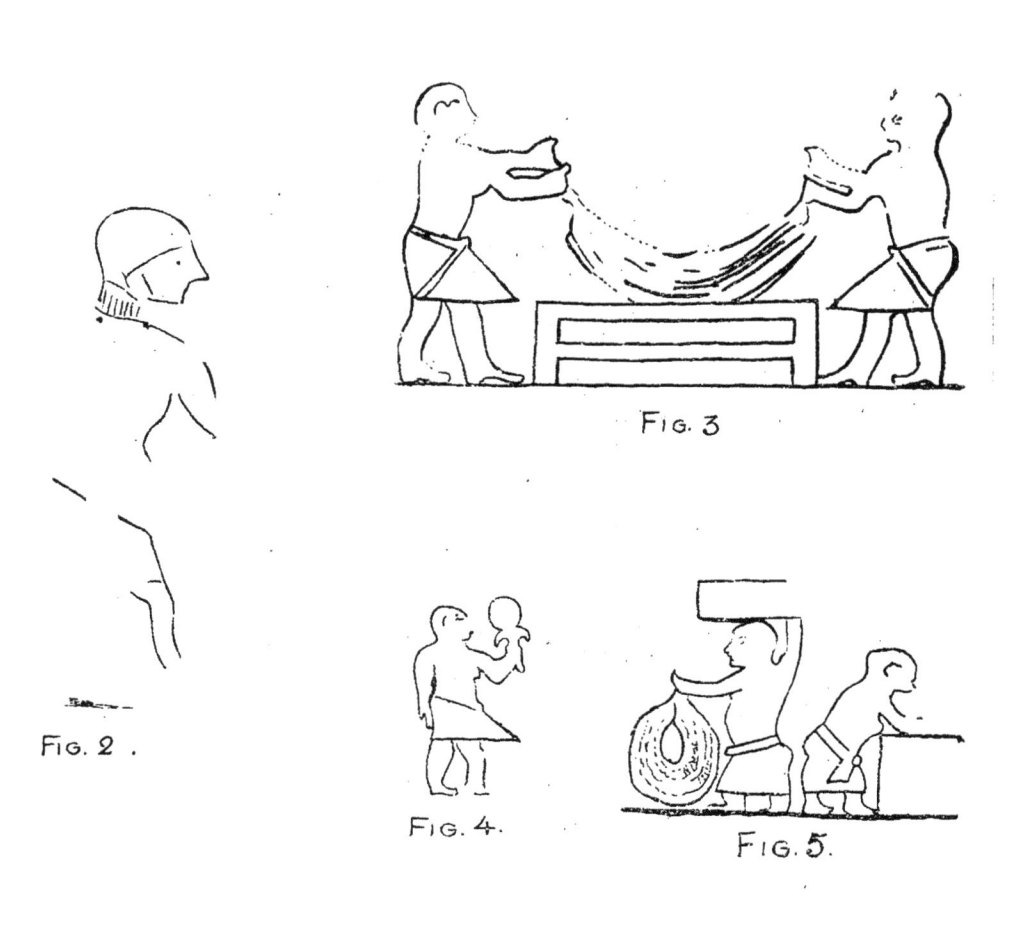

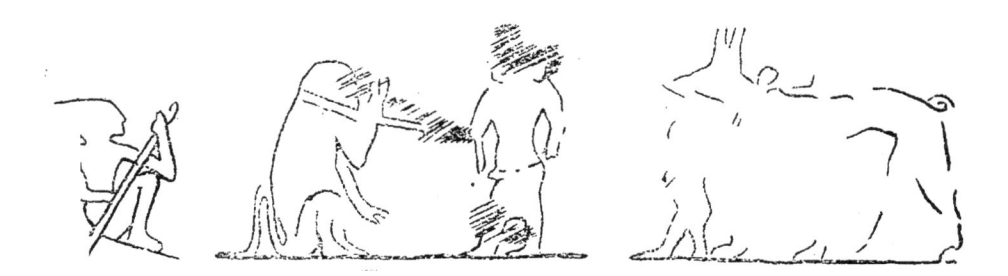

Fig. 2.

Fig. 3.

Fig. 4.

Fig. 5.

Fig. 9.

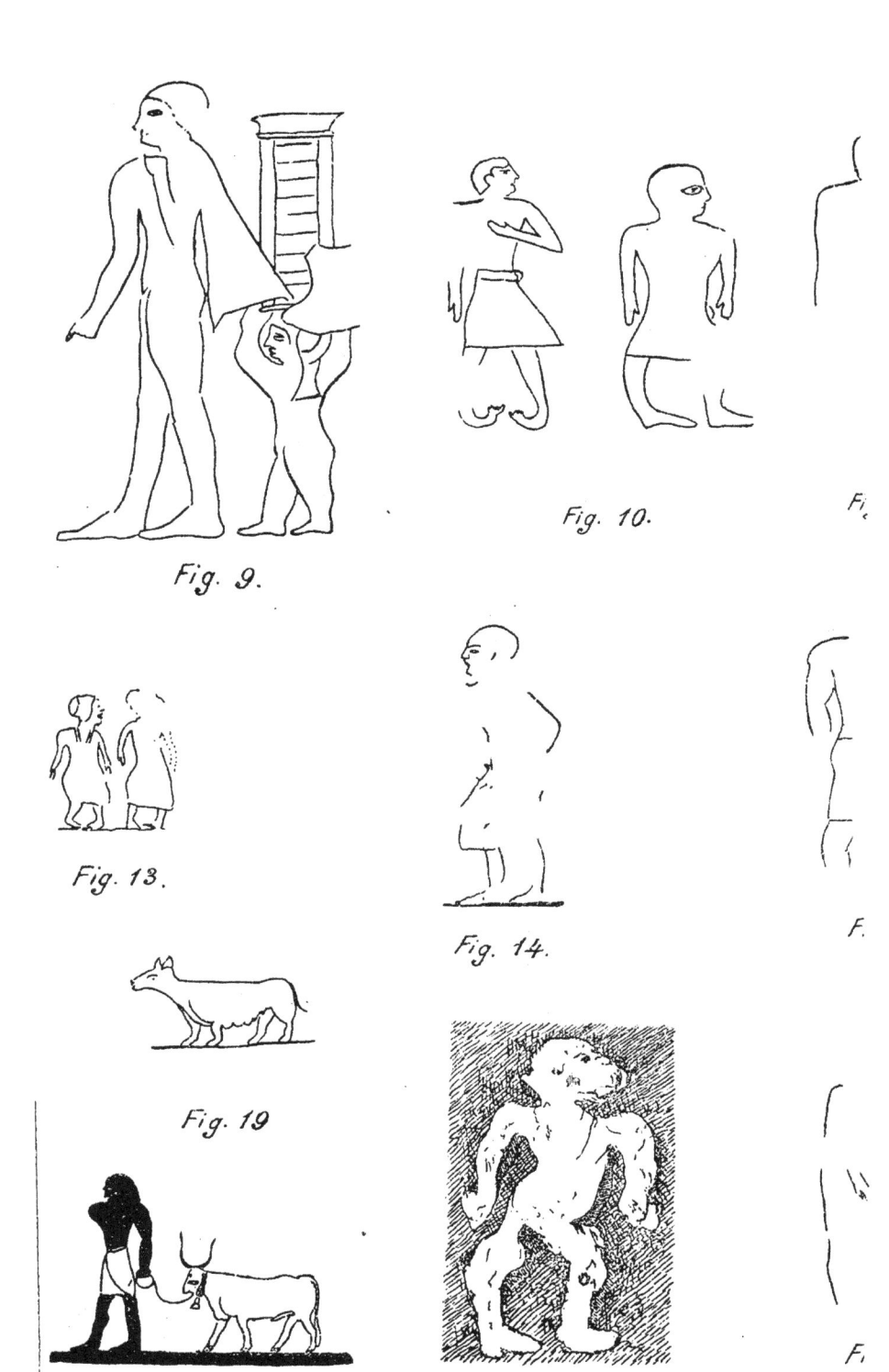

Fig. 10.

Fig. 13.

Fig. 14.

Fig. 19.

Fig. 18.

Fig. 16.

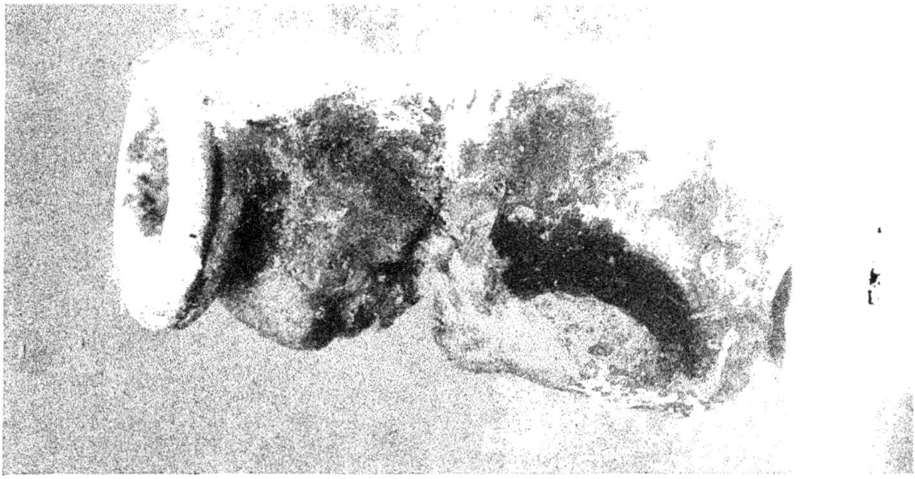

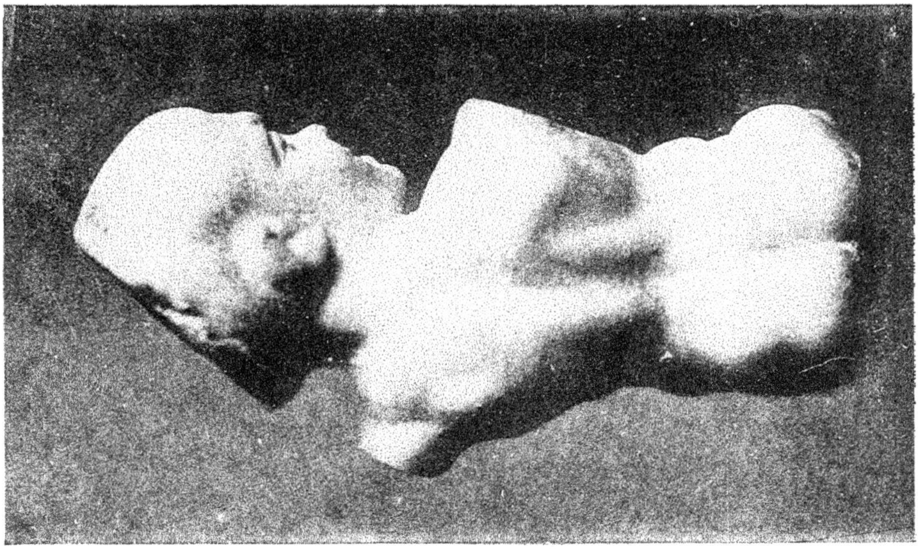

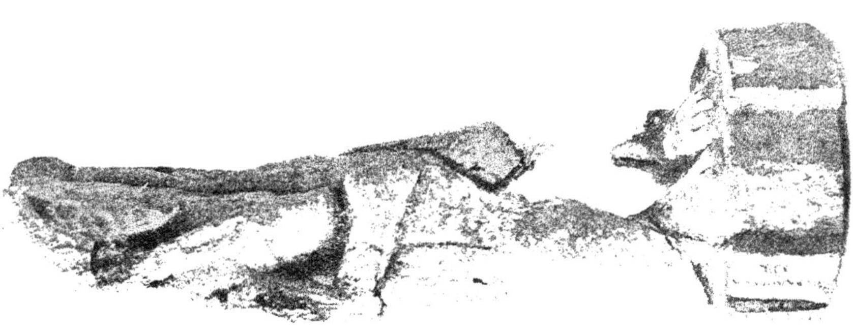

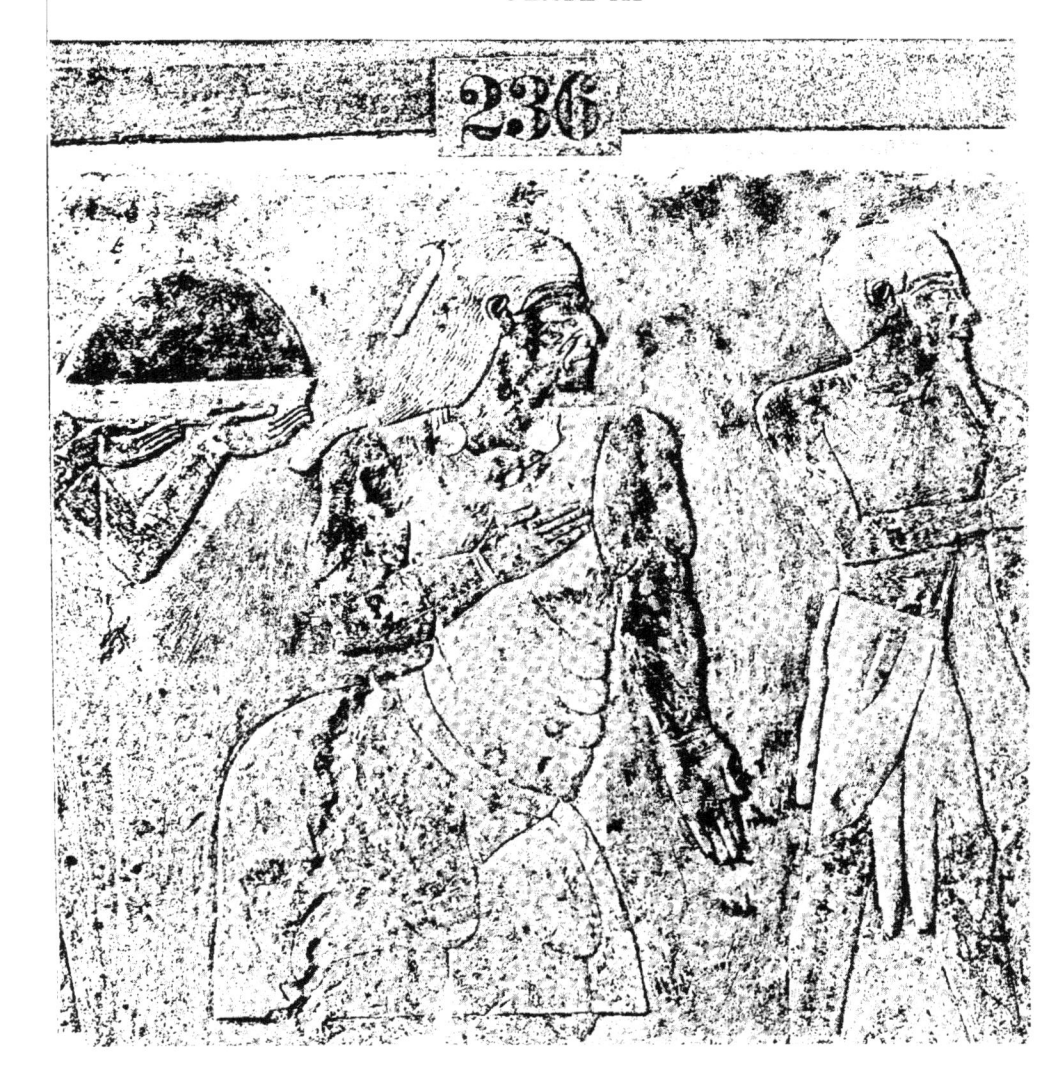

PLATE XI

236

HISTOLOGICAL STUDIES ON EGYPTIAN MUMMIES

(*Mémoires présentés à l'Institut Égyptien*, Le Caire, Tome VI, Fascicule 3 [mars 1911])

INTRODUCTION

The diseases of ancient Egyptians have been studied by several different methods.

Philologists have translated a few Egyptian papyri relating to medical subjects, and the chief interest of their studies lies in the demonstration of the existence of a medical literature and of a fairly extensive pharmacopoeia at an early period. These documents, however, are not adequate for the identification of diseases which were fatal in olden times.

Even in the "Papyrus Ebers," the most famous of Egyptian medical documents, the description of symptoms is crude, and, although the papyrus contains some information regarding the occurrence of intestinal worms and diseases of various organs, yet an indisputable diagnosis of any one disease in this work is in my opinion impracticable.

The same is partly true of the Berlin medical papyrus[1] lately edited and translated by Wreszinsky. The veterinary papyri discovered by Professor Flinders Petrie demonstrate that the old Egyptians cultivated veterinary as well as human medicine.

Another source of information regarding ancient Egyptian pathology is found in the pictures and statues representing malformed persons which have been discovered in many places. Egyptian temples and tombs contain likenesses of people with club-foot (tombs of Beni-Hassan), rickets (Kasr-el-Nil Museum), steatopygia (Ashmolean Museum). Pictures and statuettes of malformed persons, e.g., dwarfs, are common in some of the oldest tombs of Egypt, in those dating from the Greek period and the Roman occupation. I have seen figures of typical hunchbacks and several of men with cutaneous cysts (private collection).

[1] The description of facial paralysis in this papyrus is excellent.

The evidence from historical works of comparatively modern times is of little service, because, as a rule, the symptoms noted are indicative not of one disease, but of several. To take an example of comparatively recent times, the epidemic which devasted Athens and was graphically described by Thucydides, has been identified according to the diverse tastes of medical and other commentators as black typhus, smallpox, yellow fever, cerebro-spinal meningitis, scarlet fever, influenza, and ergotism complicated with typhus.

Very precious information has been obtained by the examination of skeletons. Lately a new stimulus has been given to this hitherto neglected branch of Egyptology, by the description by Professor Elliot Smith, Dr. Wood Jones, and Dr. Derry, of bones found in the Nile Valley above Assuan. Unfortunately, the inspection of skeletons reveals only the few maladies which cause osseous lesions, whereas many diseases leave no traces on the bones.

The result of the macroscopical examination of mummified organs is unsatisfactory also, as, in the process of drying, the soft parts shrank and are therefore so changed as to render pathological lesions unrecognisable (see Plates XII, XIII, XIV). Still, this method may give noteworthy results, and Professor Elliot Smith, for instance, showed me a gall-bladder which undoubtedly contained biliary calculi.

One other available method consists in the microscopical examination of mummies, which, as far as I know, has never been applied systematically. Histologists were probably repelled by the very unpromising appearance of the material. It is not easy to say, for instance, to what organ some of the brownish, dry, hard fragments found in the body cavity belong. A provisional diagnosis, as I have found to my cost, not infrequently proves incorrect. I am informed, however, that Professor Looss demonstrated the striation of mummified muscles to his colleagues, but I am not aware of any systematic work on the histological examination of mummies.

It appeared to me that if, by any process, the flexibility and original shape of the mummified tissues were restored, their microscopical structure would be recovered also, partially at least, and that pathological alterations might then possibly be demonstrated.

This paper, however, is concerned with the first two questions only, viz., the restoration of mummified tissues to their original size and the recovery of their microscopical appearance.

For the material necessary for this work I am indebted in the first instance to Professor Elliot Smith. I obtained also very valuable specimens from Professor Flinders Petrie, Sir Gaston Maspero, and from Dr. Keatinge. I take this opportunity of thanking all these gentlemen for their help, as also Mr. A. Cooper for many of the illustrations and Mrs. Alice Mary Ruffer for most of the paintings of microscopical specimens accompanying this paper.

METHODS OF EMBALMING

I do not intend to give here a full account of the various methods of embalming in successive dynasties, as a volume would be required for that purpose. It is extraordinary that, as far as I know, no such work exists and a full account has not been written of the methods of embalming the bodies discovered in the many tombs opened lately. Indeed, most of the writers on this subject are content to copy the accounts given by Herodotus and by Diodorus Siculus.

Herodotus'[1] description is as follows:

There are certain individuals appointed for the purpose [embalming], and who profess that art; these persons after any body is brought to them, show the bearers some good models of corpses, painted to represent the originals; the most perfect they assert to be the representation of him whose name I take it to be impious to mention in this matter; then they show a second which is inferior to the first, and cheaper; and a third, which is cheapest of all. They then ask of them according to which of the models they will have the deceased prepared: having settled upon the price, the relations immediately depart, and the embalmers, remaining home, thus proceed to perform the embalming in the most costly manner. In the first place, with a crooked piece of iron, they pull out the brain by the nostrils; a part of it they extract in this manner, the rest by means of pouring in certain drugs: in the next place, after making an incision in the flank with a sharp Egyptian stone, they empty the whole of the inside; and after cleansing the cavity, and rinsing it with palm wine, scour it out again with pounded aromatics: then having filled the belly with pure myrrh pounded, and cinnamon, and all other perfumes, frankincense excepted, they sew it up again; having so done, they steep the body in natrum,[2] keeping it covered for 70 days, for it is not lawful to leave the body any longer in the

---

[1] This is copied from Pettigrew.   [2] Pettigrew wrote natrum.

brine. When the 70 days are gone by, they first wash the corpse, and then wrap up the whole of the body in bandages cut out of cotton cloth, which they smear with gum, a substance the Egyptians generally use instead of paste.

The relations, having then received back the body, get a wooden case, in the shape of a man, to be made; and, when completed, place the body in the inside; and then, shutting it up, keep it in a sepulchral repository, where they stick it upright against the wall. The above is the most costly manner in which they prepare the dead. For such as choose the middle mode, from a desire of avoiding expense, they prepare the body thus: they first fill syringes with cedar oil, which they inject into the belly of the deceased, without making any incision, or emptying the inside, but sending it up by the seat; they then close the aperture, to hinder the injection from flowing backwards, and lay the body in brine for the specified number of days, on the last of which they take out the cedar oil which they have previously injected, and such is the strength it possesses that it brings away with it the bowels and inside in a state of dissolution: on the other hand, the natrum dissolves the flesh, so that, in fact, there remains nothing but the skin and the bones; when having so done, they give back the body without performing any further operation upon it.

The third mode of embalming, which is used for such as have but scanty means, is as follows: after washing the inside with syrmaea, they salt the body for the 70 days, and return it to be taken back. The wives of men of quality are not given to be embalmed immediately after their death, neither are those that may have been extremely beautiful, or much celebrated; but they deliver them to the embalmers after having been 3 or 4 days deceased: this they do for the following reason, that the workmen may not be able to abuse the bodies of these females; for it is reported by them, that one of these artificers was discovered in the very act on the newly-deceased body of a woman, and was impeached by his fellow workman.

Diodorus Siculus wrote as follows on the same subject:

When anyone amongst the Egyptians dies, all his relations and friends, putting dirt upon their heads, go lamenting about the city till such time as the body shall be buried. In the meantime they abstain from baths and wine, and all kinds of delicate meats, neither do they during that time wear any costly apparel. The manner of their burial is threefold; one very costly, the second sort less chargeable, and the third very mean. In the first, they say there is spent a talent of silver, in the second 20 minae, but in the last there is very little expense. Those who have the care of ordering the body are such as have been taught that art by their ancestors. These, showing to the kindred of the deceased a bill of expenses of each kind of burial, ask them after what manner they will have the body prepared; when they have agreed upon the matter, they deliver the body to such as are usually appointed for this office. First, he who has the name of scribe, laying it upon the ground, marks about the flank on the left side how much is to be cut away. Then he who is called the cutter or the dissector, with an Ethiopic stone cuts away as much of the flesh as the law commands, and presently runs away as fast as he can: those who are present, pursuing him, cast stones at him, and curse him, hereby turning all the execrations which they imagine due to his office, upon him. For, whosoever offers violence, wounds, or does any kind of injury to a body of the same nature with himself, they think him worthy of hatred; but those who are called the embalmers they esteem worthy of honour and respect; for they are familiar with their priests and go into the temples as holy men, without any prohibition. So soon as they come to embalm the dissected body, one of them thrusts his hand through the wound into the abdomen, and draws forth all the bowels but the heart and kidneys, which another washes and cleanses with wine made of palms and aromatic odours; lastly, having washed the body, they anoint it with oil of cedar and other things for above thirty days, and afterwards with myrrh, cinnamon, and other such like matters, which have not only a power to preserve it for a long time, but also give it a sweet smell; after which they deliver it to the kindred, in such manner that every member remains whole and entire, and no part of it changed, but the beauty and shape of the face seems just as it was before, and may be known, even the hairs of the eye-lids and eye-brows remaining as they were at first. By this means many of the Egyptians, keeping the dead bodies of their ancestors in magnificent houses, so perfectly see the true visage and countenance of those that died many ages before they themselves were born, that in viewing the proportions of every one of them, and the lineaments of their faces, they take as much delight as if they were still living among them.

The importance of these two classical accounts of the process of embalming must not be overrated. Herodotus died 406 B.C., and Diodorus Siculus 440 years afterwards. Their descriptions, therefore, though possibly true for their epoch, may not represent accurately the practice followed during the thousand preceding years or so, when embalming was a common practice.

The same criticism holds good for all the old descriptions. The only way to obtain information with regard to embalming processes, therefore, is to dissect the mummies of various dynasties. Such an attempt was made by Pettigrew[1] who gave a somewhat incomplete résumé of the literature and of the facts known at his time, and carefully described some of the mummies he had studied.

[1] *A History of Egyptian Mummies and an Account of the Worship and Embalming of the Sacred Animals by Egyptians*, with remarks on the funeral ceremonies of different nations and observations on the mummies of the Canary Islands, of the ancient Peruvians, Burman priests, etc., London, 1834.

More lately two papers on the subject have appeared: the first by Dr. Fouquet[1] and the other by Professor Elliot Smith.[2]

The two memoirs are based on the study of mummies of the priests and priestesses of Amon found at Deir el Bahri and dating from the XXIst Dynasty (1000 B.C.), and as most of my specimens come from these same mummies, I must enter more fully into the work of these observers.

Dr. Fouquet states that such a mummy when unrolled is found to be enclosed in two layers of bitumen. The legs are extended, the arms brought alongside the body or slightly crossed at the pubis. The skin is everywhere smooth and clean, absolutely shaved, except for the hairs of the head, the eyebrows, and the eyelashes. The mouth, the nostrils, the eyes, and the ears are covered with a layer of virgin wax closely applied and with resin of cedar under the wax. The closed mouth conceals the teeth, the lips are painted red, the eyebrows are painted also, and the eyelids are often adorned with kohl. The face, hands, feet, and sometimes even the whole body are painted. The body itself has sometimes kept to some extent the well-nourished appearance it had during life, the breasts alone of women are flattened and closely applied to the thorax. The neck, comparatively thin, looks even thinner on account of the face, which is artificially distended.

I have no doubt that the account given by Dr. Fouquet is correct as far as the mummies examined by him are concerned. In the fragments of the five mummies which Professor Flinders Petrie gave me, dating from some period between the XVIIIth and XXth Dynasties, and in numerous mummies of the XXIst Dynasty, I was not able to find the slightest trace of bitumen on the surface of the bodies, but the abdominal walls were covered by a thick layer of what looked like resin. Similarly, Dr. Elliot Smith says nothing about bitumen.[3] The female bodies that he examined were painted

[1] *Note pour servir à l'histoire de l'embaumement en Égypte*, communication faite à l'Institut Égyptien dans la séance du 6 mars 1896, Le Caire, 1896.

[2] "A Contribution to the State of Mummification in Egypt," with special reference to the measures adopted during the time of the XXIst Dynasty for moulding the form of the body, *Mémoires présentésà l'Institut Égyptien* (publiés sous les auspices de S. A. Abbas II, Khédive d'Égypte), Cairo, 1906.

[3] It is a peculiar fact that I have never yet found bitumen in any mummy, and my experience now extends from prehistoric to Coptic times (March, 1911).

with a mixture identified by Dr. Schmidt as yellow ochre and gum. The bodies of the men were painted either red, rose-coloured, or more usually a dull reddish or yellowish brown. This, judging from my own observations, is quite correct.

I discovered no trace of paint in mummies of later periods, nor in a Greek (?) mummy, but the face, though not the body of a Roman child, was gilded all over (see also Pettigrew, *loc. cit.*).

According to Dr. Fouquet, a ball made of rag, on which the iris was roughly painted, was placed under the half-closed eyelids. I have confirmed this observation in one case.

In another body of which I examined the eyes there was not a trace of rag. The eyeballs had disappeared, but the pedicles of the eyes (muscles) were still to be seen. In another, two artificial eyes had been inserted.

Professor Elliot Smith states that during the preliminary stages of embalming, the eyes collapsed and fell back into the orbits. Artificial eyes were then introduced in front of the remains of the real eyes, and the eyelids pulled down into a semi-closed position. The artificial eye usually consisted of a piece of linen rolled up roughly; the pupil is represented by a spot of black paint; in two cases the eye was represented by a piece of white stone with a black spot on it. In the mummy of Ramses IV, small onions were put in front of the collapsed eyes.

In two mummies of the XXVIIth–XXIXth Dynasties which I examined the eyeballs had shrunk greatly, but the eyes were uninjured, and the contents of the orbit had not been interfered with. The eyelashes were perfect. In a Roman child and in a Greek (?) mummy nothing appeared to have been done to the eyes. The orbits certainly contained no foreign matter whatever.

I also examined the eyes of several bodies of the Greek period, which had simply been buried in the sand. The eyeballs could not be recognised. On the other hand, all the muscles were unmistakable and the transverse striation easily demonstrated. The optic nerves were visible; unfortunately their microscopical structure was greatly altered by an enormous growth of moulds.

Dr. Fouquet states that some of the tissues and bandages which touched the bodies were examined by Professor Lacassagne and that he obtained the characteristic reaction of haemoglobin. On the other hand, Professor Elliot Smith writes:

> No one has a greater knowledge of all the most modern tests, chemical and biological, for blood-stains, nor a better acquaintance with those methods in medico-legal practice than my colleague Prof. Schmidt of the Cairo School of Medicine. Dr. Schmidt has examined large numbers of pieces of stained cloth and pieces of highly vascular tissues from a large series of mummies; he tells me that he has been utterly unable to recognise the presence of haemoglobin, although the tests in use now are immeasurably more delicate and sure than those used 10 years ago. All the reddish stains on linen were found to be due to resin.

I can only agree with Professor Elliot Smith and Professor Schmidt. I have repeatedly tried to get blood reactions from tissues of mummies, but always unsuccessfully. Although I have examined many hundred specimens, I have never demonstrated undoubted red blood corpuscles. In one case only did I see some brownish bodies which certainly resembled red blood corpuscles, but I could not identify even them with certainty.

METHODS OF PRESERVING THE DEAD

We may now give a general account of the treatment to which the body cavities and the viscera were subjected after death.

I shall limit myself almost wholly to the method of embalming which was used during the XXIst Dynasty, and hence, I cannot do better than follow closely the account given by Professor Elliot Smith.

The price having been agreed upon, the embalmers took charge of the body, and, as the process is supposed to have taken at least seventy-two days to carry out, the body was probably carried to some special laboratory fitted for the purpose.

Considering the delay which must have ensued while the bargain was made and the body carried to the laboratory, it is not improbable that, in the majority of cases, several hours elapsed from the time of death to that of the first incision.

The embalming incision usually caused a large, vertical, fusiform, gaping wound in the left lumbar region, extending from the iliac crest, about 2–3 cm. behind the anterior superior iliac spine, to the costal margin.

It may be further forward, or extend lower down in front of the iliac spine. As a rule, no attempt was made to close the wound, which was then covered with a plate, usually of wax, but sometimes of bronze, bearing the conventional sign of the eye or *Uta*. In some cases, the gaping wound was not protected by a plate of any sort; and in two cases examined by Professor Elliot Smith the edges were brought together and kept in position by a running ligature.

In one mummy that I dissected the wound was firmly closed by a linen plug which must have been rammed in with considerable force, after the body had been well filled with earth.

The body cavity having thus been opened, the intestines, liver, spleen, kidneys, stomach, pelvic viscera, and most of the vessels were completely removed. The diaphragm having been been cut through, the lungs were freed by severing the bronchi, or, in some cases, the lower end of the trachea.

The heart was left in the body but never exactly in the normal position. Generally it was pushed upwards into the upper part of the right side of the thorax; sometimes it was left in the middle line in front of the vertebral column, or again, it is found in the left side of the chest.

In one mummy which I examined the heart had been removed by the embalmer. It had not been replaced in its proper position, however, for both kidneys filled the pericardium. Behind the liver there was a packet containing striped muscular fibre, which was probably the heart.

Sometimes only the arch and a small part of the aorta were left behind, but in one body Professor Elliot Smith found the whole aorta and iliac arteries. I also dissected out the whole of the aorta (except the transverse part), together with the iliac arteries, of one mummy.

After the viscera had been removed, both the body and the organs were put into the saline bath described by Herodotus. The various tissues of the body and the organs contain saline material and the skin shows unmistakable signs of having been macerated until all the cuticle, together with the hair, except that of the head, had peeled off. There are certainly exceptions to this rule, as in some cases I have found the epidermic cells intact and even their nuclei stained well.

The heart left in the body cavity is always well preserved. In many cases the valves are intact and it is often possible to recognise the chordae tendineae and musculi papillares. As a rule, the organ is considerably damaged, as the result no doubt of unintentional hackings inflicted on it by the operator cutting through the roots of the lungs and the oesophagus (Plate XIV, Figs. 2 and 3). The commonest injury to the heart is, as is natural, a complete opening of the left auricle, or often of both auricles; in many cases great gashes are found in one or both ventricles.

The cavities of the heart are in many subjects tightly stuffed with mud or a mixture of mud and sawdust. How this material was introduced is doubtful.

The viscera, after having been removed from the salt bath, were thickly sprinkled with coarse sawdust of various aromatic woods, and when still flexible were moulded into shape and wrapped in linen. This must have been done before desiccation, as one end of the linen bandage is almost always interwined with—and so fixed to—some part of the organ. The small intestines are usually bent upon themselves many times so as to form an elongated parcel of parallel bands.

Among these bands there was placed (when the viscus was still flexible) a wax image of one of the four genii, usually the hawk-headed Khebsennuf. Then, after being sprinkled with sawdust, the mass was wrapped in the linen bandage.

The liver is usually flexed round its transverse axis, so as to form a hollow tube open on one side, and either the upper or lower surface may form the surface of the tubular cylinder. Inside the cylinder thus prepared a wax statuette, usually the human headed Amset, is found in most cases. In other respects the liver was treated exactly like the intestines. It would appear, however, that in many cases the embalmer was unable to remove or reintroduce the liver without tearing it. In such cases he was content to replace only a fragment of the organ into the body (see further on).

Although either of these parcels may be found in any part of the body cavity, yet in the majority of subjects they occupy definite situations. The parcel of intestines is placed vertically in the abdomen against the right wall and extends from the iliac fossa to the right costal margin, and the liver lies transversely in the lower part of the thorax.

After the various parcels of the viscera had been returned to the body and had been packed tightly in sawdust or coarser fragments of wood, a large part of the abdomen and pelvis still remained comparatively empty. This region was then tightly stuffed with sawdust, and the opening in the left flank was subsequently closed.

The genital organs of women are always absent, the labia majora being the only parts of the vulva left. In only two or three cases the remains of the pudenda and the labia majora were left in their natural position. In most cases, the skin, while still soft and flexible, had been pushed back towards the anus, so as to form an apron covering the rima pudendi.

The bladder, according to Elliot Smith, is sometimes in situ.

The penis and scrotum were painted red like other parts of the body, and as a rule were wrapped separately from the limbs. In some cases the genital organs were pushed against one or the other thigh and wrapped with the limbs. In one case the penis was flattened against the perineum, so that, at a casual glance, the organ seemed to be missing. In several subjects, male and female, the pubic region was packed either with cloth or with mud.

When the viscera were returned to the body cavity, it was customary to place, along with some of the organs, certain wax or pottery models of the children of Horus. Details regarding this custom are contained in Elliot Smith's papers, and it will be sufficient to say that besides the human-headed Amset generally found wrapped up in the liver, the hawk-headed Khebsennuf with the intestines, the ape-headed Api is usually associated with the left lung, and the jackal Tuamautef with the stomach.

Flowers and other vegetable substances, especially onions, are often found among the wrappings, on the surface of the body or inside the mummy.

Elliot Smith says that the saline bath toughened the skin and the lining of the cavity, but the underlying tissues in the limbs, back, or neck were not exposed to the action of the preservative agent, and were soon reduced to a soft pulpy mass, of fluid or semi-fluid consistency. It was the custom to stuff into this pulpy mass large quantities of foreign material, so as to restore to the collapsed and shrunken members some semblance of the form and consistency they possessed during life. The foreign material varied a good deal, the ingredients chiefly used being mud, linen bandages, a mixture of mud and sawdust, or a mixture of soda and butter. The ways in which this material was introduced and the body packed have been fully described in Professor Elliot Smith's paper.

The description of the packing is of course perfectly correct, but I must point out that there is no proof that the tissues were changed into a soft, pulpy mass. I have examined several mummies, the limbs of which had not been packed by the embalmer, and I found the muscles, nerves, arteries, etc., in a very good state of preservation. Indeed, most of the histological details were plainly visible.

A good deal of interest attaches to the "natron" bath in which the bodies were immersed for seventy days, and some controversy has taken place with regard to its chemical constitution. Analyses of the mineral salts from mummies have given but doubtful results.

According to Mr. A. Lucas, the inorganic substances used by embalmers were essentially of two kinds: namely "natron" and common salt. Natron is the natural soda found in Egypt, chiefly in the Wady Natroun, and is essentially a mixture of sodium carbonate, sodium chloride, and sodium sulphate in varying proportions. It contains also a certain amount of clay and calcium carbonate. Mr. Lucas found that of two samples of natron discovered in Canopic jars in the tomb of Iaa at Thebes, one was crude natron of pure quality, such as occurs in many parts of Egypt, and the other a mixture of crude natron and coarse sawdust. Several other observers have found natron in the bodies of wrappings of mummies. The resinous material from mummies also contains a large amount of natron.

On the other hand, Professor Schmidt of Cairo is of opinion that the inorganic material used for packing was not natron but common salt. His results may be summed up as follows:

Mummies contain volatile and nonvolatile fatty acids, albuminous substances, cholesterin, and traces of unaltered fat. Specific

HISTOLOGICAL STUDIES ON EGYPTIAN MUMMIES

human antisera (whether obtained by the injection of blood or muscular tissue) produce no precipitate in mummy tissue. The presence of haemoglobin cannot be demonstrated by any method.

He does not deny that natron was used, but considers that it was only used for packing, as, for instance, in the mouth, and in that case it was mixed with fat, e.g., butter to form a paste.

He maintains that the fatty acids are derived not from the fat of the body only, but from the albuminous material, and that during mummification fixed fatty acids were formed which, later on, were converted into volatile fatty acids. He bases this hypothesis on the fact that the older the mummy, the greater the amount of volatile fatty acids as compared with the quantity of fixed fatty acids.

Schmidt found a large quantity of higher fatty acids in the natron used for packing. He is of opinion that the volatile acids present in this natron were not due to the decomposition of some fat added. but originated in the body fat and tissues. He has found, for instance, the higher fatty acids in the spleen and liver, which had never been in contact with natron.

Schmidt summed up his opinion as follows:

We see that the old Egyptians worked with very simple methods. The following are the only important parts of their process: 1st: removal of the most easily putrescible viscera, 2nd: the salt bath, 3rd: thorough drying of the corpse in the air, and 4th: the rolling of the body in bandages.

Modern researches on the microscopical changes taking place in putrefying or mummifying tissues help us very little, for the microscopical appearance of putrefying organs has not been the subject of many careful investigations.

The appearance of putrefaction in nervous tissue shows itself first in the axis cylinder and nerve fibres, which break up into fragments. The nervous cells of cerebral and peripheral ganglia resist for a long time.

In the lungs, the epithelial lining of the alveoli and bronchi is first affected. This is loosened and finally disappears totally. The elastic tissue long remains unaltered.

The epithelium cells of the liver, kidneys, and stomach become opaque and lose their nuclei. The epithelium cells of the kidney— especially those of the contorti—fall off, and chronic nephritis may then be simulated. The connective tissues of all organs keep their nuclei longer than the epithelium cells.

The unstriated muscular fibres retain their characteristic appearance for a long time, and so do the striated muscular fibres which lose their striation only slowly. The heart fibres show their characteristic arrangement, and the structure of kidney and liver is no longer recognisable.

The state of the stomach gives no valuable information, as self-digestion varies considerably.

It is stated that in contradiction to putrefying organs, dried (mummified) tissues retain their characteristic structure for a much more extended period.

ON THE FORMATION OF ADIPOCERE (?) IN MUMMIFIED ORGANS

I attempted to soften entire organs of mummies of the XXIst Dynasty by placing them in a solution of 1 per cent formol, containing 1 per cent carbonate of soda. Some organs, e.g., lungs, swell up considerably, and their characteristic spongy structure becomes evident. The liver never swells up to any extent, whereas the kidneys become considerably larger and softer. When the carbonate of soda-formol solution extracts no more colouring matter, it is replaced by a 5 per cent solution of formol, in which the organs may remain indefinitely.

Not infrequently a curious change is observed to have taken place, especially in the lungs. After the mud and vegetable matter have fallen to the bottom or floated off, the organ, or part of it, is found to be converted into a snow-white, somewhat brittle and stiff substance. The pleura and the parts immediately underlying it appear to be specially affected. I presume that this white substance is adipocere or some substance closely resembling it.

I have never seen this change in the liver, and only once in the two kidneys of one mummy. One of these showed small patches of adipocere (?), whereas the other was almost snow-white. The stomach of one mummy, though it had kept its shape fairly well, was completely converted into adipocere. The intestines of another had been almost wholly changed into rigid white strands by the same process.

I have seen indications of a similar change in Roman and Greek bodies, which had been simply buried in sand. In these, the change occurs in the shape of small white patches scattered over the intestines, lungs, heart, and kidneys, which have a curious resemblance to miliary tuberculosis.

Microscopically one sees nothing except an amorphous substance staining faintly with haematoxylin. Here and there, however, one finds places where the structure of the organ is preserved.

METHODS OF HISTOLOGICAL EXAMINATION

The naked-eye appearance of the tissues will be described as we treat of each; for the present it will be sufficient to say that most mummified organs are hard to the touch, brownish in colour, and often very brittle.

Even in the damp heat of an Alexandria summer, when the temperature of my laboratory seldom fell below 30° C., most of the mummified pieces underwent but little change. Some pieces of intestines alone became soft and pliable and gave off a distinct musty odour. An exception must also be made for the skin, muscles, and internal organs of some mummies of the XVIIIth–XXth Dynasties, which, though stiff, had a peculiar soft, soapy feel.

A satisfactory microscopical examination of organs in such a condition is not possible, not only on account of the brittleness of the tissues, but also because the microscopic structure is obscured by an opaque, dark-brown colouring matter with which the tissues are saturated. Further, the larger amount of the closely adherent "packing," e.g., mud, charcoal, sand, and sawdust, increases the difficulty.

The objects to be attained were: (1) to soften the tissues in order to render them less brittle, (2) to remove the colouring matter, and (3) to bring back consistency sufficient for histological examination.

Microscopical sections had to be prepared, as except in the case of muscular fibres all other methods, such as teasing, etc., proved useless for the reasons already stated.

I need not enumerate all the reagents I employed together and seriatim. The main difficulty was that reagents such as alkalies, neutral, alkaline and acid salts, mineral and organic acids, glycerine, formol, acetone, alcohol, chloroform, ether, etc., whether employed together or alone or in solutions of different concentrations, either softened the tissues too much or not enough, and the invariable result was failure. After many attempts the following stock solution proved most useful:

	c.c.
Alcohol	30
Water	50
5 per cent carbonate of soda solution	20

In some cases instead of water and alcohol a 1 per cent solution of formol was used.

Although this solution generally gives good results, yet the details of the process must often be altered. The time during which the tissues remain in this solution, and the percentage of alcohol and carbonate of soda require modifying according to the size and consistency of the tissue to be studied. The harder and larger the tissue, the more carbonate of soda required, and the longer the time during which the tissue must remain in the liquid. The process, therefore, is delicate, empirical, and requires constant watching. On the whole, it is better to soak small pieces (3–5 mm.) in dilute solutions of carbonate of soda, rather than larger ones in stronger solutions.

Within two minutes of placing the tissue in the softening solution, a brownish-yellow colouring material begins to dissolve out. This does not diffuse readily throughout the fluid, but falls to the bottom of the beaker; so that for hours and days even, the lower layer of fluid resembles a strong solution of iodine, the supernatant liquid remaining almost colourless. This brown colouring matter is thus extracted not only from organs which had been removed from the body during the process of embalming and then replaced, but also from muscles, blood vessels, etc., which had been left in situ; and even, though in lesser quantity, from the heart. The muscles appear to contain a great deal of it. During this process, a certain quantity of mud, sand, sawdust, etc., drops off the tissue and can then be mechanically removed.

The tissues, especially the internal organs, after remaining in the fluid for a few hours, sometimes become so soft that the slightest movement of the vessel may entirely break up the material. Even the removal of the fluid by careful decantation or by means of a pipette is not infrequently disastrous, as the flow of liquid may suffice to disintegrate the fragment, or the tissue may run up the pipette as a sticky, oily, brown fluid containing a few shreds.

The difficulty is obviated by placing the piece which is to be softened on a small wire-platform, and adding softening fluid until the layer of reagent above and below the tissue are about equal. When the tissue is softened sufficiently, the lower third of the fluid, containing most of the colouring matter, is pipetted off and replaced by absolute alcohol. The same process is repeated on three consecutive days, and on the fifth day the tissue has become so firm that all the fluid can be poured off and replaced by absolute alcohol, or acetone.

Under the influence of the solution the mummified pieces become of grey colour and somewhat transparent, as if they had been plunged for some hours in a clearing fluid, e.g., turpentine or oil of cloves. A certain amount of differentiation is then noticeable: the mucous membrane of the intestine stands out from the muscular layer, the liver tissue from the Glisson's capsule, the pleura from the lung; but as alcohol is added, all differentiation disappears, and every tissue, though remaining pliable, becomes opaque again and of a dirty-grey colour.

The material is now plunged in chloroform. Sometimes this liquid extracts a further quantity of colouring matter; at other times a precipitate is formed. Embedding in paraffine, carried out in the usual manner, then follows, and the pieces are ready for cutting. Very thin sections (one division of Minot's microtome) are easily obtained, but present no advantages. The famous dictum attributed to Virchow "nur so dick wie möglich" is certainly true for this work. For staining, acid and basic dyes are equally useful. The best colorations are obtained with a dilute solution of Böhmer's haematoxylin or a 0.5 per cent solution of acid fuchsine. After staining, the sections are dehydrated, cleared, and mounted in Canada balsam in the usual manner.

HISTOLOGICAL EXAMINATION OF THE SKIN

I obtained from the Museum in Cairo particles of skin of the bodies of the Hearst collection, which, I am informed, are between eight thousand and twelve thousand years old. The tissue was extremely fragile and disappeared almost entirely in the ordinary softening solution. The skin could be prepared for section by using a solution containing only 0.25–0.50 per cent of carbonate of soda. In such preparations the epidermis had completely disappeared but the dermis had retained its peculiar structure fairly well. The extraordinary part, however, is that many of the nuclei of the subcutaneous tissues still stained darkly with haematoxylin (Plate XVI, Fig. 6). The amount of material at my disposal was so small that I was not able to get many preparations.

Before the body was put up into the macerating solution (soda bath) by the embalmers, each nail of both hands and feet was carefully secured by a piece of string wound in a circular manner round the finger or toe, so that when the epidermis peeled off, it did not carry the nails with it. The impressions left by these pieces of string are visible in almost all cases, and it often happens that the string is left in position on one or more fingers or toes. In most cases, however, the string was removed when the body was taken out of the salt tank. Professor Elliot Smith gives various photographs illustrating this, but as I shall show presently, in many cases the epidermis, especially that of the toes and hands, is practically normal.

Several pieces of skin from the front of the chest and fingers of various men and from one woman were examined. The whole finger of one mummy was macerated for a fortnight in 90 per cent alcohol, containing 3 per cent of pure nitric acid, then transferred to pure alcohol, which was repeatedly changed until all the acid had been washed out.

The skin before being prepared is yellowish white, very hard, and brittle, so hard indeed as often to break the edge of the knife (Plate XIII, Fig. 3). When broken across, the fractured surface is smooth and glistening; the muscles below dark-brown, hard and glistening, with a distinctly resinous fracture. The connective tissue, fat, etc., between the muscle and skin are not recognisable. Under the influence of the softening solution, the skin of the chest and mammae separate into two layers; the first is composed of the muscles and the greater part of the connective tissue, which sink to the bottom of the vessel, and the second of the dermis which floats on the surface. The latter is exquisitely smooth, soft and much resembles yellow wash-leather, except that it is not so pliable.

The epidermis on the fingers is well preserved, and long thin strips of yellow colour float off when the finger is allowed to soak in the acid alcoholic solution. These prove to be layers of horny scales, which, though somewhat thinned out, are easily recognisable (Plate XVI, Fig. 4).

The rete mucosum of the skin of chest and mammae is almost completely gone (Plate XVI, Fig. 2). I at first attributed this state of things to the effect of the salt bath, but that it cannot be wholly due to this is proved by the fact that the epidermis of bodies which had certainly never been placed in this bath had also fallen off. This shedding of the epidermis did not take place in the softening solution used by me, for some of the extraneous material in which the skin had been packed (bits of bandages and sawdust, etc.) was still in contact with the corium (Plate XVI, Fig. 2a). The few epithelium cells which are left behind are usually found in the depressions between the papillae, forming the somewhat wavy free border of the preparation.

The outermost layer of the corium of the chest and mammae is represented by wavy homogeneous tissue with no particular structure. Its texture, however, is closer than in the parts below and it stains intensely. The deeper parts of the corium and the connective tissue below form a loose network; so loose indeed as to show that a good deal of the original connective tissue has disappeared (Plate XVI, Fig. 2).

Some preparations are riddled with almost circular holes, which, as their walls have no particular structure, must have been formed post mortem. Some of these cavities extend to the outer edge of the preparation and open out on the surface. I suggest that they are due to gas bubbles formed during the process of putrefaction.

In preparations of the chest and mammae, sweat glands and other glands cannot be identified with certainty. Well-defined blood vessels are not rare, and the fat, loose connective tissue and voluntary muscles of some of the deeper parts of the skin are beautifully preserved. Nuclei can be demonstrated in the connective tissue; and so dense is this underlying tissue still that, as has been described already, it often separates from the dermis and sinks in the softening fluid.

The skin of the fingers is in an astonishingly good state of preservation. The layer of horny tissue which floats off in acid alcohol when washed, stained, and mounted, shows individual horny cells plainly (Plate XVI, Fig. 4). The other microscopical appearances of the skin in this region are easily seen, and although the epidermic cells are occasionally absent, yet the epidermic layer is often complete over large surfaces.

The epidermis does not stain very readily and the cells remain of a yellowish colour, whereas their nuclei turn a pale red in acid fuchsin and greyish mauve in haematoxylin (Plate XVI, Fig. 1).

Under a high power the contours of some of the cells are sometimes distinct; the lowest cells are occasionally pigmented, and the pigment varies from light yellow to brown. Distinct granules are generally absent, the pigment being usually diffused through the cell.

The papillae and the dense connective tissue of the corium stain brightly and nuclei are not infrequently seen (Plate XVI, Fig. 1).

The wavy elastic fibres greedily absorb acid fuchsin.

The deeper connective tissue and the fat are in a remarkably good state of preservation, although, except occasionally, no nuclei are evident.

The sweat glands are not always easily found, owing to their being greatly compressed by the connective tissue. Sometimes, however, they are unmistakable and form a yellowish-green streak lined by the nuclei of the epithelium cells (Plate XV, Fig. 3). Their ramified endings, though somewhat flattened, are distinct and the epithelium cells show the same staining reactions as those of the epidermis (Plate XVI, Fig. 3).

The arrangement of the fat and connective tissue is well seen in Plate XVI, Figs. 1, 2, 5, 7.

In contrast with the dry and resinous state of the skin of the mummies of the XXIst Dynasty which had been carefully packed with rags, mud, and sand, the skin of the mummies of the XVIIIth–XXth Dynasties, which were given me by Professor Petrie, was almost soft and flexible. It was possible to strip off the skin from the subjacent muscles, and a subcutaneous layer of yellowish fat was still present. The limbs of these mummies had not been packed, nevertheless the muscles, cartilages, ligaments, and nerves were in an extraordinarily good state of preservation. The microscopical appearances were identical with those of the skin of the chest and mammae which have just been described; the horny layer had completely disappeared.

The skin of a Greek mummy[1] dating from about 300 to 400 B.C. was fairly soft. After lying in Alexandria for some months it became soapy to the touch and was easily dissected from the underlying tissues. Histologically, its structure was similar to that of the skin of the chest and mammae of the XXIst Dynasty.

I had an opportunity also of examining the skin of a Roman child which had been buried in the sand. The face was gilded, but no incision was found, and all the organs, including the brain, were in situ. The skin was rather soapy to the touch, soft and pliable, and large pieces of it were stripped off. Its microscopical structure was identical with that of mummies of the XXIst Dynasty.

I also examined the skin of a child probably belonging to the Greek period. This had been buried in the sand, but there was absolutely no sign that it had ever been touched by the embalmer. The skin was fairly soft and dry. The whole of the epidermis of the soles of the feet and toes was almost completely detached so that it could easily be removed with a forceps. Microscopically the epidermic cells were plainly seen, but the sections of the skin were not very satisfactory.

The skins of several heads which had been buried in the sand at Mellawi were well preserved, and so dry that in spite of a prolonged stay in the softening solution they never swelled up to a great extent.

[1] This mummy was given me by the Museum authorities. I was told that it belonged to the Greek period, but it was prepared exactly the same way as the mummies of the XXIst Dynasty. Its limbs had not been packed in any way. The body was undoubtedly that of an Egyptian.

The hairs and follicles were easily seen. The epidermic cells of the scalp had not been shed and were represented by a thin, darkly staining fringe. The date at which these people lived is uncertain, though the bodies were certainly more than two thousand years old.

From the appearance of the skin I conclude that most probably putrefaction had not gone very far before the bodies were either buried in the sand or steeped in the pickling solution. With the onset of putrefaction the epidermis is raised and ultimately falls off. This process starts in the regions nearest the abdominal cavity, viz., the abdominal walls, the skin of the chest and back, and shows itself last near the extremities, i.e., toes and fingers.

Considering that the epidermic cells had disappeared on the chest, it is possible that putrefaction had just started before burial, or before the bodies were placed in the natron solution. It was certainly not very far advanced as no micro-organisms were seen.

The observation of Professor Elliot Smith to the effect that in some mummies each nail was securely tied to the finger, seems to show that the epithelium was often shed in the "natron" solution and that this had some caustic property. On the other hand, the fact that the skin including the epidermis of certain bodies was almost normal shows that the "natron" cannot always have had a very powerful macerating effect.

MUSCLES

These muscles are as dry as tinder and flake off easily. They much resemble dry camomile leaves and, like the latter, can easily be crushed to powder between the fingers. They dissolve entirely in the ordinary softening solution, but their structure is made evident by placing them in 30 per cent alcohol containing only a trace of carbonate of soda. A small fragment is then teased out under the microscope from time to time, when after an hour or two the transverse striation of the muscular fibres and the sarcolemna are demonstrable as a rule. The striation is regular, though owing to the great shrinkage of the muscle the transverse bands are of course much smaller than in the muscles of modern times (Plate XVII, Fig. 2).

The voluntary muscles examined were the great pectoral, diaphragm, cremaster, and finger muscles, and all proved equally good objects for histological examination.

Their appearance is very deceptive, as sometimes they resemble a lump of resin, so that the diagnosis between the muscles and resin by the naked eye is not infrequently almost impossible. As an instance, I may relate that the first muscular fibres which I ever saw were found while examining under the microscope a small particle of what I had thought to be resin. Such a muscle is of stony hardness and brittle. When broken across it shows a smooth, dark-brown, shiny, and glistening surface. In other cases the muscle is pale yellow, fibrous in appearance, and thin strands can then be easily teased out. This was especially so in mummies of the XVIIIth-XXth Dynasties, in which the limbs had not been packed.

For purposes of demonstration, small fragments were macerated in a very weak solution of caustic potash (0.5–0.01 per cent) and then teased. The teased fibres were stained with eosin or acid fuchsin, washed in water, alcohol, xylol, and mounted in Canada balsam (Plate XVII, Fig. 2). Unstained preparations, however, show histological details quite as well if not better than stained slides.

The fibres appear to be somewhat stiffer and thinner than normal. The transverse striation is conspicuous throughout the whole length of the fibre. The perfectly stained transverse bands are certainly not as wide as those of modern muscles. No doubt the shrinkage due to a desiccation lasting nigh on three thousand years has not been compensated by a few hours stay in alkaline fluid. Nuclei are never seen.

The sarcolemma is often noticeable and forms a thin transparent membrane, specially well seen where, during manipulation, the fibre has been twisted or torn (Plate XVII, Fig. 3). The striation is also obvious in sections, provided these are nearly parallel to the long axis of the muscle, which is seldom the case. The muscle then often looks as if it were breaking into discs, and this is especially marked in sections on the cremaster muscle.

In transverse sections, the perimysium stains readily and deeply, and its prolongations between the fasciculi are easily demonstrated.

The endomysium is visible if the section is deeply stained and shows as thin, dark strands, so fine and sharp that they look as if they had been painted in with a pen dipped in the darkest blue ink. On the whole, although sections of muscles both longitudinal and transverse give excellent pictures of peri- and endomysium, yet the teasing method is to be preferred when the object in view is to demonstrate the traverse striation.

I may mention that I found striated muscular fibres in the contents of the intestinal canal of a mummy of the XXIst Dynasty. It is not a little astonishing that these muscular fibres, which had probably undergone a certain amount of digestion, should have kept their structure for over three thousand years.

The muscles of the limbs of Greek and Roman mummies are hard, fibrous, and by no means brittle. They can be teased out almost as easily as fresh muscles. A large amount of colouring matter dissolves out in the softening solution and the tissue becomes soft and pliable. The striation is then easily demonstrated. On the whole, these muscles are as perfect as those of the XXIst Dynasty, although no preservatives whatever appear to have been used for the muscles of the limbs of these Greek and Roman mummies. Similarly I found that the muscles of Egyptian mummies of the XVIIIth and XXth Dynasties, which had been simply dried, gave beautiful histological pictures.

NERVES

Excellent results were obtained by making transverse sections through the finger. The whole finger was macerated for a fortnight in 90 per cent of alcohol containing 3 per cent of pure nitric acid, then transferred to pure alcohol, which was repeatedly changed until all the acid was washed out.

The digital nerves are in a very fine state of preservation and easily identified, not only by their position with regard to the digital arteries and other structures, but also by their characteristic histological appearances. The funiculi have a wavy aspect, which is less marked than in fresh tissue, and as the connective tissue always swells up rather unequally under the influence of the softening solution, blank spaces are often left between the connecting fibres:

Similarly, owing to shrinkage, the funiculi do not always fill up the spaces between the septa formed by the epineurium (see Plate XVII, Fig. 1). In some cases, however, the sections are perfect, and no blank spaces are left.

The endoneurium, on the other hand, is excellently preserved, and in consecutive serial sections not a fibre is missing, and the blood vessels even are unaltered. The outer or primitive sheath of the nerve fibre is so closely applied to the endoneurium that it cannot be separately demonstrated.

Under a low power, the interior of the nerve fibre has a peculiar glistening appearance, which it was almost beyond the artist's power to reproduce. Under a high power, however, the tube is seen to contain a greenish-yellow substance, which stains best with haematoxylin (Plate XV, Figs. 1 and 2), and acid fuchsin, and evidently represents the medullary sheath. In many of the nerve tubes, a dot staining deeply with both dyes probably represents the axis cylinder (Plate XV, Fig. 2, and Plate XVII, Fig. 1). The number of these dots varies greatly, some sections showing them in almost every fibre, whereas in other preparations they are very rare.

Nerve trunks were obtained by dissection from mummies of the XVIIIth–XXth Dynasties. The whole limb was immersed in solution containing formol 0.5 per cent, carbonate of soda 1 per cent, and water to 100. The skin after a day or two became soft and flexible and was then stripped off and the limb replaced in the solution. After a few days, nerves, muscles, ligaments, etc., were dissected out.

The nerves especially are in a very fine state of preservation, and can be followed almost as easily as in a fresh specimen. For histological examination, small fragments of nerves are placed in 30 per cent alcohol for twenty-four hours and afterwards hardened and cut in the usual manner. The nerves present the same appearance as those described above, except that the axis cylinders are not visible as a rule; the medullary sheath on the other hand is very conspicuous.

These nerves are in no better state of preservation than those of mummies of the XVIIIth–XXth Dynasties.

BLOOD VESSELS

The state of the blood vessels varies exceedingly, probably owing to their having been subjected after death to widely different influences according to their position in the body.

Clearly, the chemical processes (putrefaction, autolysis) modifying the anatomical structure of blood vessels after death were not as active in the peripheral parts of the body, as for instance fingers and toes, as in a large internal organ, e.g., liver. As several hours undoubtedly passed between death and the removal of the organs from the body and the immersion in the pickling solution, some putrefactive changes may have taken place in all internal organs, especially during hot weather; and this must have been the case also to some extent with the skin, especially the skin and subcutaneous tissue of the trunk.

On the other hand, the putrefactive bacteria and their products probably never reached the tissues of the extremities, which therefore were almost sterile when the body was placed in the pickling solution.

After the removal of the organs, the large vessels of the neck near the heart were filled with mud and sand and are considerably damaged in consequence. It appears to me doubtful whether in some mummies the pickling solution ever reached the heart, as the consistency of this organ often differs entirely from that of other muscles. The muscles of the heart may crumble to dust when pressed between the fingers, and when carefully broken they show a granular, dull-grey, fractured surface, even when the other muscles of the body are of stony hardness and show a glistening, brown, resinous fracture. The consistency of the vessels of the neck may resemble that of the heart, whereas the lower part of the thoracic aorta is entirely different, its fractured surface resembling that of muscle.

Elliot Smith has pointed out correctly that the aorta was generally removed in mummies of the XXIst Dynasty. I have found this vessel, however, in mummies of the XVIIIth–XXth Dynasties and also in a Greek (?) mummy. The aorta was absolutely collapsed and would certainly not have been found, surrounded as it was with packing (sawdust and mud), had the whole mummy not been placed in the softening solution. All the coats of the vessel could be easily demonstrated under the microscope (Plate XVIII, Fig. 3).

The intima of the large veins and arteries near the heart is not to be seen as a rule (Plate XVIII, Fig. 2), having probably been torn off when these vessels were forcibly filled with sand or mud. The adventitia of these vessels is not well seen and the middle coat is often represented by very thin annular fibres only, which probably correspond to the muscular coat (Plate XVIII, Fig. 2).

In the pickling solution, organs such as intestines were quickly saturated with natron and the putrefactive changes were arrested. On the other hand, the internal parts of larger and thicker organs, as for instance liver and kidneys, were not impregnated with salt for a considerable time, if indeed the salt ever penetrated them deeply. It certainly seems to me doubtful also whether the salt ever reached the deeper part of the limbs, notably of the extremities.

The question is only to be settled by experiment; but in any case, it is evident that the action of the salt on blood vessels varied according to the anatomical position of the blood vessels. Similarly, the autolytic processes must have produced more or less effect on the arteries and veins according to the size of the organs in which the vessels were embedded. Lastly, the internal parts of the liver and kidneys dried much more slowly than the more superficial organs, and these organs themselves, owing to their size and structure, were desiccated much more slowly than other tissues.

Considering, therefore, that all the processes tending towards the production of alterations in the blood vessels were more marked in the larger organs, we should expect (leaving the heart and the arteries and veins of the neck out of consideration as having been subjected to a special form of treatment) that the state of preservation of blood vessels would vary according to the size of the organ containing them.

On the whole, the facts are in accordance with theoretical considerations. In the largest organ, the liver, the portal system has almost wholly disappeared; and though the hepatic system shows less profound alterations, yet often enough the larger veins are represented by a few shreds of tissue only (Plate XIX, Figs. 2 and 3).

The blood vessels of the parenchyma of the lungs are very distinct. This is probably due to the fact that the lungs do not putrefy as quickly as the abdominal organs and that, owing to their loose, spongy structure, the salt solution penetrated them rapidly and the organs dried quickly afterwards.

The vascular system of the stomach and intestines is often well preserved. The three coats of the arteries, for instance, are evident. Here the satisfactory result is probably due to the thorough and rapid penetration of the pickling solution, and the ulterior quick desiccation of the thin tissues.

The vessels of the extremities, i.e., fingers, are most interesting; the adventitia and media are well-nigh perfect, the intima alone showing signs of disintegration (Plate XVIII, Fig. 4). Similarly, the small blood vessels of the testis, of nerves and muscles are in excellent condition.

HEART

In mummies of the XXIst Dynasty the heart is always shrunk to an extraordinary extent (Plate XIV, Figs. 2 and 3). The organ depicted here, for instance, measures 5.5 cm. in length, 4 cm. in breadth, and 5.5 cm. in depth, and weighs 26 gm. It is is obviously torn or incised along both its anterior and posterior surfaces. The ventricles are very well preserved, but the auricles with the origins of the larger veins are collapsed and shrunk, and are invaginated into the ventricles. Prolonged desiccation and consequent shrinking have thrown all the surface of the heart into deep wrinkles, and the whole organ is as dry as tinder, requiring very careful handling if it is to be kept intact. Fragments chip off readily and crumble to dust under very slight pressure.

Several attempts were made to restore such a mummified heart to its former shape by leaving it for some time in the softening solution. Apparently, all the connective tissues had disappeared during centuries of drying, for after a few hours the muscular bundles fell apart. These were of a pale-yellow colour, and as transparent as if they had been soaked in some clearing reagent such as xylol. A good deal of sand which had obviously been contained in the heart and blood vessels dropped to the bottom of the vessel.

The tricuspid, mitral, and aortic valves were intact and fairly tough, though as thin as the flimsiest tissue paper.

As Professor Elliot Smith pointed out, the heart was generally left in the body cavity of mummies of the XXIst Dynasty. In a mummy of the XVIII–XXth Dynasties, however, I found that it had been removed. Within the pericardium there was a largish bundle containing both kidneys, and behind the liver I found a small packet, containing a bundle of muscular fibres. This probably represented the heart, the embalmer having evidently made a mistake and put the kidneys in the wrong place.

Under the microscope hardly any connective tissue remains between the muscular fibres, so that in many sections none can be demonstrated.

The muscular fibres are normal in so far that the transverse striation and the individual fibres are readily shown, whether running parallel or crossing one another. These are considerably shrunk both longitudinally and laterally. The striation lines are much closer to one another than in the normal human heart and the fibres themselves are correspondingly narrowed.

In the bodies of Roman and Greek children buried in the sand, the heart is of course in situ. The microscopical examination of the muscular fibres gives no better results than in the older mummies. The valves appear normal and are readily demonstrated when the heart is properly softened. The only difference is that the organ does not fall to pieces, as is the case in mummies of the XXIst Dynasty, and that the connective tissue can be demonstrated.

LIVER

The liver, owing to its bulk, necessarily dried very slowly and therefore underwent profound changes. The organ represented in Plates XII and XIII had evidently been compressed into the form of a tube, and either before or after drying, part of the organ had been torn away. It measured 22.5 cm. in its longest and 7 cm. in its broadest diameter, and it was nowhere more than 4 cm. thick. It weighed 300 gm. with its bandages.

We must remember in this connection that the incision through which the liver was extracted measured not more than 5 inches as a rule, and it is very difficult to understand how the embalmers removed this enormous organ through this comparatively small opening. The liver was frequently damaged, and the embalmers did not always take the trouble to replace the whole of the organ into the body cavity. The liver depicted here is the most perfect I have ever seen and almost an exception. In other cases the organ was represented by a few ounces of tissue only, the rest having completely disappeared.

The liver of the Greek mummy was fairly perfect, but nevertheless a large part, viz., the quadrate lobe, the gall bladder, all the hepatic vessels, and caudate and Spigelian lobes had been torn away.

Fragments of five different livers were examined. These were as hard as stone and when broken across expose a mahogany-brown, smooth, glistening surface. In the softening solution they showed, as a rule, a marked tendency to fall into minute fragments, and the slightest movement of the vessel caused the tissue to break up into a flocculent precipitate. Much of the hepatic substance had disappeared, and even when treated with the greatest care, the fragments formed small laminae which readily separated from one another. After many failures large pieces of tissue were prepared for microscopical examination by carefully adding absolute alcohol drop by drop to the softened fragments. The bile ducts had completely or almost completely disappeared. In two livers not a trace of such a channel remained. In a third a few bile ducts were observed, these probably owing their escape from destruction to the dense connective tissue (cirrhosis) surrounding them. The typical arrangement of the lobule, with its cells radiating from the hepatic vein, was still evident (Plate XIX, Figs. 2 and 3), but in almost every section cells were missing here and there, or had been converted into a thin reticulum without any definite structure (Plate XIX, Fig. 1). This is evidently a post-mortem change due possibly to putrefaction, or more probably to autolysis.

The state of preservation of the hepatic cells varies a good deal, sometimes even in sections of the same organ. In some, the cells are converted into slender, almost homogeneous strands, and so thin as to simulate fibrous tissue. In other parts of the same organ the cells are much larger, their lateral borders run into one another, leaving but little space between them. As a rule, owing to the long desiccation that they have undergone, they form a network with almost homogeneous branches.

Examination of the plate (Plate XIX, Fig. 3) shows that in many places several layers of cells have been depicted, the superficial appearing more darkly stained than the deeper ones.

The drying process has evidently reduced the size of the individual cells so much that, however thin the section (and this one was only one micromillimeter thick), several layers of cells are exhibited. Nevertheless, in each preparation, however imperfect the state of the organ, there is seldom any difficulty in recognising the typical arrangement of the liver cells.

Occasionally the hepatic cells are in a much better state of preservation. In one liver of the XXIst Dynasty, not only can individual hepatic cells be recognised, but the nucleus of each is perfectly plain (Plate XIX, Fig. 3). The blood vessels of this organ are in a very fair state of preservation.

As a rule, the state of the vascular system is very unsatisfactory, and the blood vessels are often represented by empty spaces only (Plate XIX, Figs. 2 and 3); here and there, torn and very imperfect fragments of the walls of the artery are found. The portal system throughout appears to have suffered most, not a trace of it remaining in many sections. The hepatic veins are sometimes in a better state, though in the majority of lobules the walls of the veins have either disappeared altogether, or are represented by a few shreds only. In no other organ is the vascular system in such an advanced state of disintegration.

The livers of these children were in an almost perfect state of preservation, and histologically, bile ducts, blood vessels, cells, and connective tissue were almost normal.

I have examined the gall bladder of a child of the Greek period, the histological structure of which was almost perfect.

LUNGS

The lungs of the ancient Egyptians were apparently dried in different ways. Sometimes each lung when still pliable was folded, and the jackal-headed figure Tuamautef placed in the tube thus formed. The pleura, though wrinkled by desiccation, is sometimes easily demonstrated. Such lungs were certainly not bound to the costal pleura by any strong adhesions, for had this been the case, the organs would have been torn during the process of removal. On the contrary, they are perfect. The small deficiencies in the pleura which I have observed were probably produced post mortem, and through the little holes so formed the spongy, reticular tissue of the lungs was evident. One of these lungs, which seemed complete, measured when dried 19 cm. in length, 44 cm. in breadth, and 2 cm. in depth.

Lungs were undoubtedly often dried flat, and this was certainly the case with one of the organs depicted in Plate XIV. Here the root of the lung is plainly recognisable, although the main bronchi, pulmonary artery, and vein cannot be separated. Some parts of this organ are riddled with small black holes, which I take to have been caused by insects.

What I have said about the difficulty of extracting the liver and the probability of the organs being torn when removed applies to the lungs, though to a less degree.

If the organ be stripped as much as possible of its bandages and placed for several days in the softening solution of formol and carbonate of soda, the whole can be made perfectly soft. The time during which the solution must be allowed to act varies with each lung. The process therefore must be watched very carefully, as, if kept too long in the fluid, the entire organ is spoilt. After a period varying from two days to a week or longer, the solution is decanted off and replaced by a 1 per cent formol solution. This is changed on several days and when all the colouring matter has dissolved out, the lung can remain for an indefinite length of time in a 5 per cent formol solution. In some cases I used 30 per cent and then 60 per cent alcohol, but the results obtained were not encouraging. Very often it is clear that the embalmer only wrapped a small portion and sometimes not more than a third of the organ, and that the rest of the bundle consists of mud and vegetable matter. Evidently, therefore, the organ had been badly torn during removal.

I have already alluded to the curious tendency possessed of these organs to produce adipocere (?) and I need not describe its formation again.

The parenchyma of the lung is as a rule in a very good state of preservation. The alveolar structure of the organ is easily seen, though of course the fine details have disappeared (Plate XX, Figs. 1 and 2). The walls of the bronchi, with the exception of the mucous membrane, are much shrunk but well preserved, and the cartilages of the larger bronchi are almost perfect in places. A few cartilage cells may be absent or may have shrunk to a mere point, but as a rule they are well seen. Two cells lying in the same space are often distinguishable. In a few sections the nuclei are still visible (Plate XVIII, Figs. 5a and b).

The microscopical structure of the pleura and diaphragm is beautifully seen in transverse sections. These tissues and the muscular fibres of the diaphragm especially are so typical that it is almost impossible to believe that the material dates from three thousand years. This excellent condition I attribute to the thick layer of mud which lined the entire pleural cavity of this particular mummy.

The lungs of the Roman child were represented by a granular, soapy-feeling mass lying at the back of each pleura. No particular structure could be demonstrated. The lungs of the Greek child will be described in another paper, dealing with pathological changes in mummies.

KIDNEYS

Sometimes both kidneys were left in situ and they may easily escape notice unless the whole mummy be softened. I have found them in a mummy of the XVIIIth–XXth Dynasties, and once I have seen the stomach wrapped up in the same parcel as the two kidneys.

The shape is well preserved, and the hilus, for instance, and sometimes even the ureters can be recognised. Occasionally, again, the suprarenal capsule is still attached to the kidney.

Good sections of the kidney are easily obtained, as the softened organ does not fall to pieces as rapidly as other viscera. The capsule of the kidney is practically perfect.

The general histological structure of the organ is readily seen and the characteristics of every region are distinct (Plate XXI, Figs. 1 and 3). The various parts of the organ, however, expand somewhat unequally; the cortex swelling up less than the medulla, so that the glomeruli and the tubuli contorti are generally more distinct than the straight and connecting tubules. The glomeruli are occasionally somewhat angular in shape and stand out prominently from the surrounding tissue (Plate XXI, Fig. 1). Their characteristic structure has disappeared, for long mummification has converted them into a finely reticulated, spongy-looking mass, in which the epithelium cells and blood vessels are matted together (Plate XXI, Fig. 4). In some kidneys not a single glomerulus has been destroyed.

The tubes of the cortex are complete, though the lumen of the tubes is often closed. Under a high power the individual cells are not recognisable (Plate XXI, Fig. 3). The whole tube forms strands staining faintly with haematoxylin. The connective tissue between the tubuli contorti is often very prominent, standing out in sharp contrast to the faintly staining and sometimes yellow-coloured epithelium cells.

In other cases the epithelium layer is conspicuous and the connective tissue almost invisible. If such sections be floated through alcohol into water, the currents set up wash out the epithelium cells and the connective tissue becomes apparent (Plate XXI, Fig. 5). The reason why the connective tissue is hidden until the epithelium cells have been washed out, is that both, having lost their specific chemical properties, stain almost exactly alike.

The large and medium-size blood vessels persist, and in some cases they can be recognised by their general characteristics only; the details of their microscopical structure have disappeared (Plate XVIII, Fig. 1). The arteries, but not the veins, are contracted, and their coats are converted into homogeneous tissue, showing no differentiation. In other kidneys, however, the blood vessels are almost perfect, even as regards the details of their histological structure.

I have already pointed out in another paper ("Remarks on the Histology and Pathological Anatomy of Egyptian Mummies,"

Cairo Scientific Journal, Vol. IV [January, 1910], No. 40) how often one finds evidence of disease in these organs.

INTESTINES

I have examined two parcels of intestines given me by the authorities of the Medical School in Cairo. The interstices between the intestines were filled with earth and sawdust, and I had great difficulty in removing this foreign matter. In spite of every possible care, I never succeeded in unfolding the coils of the intestines, and I am still unable to say whether the whole or only part of the intestines was placed in the abdomen. I should feel inclined to think, however, that neither of these parcels contained more than half the length of the intestines. The difficulty was increased by the fact that a large part of the guts in one case had been transformed into that peculiar substance for which I have provisionally used the name of adipocere.

Professor Elliot Smith kindly gave me some small pieces of intestine. In Cairo these fragments were hard, dry, and brittle, but after being kept a few weeks in the moist heat of my laboratory at Alexandria during the summer, they became somewhat softer, more pliable, and gave off a distinctly musty odour.

Small pieces swell up quickly in the softening solution, and the muscular and mucous coats are then recognised even with the naked eye, though under the influence of absolute alcohol all differentiation disappears. Microscopical preparations are easily obtained, and the various layers entering into the formation of the intestinal walls are distinctly seen. Plate XXII, Fig. 1, is an exact representation under a low power of an almost complete oblique section through the walls and part of the lumen of the intestine. At (a) the annular muscular coat is depicted. The longitudinal coat of muscular fibres is well preserved also, but is not included in the picture so as to keep the latter within reasonable limits. The submucous tissue between (a) and the muscularis mucosae (b) is fairly well preserved, but in other sections it is altogether absent. The muscularis mucosae (b) is always present and the glandular layer when examined under a low power looks like an open meshwork. The lumen of the intestine is shown bounded by a thin, dark line, which doubtless represents the layer of columnar epithelium.

The lumen of the intestine is always empty in microscopical sections, but on macerating small pieces of intestine in dilute caustic potash and centrifugalising, one finds in the centrifugalised residue débris of partially digested muscular fibres and vegetable cells. In one case I saw granules which gave all the histological reactions of starch.

Examination under a high power is instructive also. Plate XXII, Fig. 3, shows part of a section passing through the annular fibres. The longitudinal striation is present; but in the process of drying the fibres shrank greatly and most of them did not expand again to their natural size in the softening solution. The result is that a kind of reticulum has been formed, and owing to the deficient longitudinal expansion, the fibres remained somewhat angular.

Plate XXII, Fig. 2, represents sections of part of the glandular layer of the intestines. Generally the structure is typical, but here again, owing to deficient expansion, the glands are peculiarly angular. I thought at first that the darkly staining strands round the lumina of the tubes were composed of connective tissue only, but further examination showed that they really consisted of dried epithelium cells, which had not expanded again. They resemble somewhat the insufficiently swollen epithelium cells of some mummified livers and kidneys.

I only obtained a very small piece, about an inch, of the colon of a body of the Hearst collection, in which I saw the transverse and longitudinal muscular fibres. The muscularis mucosae had apparently completely disappeared.

On opening the body, the intestines were all found lying in the abdominal cavity and looked exactly like brown tissue paper. They were removed bodily, and when placed in the formol and carbonate of soda solution, they became again beautifully soft. After a time, although slightly yellowish in colour, they looked almost normal. They were found to be empty from end to end. Microscopically the peritoneal and muscular coats were readily demonstrated, but the mucous membrane appeared to have completely disappeared.

The intestines of that child much resembled those of the Roman child, except that the whole rectum and large intestine, as far as the top of the sigmoid flexure, was filled by an enormous mass of material. So distended was the rectum that it filled practically the whole of the pelvis. It is difficult to believe that this was the normal condition of things, and it is probable that there had been complete intestinal obstruction, although no stricture nor cause for that obstruction could be discovered. The rest of the intestines were quite empty. Microscopically the state of the intestines was exactly that of the Roman child.

My friend Mr. A. Lucas kindly analysed the contents of the rectum for me and found the following chemical composition:

	Per Cent
Fatty matter	28.1
Vegetable tissue (not identified)	26.6
Mineral matter (insoluble in water), chiefly phosphates	5.2
Sodium chloride	9.8
Organic matter (soluble in water, not identified)	14.0
Organic matter (soluble in alcohol, not identified)	16.3
	100.0

The extraordinary fact is the amount of sodium chloride, which is far larger than is usually contained in faeces. In this connection one must remember that this salt was a favourite ingredient of medicines and enemata of the old Egyptians.

STOMACH

I have only examined one stomach histologically. It was as hard as stone and when broken across showed a distinctly resinous fracture. Microscopically the muscular coats were easily seen, though the mucous membrane had completely disappeared. This may have been due to autodigestion before death. (Plate XIII, Fig. 1.)

TESTICLES

In one mummy of the XXIst Dynasty the left testicle could not be found at all, and its place was filled by a quantity of earth which had been pushed in from above. Whether it was really absent during life, or whether it had been torn away by the embalmer, I could not make out. The testicle on the other side was surrounded by sawdust and earth, and it was only with the greatest difficulty that I found part of it together with shreds of the cremaster muscle. The microscopical sections obtained are represented by Plate XVIII, Fig. 6. The spermatozoa and other cells had entirely disappeared and were replaced by a very small quantity of a yellowish, almost homogeneous substance.

In the Greek mummy before mentioned the testicles were found, as the scrotum had not been packed at all. They were very badly preserved and all that could be made out for certain were the septa between the lobes. Altogether the result of the examination of the testes was not very satisfactory.

MAMMARY GLANDS

The mammary glands of women were sometimes not packed and therefore lie flattened and dried against the chest wall. The only mammae I examined were those of old women in which the glandular structure had almost wholly disappeared. The alveoli were recognisable in places, the epithelium cells forming thin, dark strands lining them. Strangely enough, the connective tissue showed beautiful nuclei (see Plate XXII, Fig. 4).

SUMMARY

The object of this work was to ascertain the state of preservation of mummies, with the ulterior object of studying pathological changes histologically. The question now arises, whether one is justified in hoping that histological methods are likely to be of assistance in the elucidation of the pathology of ancient Egyptians. My studies show that the general arrangement of the anatomical elements entering into the formation of tissues and organs of mummies of the XXIst Dynasty, and of dried bodies, is well preserved, as the chief microscopical characteristics of the skin, breast, lungs, liver, kidneys, testicles, heart, intestines, stomach, blood vessels, and muscles are easily recognised. Indeed, none of my numerous competent visitors had any difficulty in diagnosing from what organs the microscopical slides shown to them had been prepared. On the other hand, however, many cells have undergone important alterations; and the nuclei, for instance, can no longer as a rule be differentiated by staining methods. There are exceptions to this rule, for some nuclei are noticeable still, as in the epidermic layer of the skin, the connective tissue of the female breast, the adenoid tissue of the intestine, and the cells of some livers and kidneys. Moreover, there is reason to think that the nuclei are really better preserved than I imagined and that an improved technique will reveal their presence more often.

The histological details of the cells of most organs have also almost entirely vanished; this is specially well marked in the liver and kidneys, where the individual cells are often undistinguishable. On the other hand, the histological characteristics of certain blood vessels, of the nerves, of the heart, and especially of muscle, are surprisingly well preserved.

I think therefore that the microscopical examination of mummies may reveal changes due to infiltration of tissues by: (1) new growths, (2) infective granulomata, (3) animal and vegetable parasites, (4) inflammation, (5) proliferation of connective tissue (cirrhosis), (6) atheroma and calcification, but that there is little hope of recognising diseases in which the chief lesions are seen in the cells of organs and tissues.

An attempt may now be made to answer another question, partly at any rate. Does the histological structure of mummies give any indication with regard to the method of preservation of the body and organs in the XXIst Dynasty?

In describing the blood vessels, I drew attention to the fact that as several hours elapsed between the time of death and the removal of the organs from the body, a certain amount of decomposition must necessarily have taken place.

When enumerating the details of the histology of the skin, the difference in the state of preservation between the skin of the trunk and that of the extremities was insisted on. This difference is probably due to cadaveric putrefaction, always beginning earlier and being more marked in the trunk than in the extremities.

The exact nature of the pickling solution has not been ascertained, but I feel inclined to think it contained a large quantity of chloride of sodium.

Strong solutions of chloride of sodium have a light macerating action, and the salt extracting water from the tissues causes the latter to shrink, and diminishes or even abolishes putrefaction. Indeed, chloride of sodium has been used from time immemorial for preserving foodstuff. On the other hand, natron is used in histology chiefly for the preparation of alkaline solutions of dyes, and for the maceration of tissues. A weak solution of such a salt would not preserve tissues, while a strong one would macerate them past all recognition.

It appears to me probable that the solution used was one of "natron," but that this "natron" consisted chiefly of sodium chloride with a small admixture of carbonate and sulphate of soda. It would be interesting to ascertain whether samples of "natron" with such a chemical composition are still to be found in Egypt.

After the organs were removed from the pickling bath, the dryness of the atmosphere alone probably sufficed in some cases to preserve the organs indefinitely. Mr. Quibell writes:

> Bodies in an extraordinarily good state of preservation, dried and very light, but with the skin complete and flesh dried in whisps (something like Bombay duck) have been found in archaic cemeteries by many people (myself among them), and as far as I know, there is no proof of a preservative having been used.

I have myself seen in the desert of Sinai the hind quarters of a camel in a perfect state of preservation, having been simply dried by the sun. The desiccation in this case must have taken place rapidly, as otherwise the flesh would certainly have been eaten by the few leopards and the many hyenas and jackals which roam about the desert.

What share these various processes had respectively in producing the described result, we can only guess. Probably the most powerful factor in preventing decomposition was[1] the dryness of the climate. The tombs, where most of the bodies were discovered, are rock-hewn tombs and far above the level of the Nile flood. The heat during the day, even in winter, is intense, and though the nights are often very cold, nevertheless the climate throughout the year is always dry, the rainfall being almost nil. It seems quite evident that incipient putrefaction would be arrested very soon for want of water.

[1] The following remarks apply only to such mummies as have been studied in this paper and not to all Egyptian mummies.

Desiccation alone, however, would not account for the good state of preservation of mummies removed to the hot, steamy atmosphere of Lower Egypt. In such cases the acid reaction and the packing of mud and sawdust would absorb all moisture and prevent putrefaction. It must be remembered also that under certain circumstances mummified organs undergo putrefaction. Thus, pieces of intestine removed to Alexandria gave off a musty odour and when suspended in dilute alkalies proved a good cultivating medium for bacteria. A dried head which I bought at Luxor and which was there quite sweet, became putrid in Lower Egypt. Mr. Quibell writes:

I have found a body of the Old Empire in a state of putrefaction and very unpleasant. The body had dried rapidly and been preserved for many centuries until the rise of the level of the country, or exposure to damp from showers after some denudation of the surface, had started the process of decay again.

On the other hand, human bodies when once well dried may be exposed to the atmosphere for considerable periods without putrefaction taking place. I have in my laboratory the body of a Roman child which had been simply dried in the sand. This has remained quite sweet; the only change that has taken place in a period of more than a year is that the skin has become softer and somewhat soapy to the touch. The strange part of it is that no insects (ants, etc.) have attacked it. The temperature of this laboratory varied between 56° and 100° F.; for four months it seldom went below 75° F. and was generally above 80° F. In the summer the air was saturated with humidity.

The methods, therefore, used by the Egyptians of the XXIst Dynasty for preserving the bodies of their friends were of the simplest; namely, pickling in salt solution and filling up with sand or mud to absorb moisture. These methods were sufficient to preserve the histological structure of the tissues.

The observations on which this paper is based were made more than two years ago. Dr. Willmore showed some of the sections at the British Medical Association in July, 1908, and I demonstrated them at a meeting of the Cairo Scientific Society in December of the same year.

The paper and the illustrations accompanying it were finished more than one year ago, but the publication was delayed until the Institut Égyptien very generously offered to bear the greater part of the expense. I may be permitted, therefore, to offer my best thanks to the members of the Institut for their kindness and generosity.

The delay has been in some measure an advantage. It has enabled me to control my work over and over again, and I have found no reason to alter this account of my observations. Indeed, the hope expressed in this paper that histological investigations would add to our knowledge of the pathology of ancient Egypt has since been fulfilled.

DESCRIPTION OF PLATES XII–XXII[1]

(For all particulars see text)

PLATE XII

FIG. 1.—Liver, drawn exactly natural size, from actual measurements. The liver is folded upon itself and contains in the cavity so formed a statuette of the human-headed Amset.

FIG. 2.—Liver (drawn exactly to scale) seen in profile.

PLATE XIII

FIG. 1.—Part of stomach, drawn natural size. It was packed in sawdust.

FIG. 2.—Stomach. Fracture showing resinous surface, though it contained no resin.

FIG. 3.—Fractured surface of skin of chest and subjacent muscle. It has a resinous appearance, though it contained no resin whatever.

FIG. 4.—Roll of intestines. Drawn from measurement and reduced to ¾ size. It contains a small figure of the hawk-headed Khebsennuf.

PLATE XIV

FIG. 1.—Lung, drawn natural size. The lung has been dried flat.

FIGS. 2 and 3.—Heart natural size. Anterior and posterior surfaces.

PLATE XV

FIG. 1.—Nerve of finger. Haematoxylin. The medullary sheath is well seen. (Leitz, Oc. 1, ×1/12.)

FIG. 2.—Another section of nerve. Two axis cylinders are seen. Same staining and magnification as preceding one.

[1] The figures are from mummies of the XXIst Dynasty, unless othewise stated.

Fig. 3.—Skin of finger. Sweat glands are evident. Nuclei are seen also. Eosin. (Leitz, low power.)

Fig. 4.—Kidney. The epithelium cells have been converted into a yellow homogeneous substance. Haematoxylin. (Leitz, Oc. 1, ×1/12.)

PLATE XVI

Fig. 1.—Skin of finger. Haematoxylin. Notice how well the nuclei have been preserved. (Leitz, Oc. 1, ×1/12.)

Fig. 2.—Skin of chest. Notice contrast with preceding one, almost all the epithelium cells having disappeared. Some of the packing material is still adherent to the surface. (a) packing material; (b) corium; (c) subcutaneous tissue. Haematoxylin. (Leitz, low power.)

Fig. 3.—Skin of finger. Transverse section of sweat glands. Nuclei still visible. (Leitz, Oc. 1, ×1/12.)

Fig. 4.—Epidermic cells of the skin floated off after maceration. Haematoxylin. (Leitz, Oc. 1, ×1/12.)

Fig. 5.—Section through a nerve. (Low power.)

Fig. 6.—From the subcutaneous tissue of a body (not mummified but dried in the sand) about 8000 B.C. No anatomical structure recognisable except nuclear masses staining with haematoxylin (nuclei). (Leitz, Oc. 1, ×1/12.)

Fig. 7.—Subcutaneous tissue of mammary gland. Haematoxylin. (Leitz, Oc. 1, ×1/12.)

PLATE XVII

Fig. 1.—Small digital nerve. Haematoxylin. (Leitz, low power.)

Fig. 2.—Teased muscle of arm, mounted in Canada balsam. Eosin. (Leitz, Oc. 1, ×1/12.)

Fig. 3.—Somewhat diagrammatic representation of muscle fibre teased in normal salt solution. At (a) the sarcolemma is visible. (Leitz, Oc. 1, ×1/12.)

PLATE XVIII

Fig. 1.—Small renal vessel. Eosin. (Leitz, Oc. 1, ×1/12.)

Fig. 2.—Large vessel of neck in very bad state of preservation. Eosin. (Leitz, Oc. 1, ×1/12.)

Fig. 3.—Middle coat of aorta. Eosin. (Leitz, Oc. 1, ×1/12.)

Fig. 4.—Small digital artery. All the coats of artery can be seen. Haematoxylin. (Leitz, Oc. 1, ×1/12.)

Fig. 5.—Cartilage cells of the trachea. At (a) two cartilage cells in same space. At (b) the nuclei are still seen. Eosin. (Leitz, Oc. 1, ×1/12.)

Fig. 6.—Testicle. The spermatozoa have entirely disappeared. Haematoxlin. (Leitz, Oc. 1, ×1/12.)

PLATE XIX

Fig. 1.—Liver in which nothing can be seen but a thin reticulum. Haematoxylin. (Leitz, Oc. 1, ×1/12.)

Fig. 2.—Liver, better preserved than the last. Haematoxylin. (Low power.)

Fig. 3.—Liver, showing rows of cells and central vessel at (a) with shreds of vessel wall. Haematoxylin. (Leitz, Oc. 1, ×1/12.)

Fig. 4.—Well-preserved liver cells showing nuclei. Haematoxylin. (Leitz Oc. 1, ×1/12.)

PLATE XX

Fig. 1.—Lung. Eosin. (Leitz, Oc. 1, ×1/12.)

Fig. 2.—Another lung. Haematoxylin. (Low power.)

Fig. 3.—Section of another lung; alveoli greatly distended and full of foreign material. Eosin. (Leitz, Oc. 1, ×1/12.)

PLATE XXI

Fig. 1.—Section of cortex of kidney showing tubuli contorti and glomeruli. Haematoxylin. (Low power.) The dark spots in the glomeruli are not nuclei, but irregular, more darkly stained shreds of tissue.

Fig. 2.—Epithelium layer of tubuli contorti, very highly magnified. (Leitz, Oc. 3, ×1/12.)

Fig. 3.—Straight tubules. (Low power.)

Fig. 4.—Glomerulus. (Zeiss, Oc. 3, ×1/12.)

Fig. 5.—Connective tissue of kidney, from which epithelium has been washed out. (Low power.)

PLATE XXII

Fig. 1.—Section of fold of intestine. Haematoxylin. (Low power.) (a) muscular coat; (b) submucous layer; (c) glandular layer and muscularis; (d) lumen of intestine. At (a) in the lower part of the intestine the muscular layer has become kinked and folded on itself. The artist faithfully reproduced what he saw, and I thought it preferable not to retouch the picture in any way.

Fig. 2.—Oblique section through glandular layer of intestine. (a) glands; (b) part of submucosa showing nuclei. (Leitz, Oc. 1, ×1/12.)

Fig. 3.—Smooth muscles of intestine. (Leitz, Oc. 1, ×1/12.)

Fig. 4.—Connective tissue of breast of woman showing nuclei. (Leitz, Oc. 1, ×1/12.)

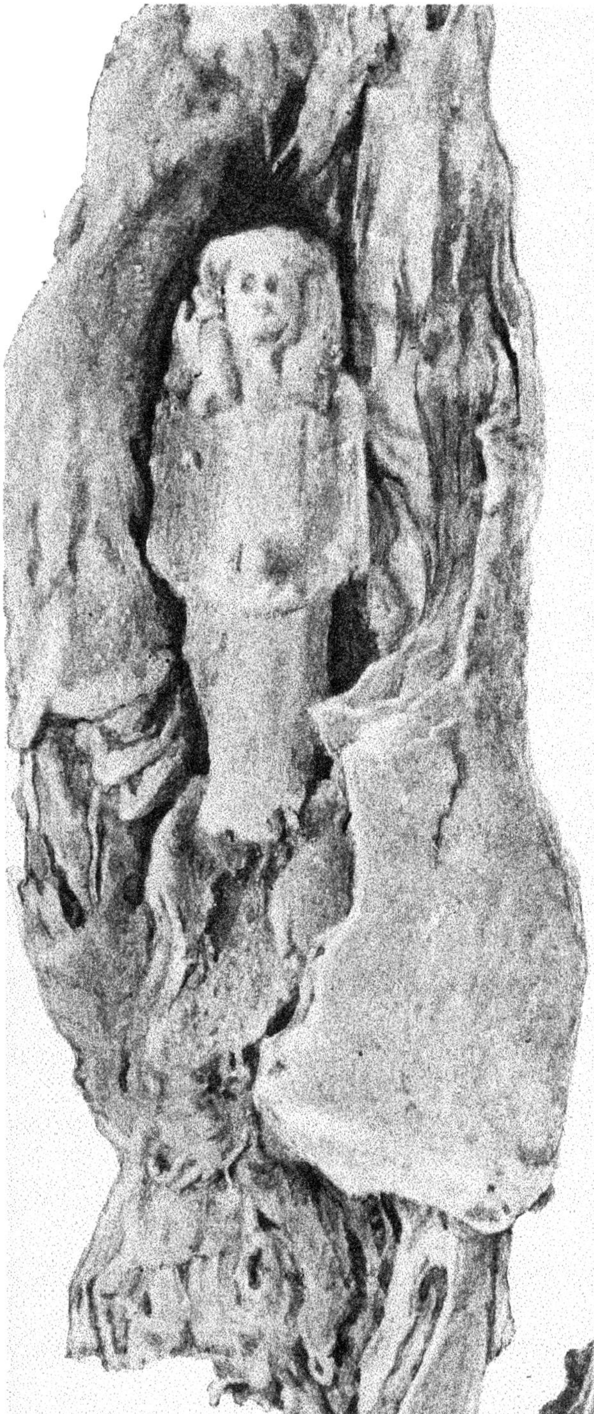

FIG. 1

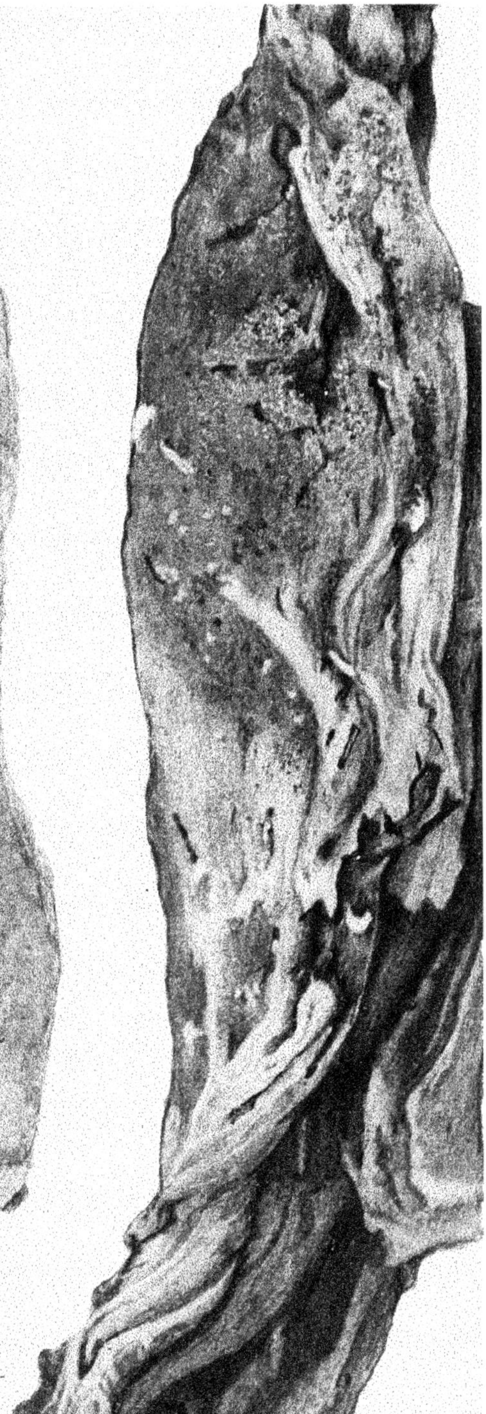

FIG. 2

PLATE XIII

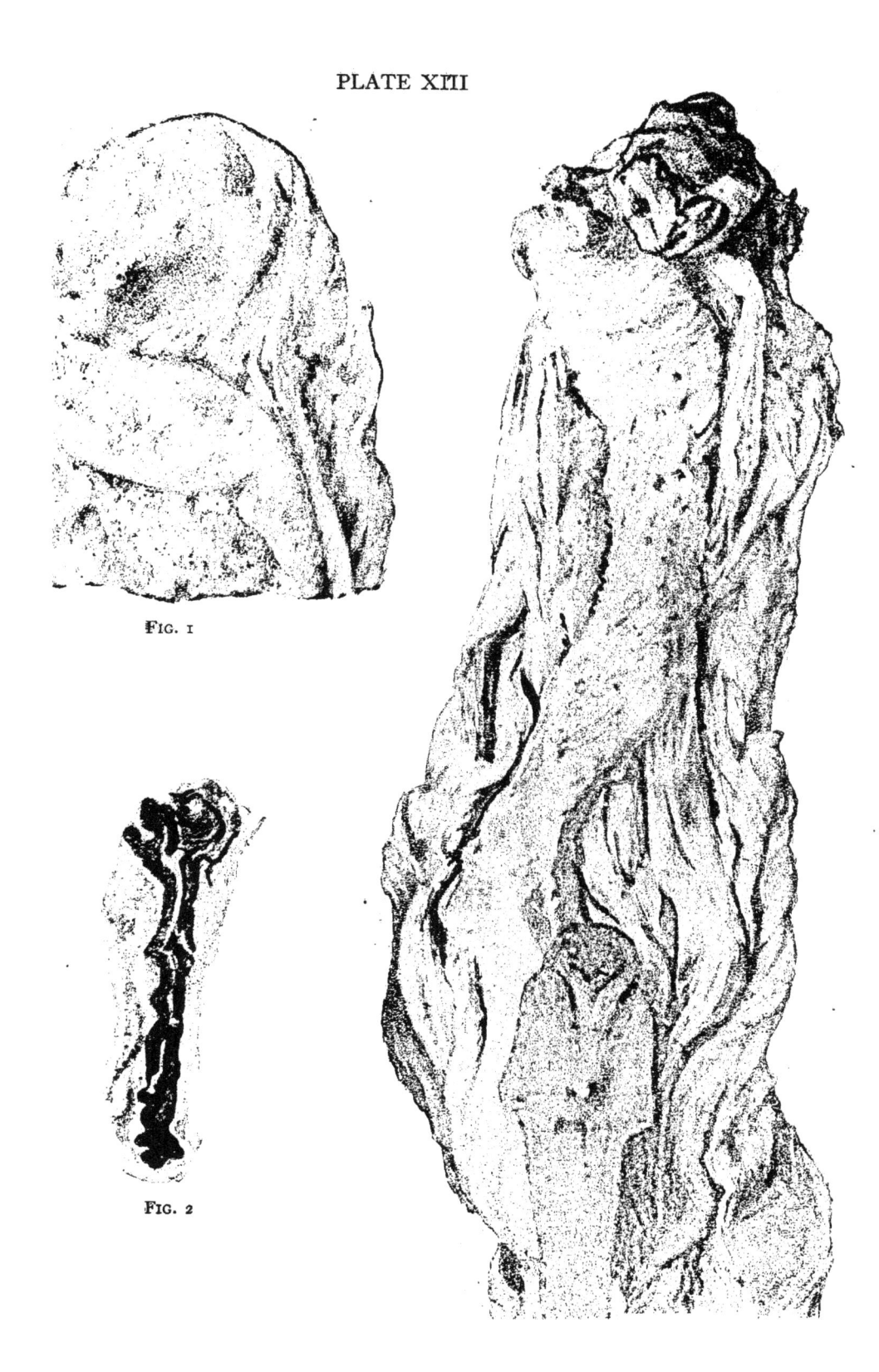

FIG. 1

FIG. 2

FIG. 2

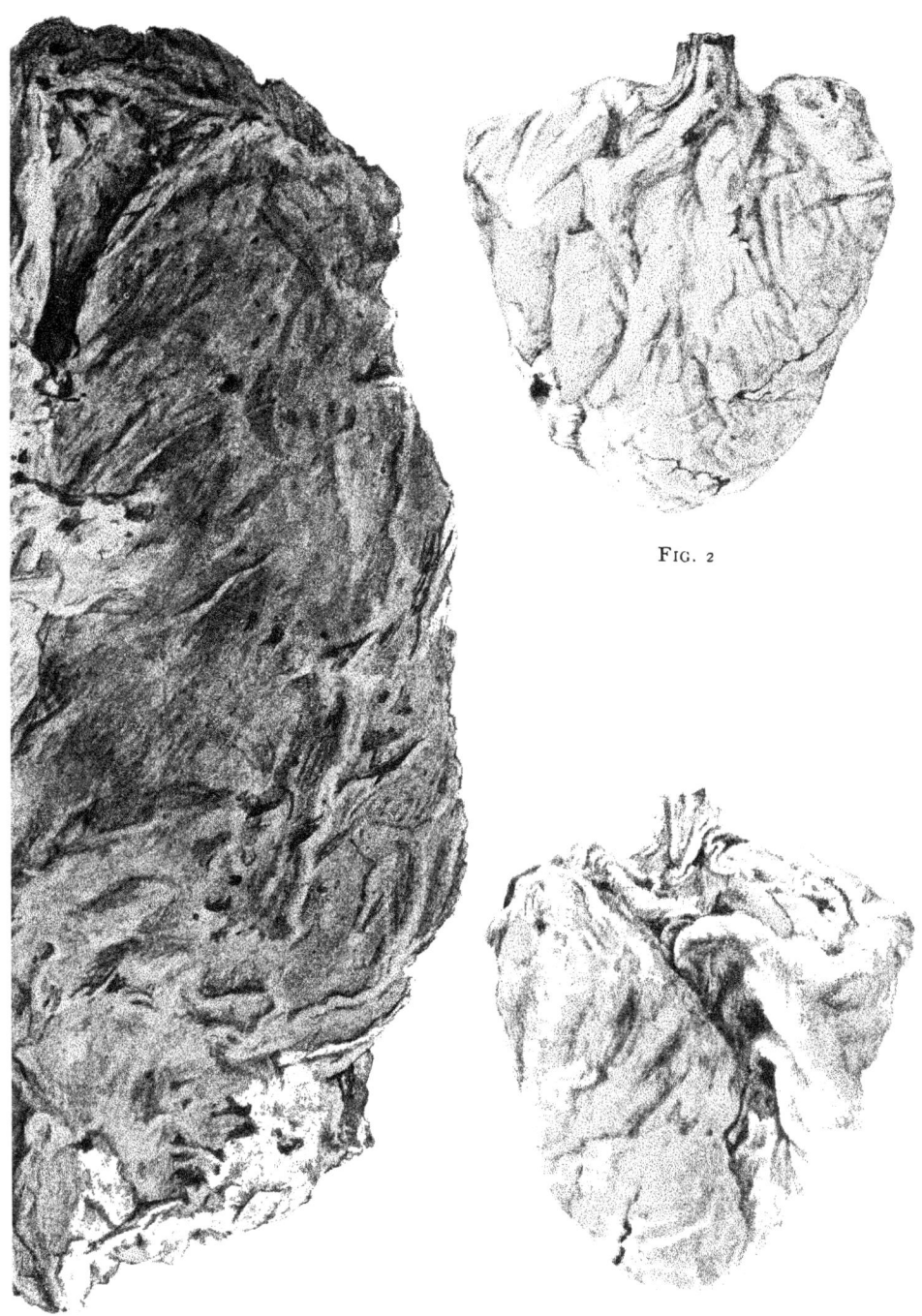

FIG. 1

FIG. 3

PLATE XV

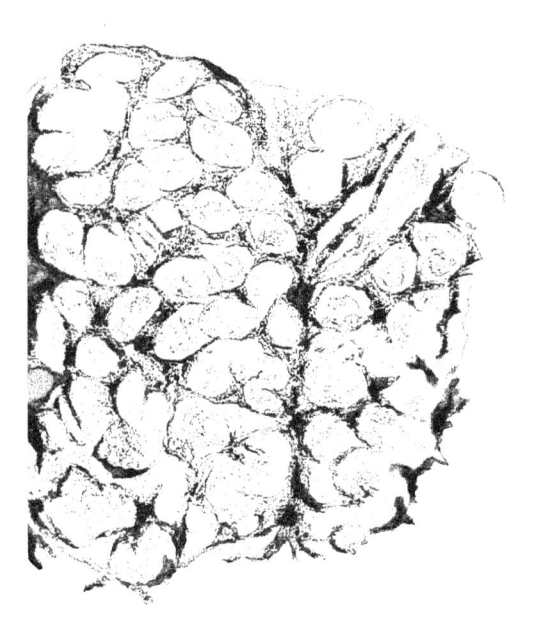

Fig. 1

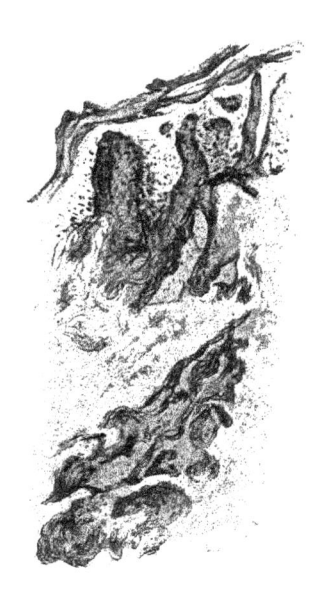

Fig. 3

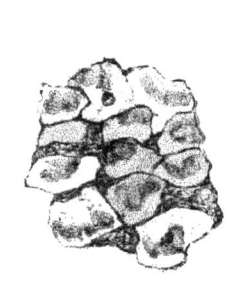

Fig. 2

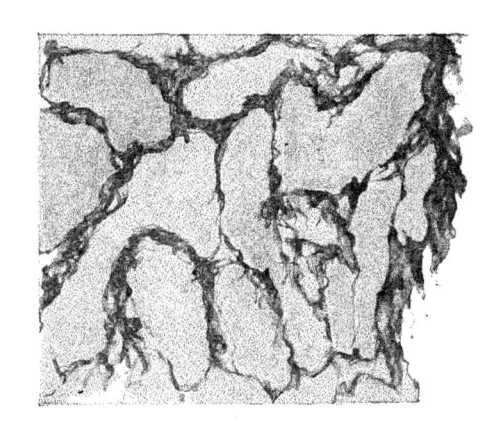

Fig. 4

a

Fig. 1

a
b
c

Fig. 2

Fig. 4

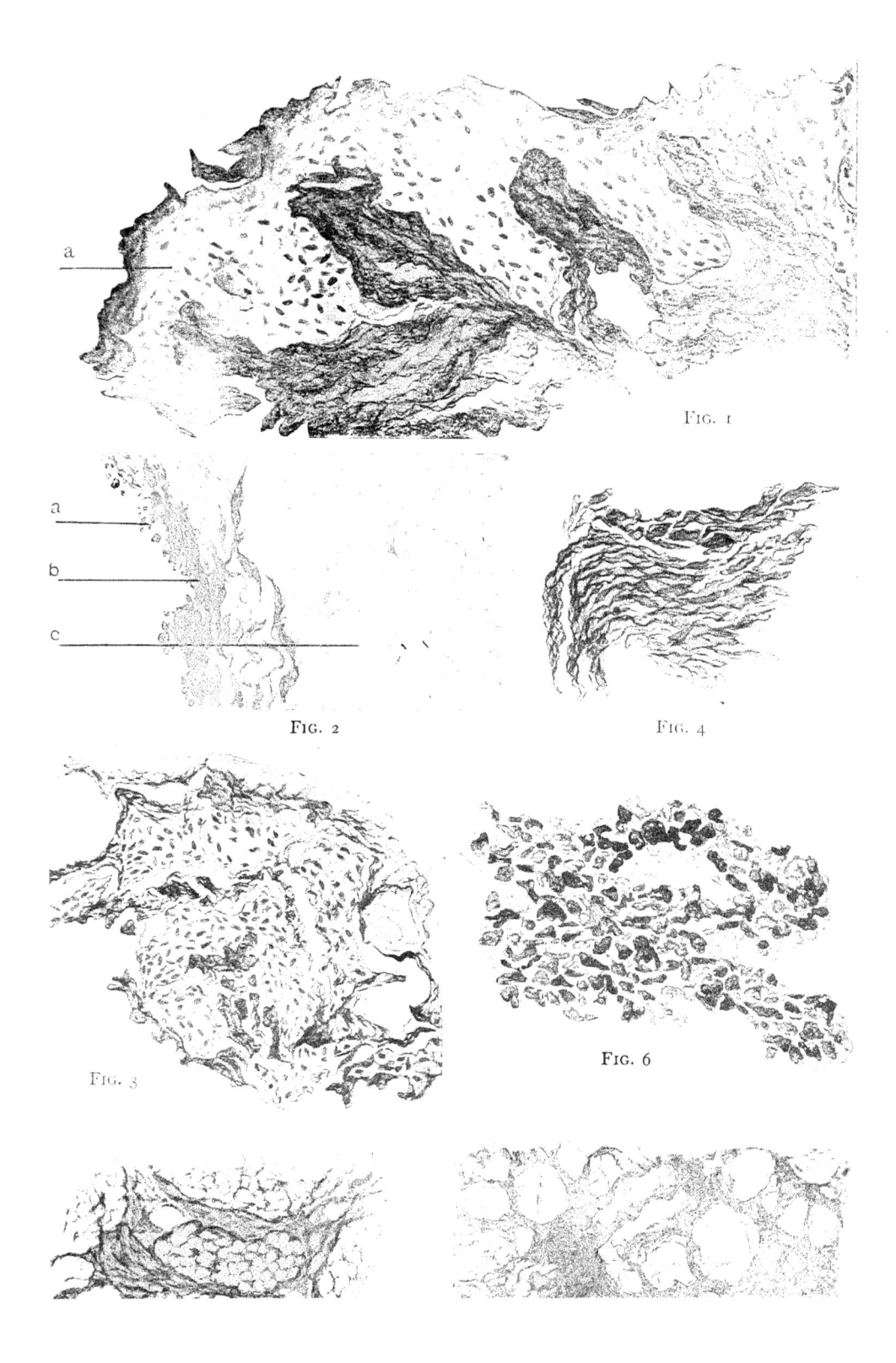

Fig. 3

Fig. 6

PLATE XVII

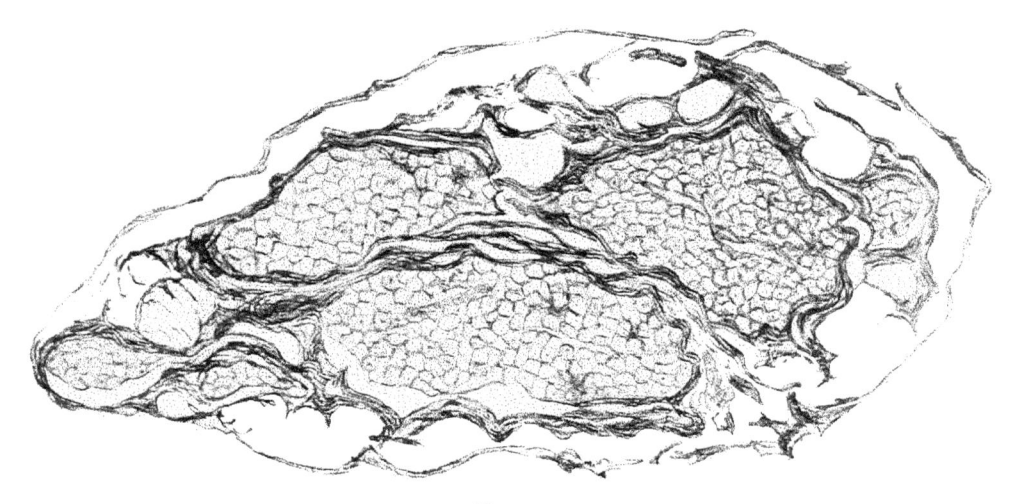

Fig. 1

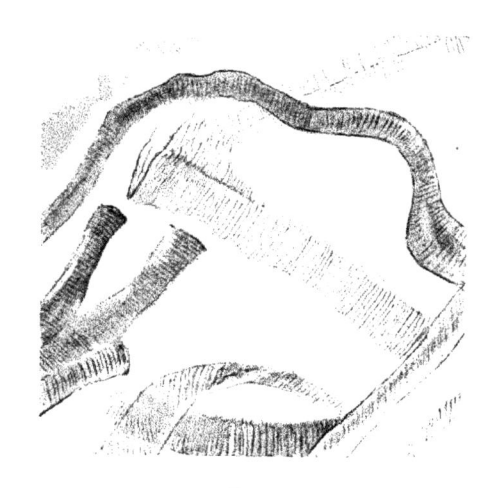

Fig. 2

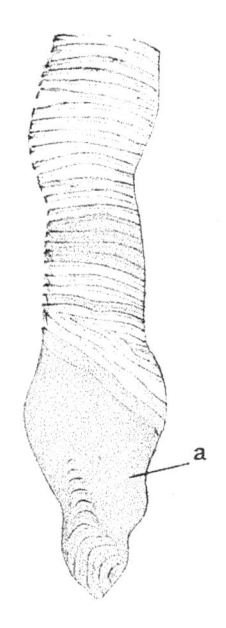

Fig. 3

FIG. 1

FIG. 2

FIG. 3

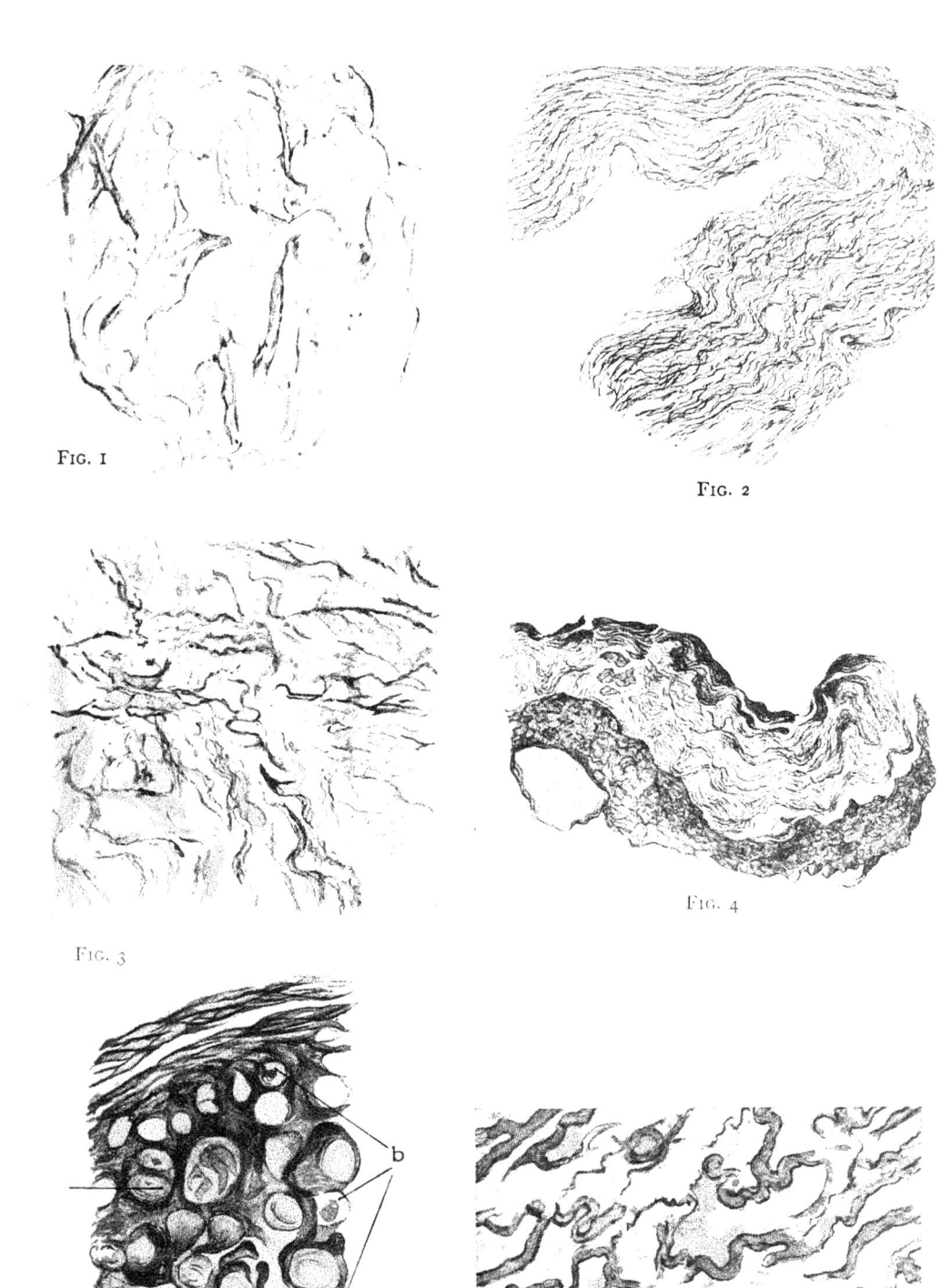

FIG. 4

b

PLATE XIX

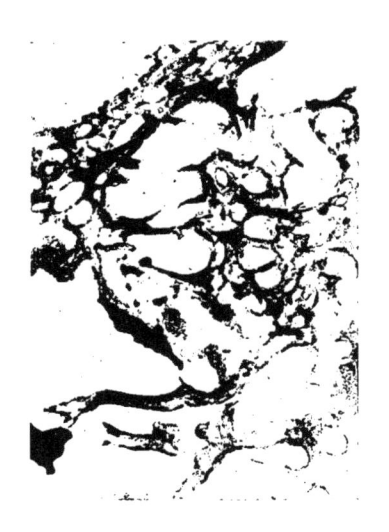

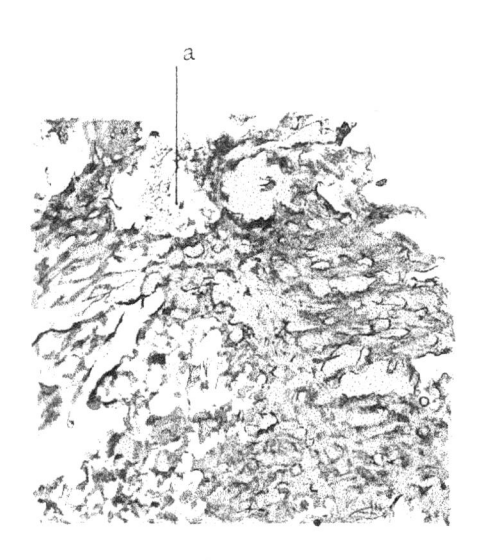

Fig. 1

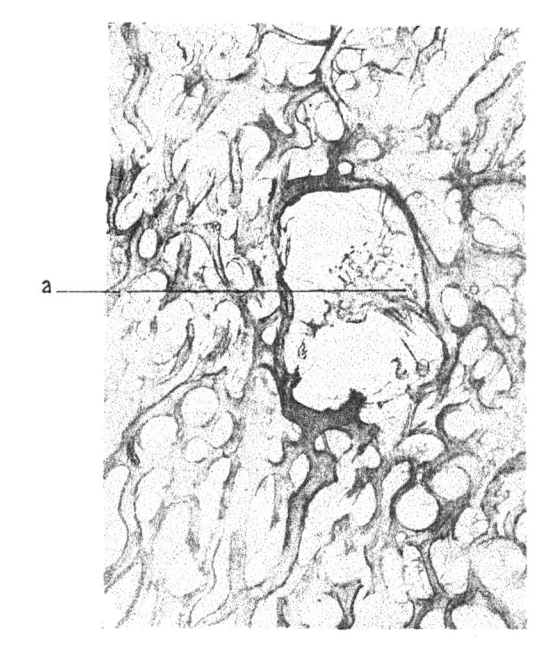

Fig. 2

Fig. 3

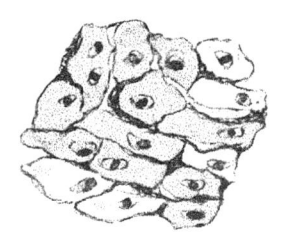

Fig. 4

Fig. 1

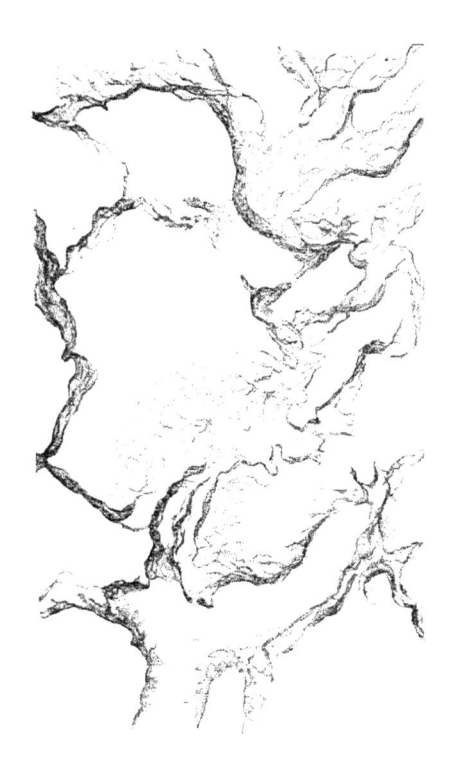

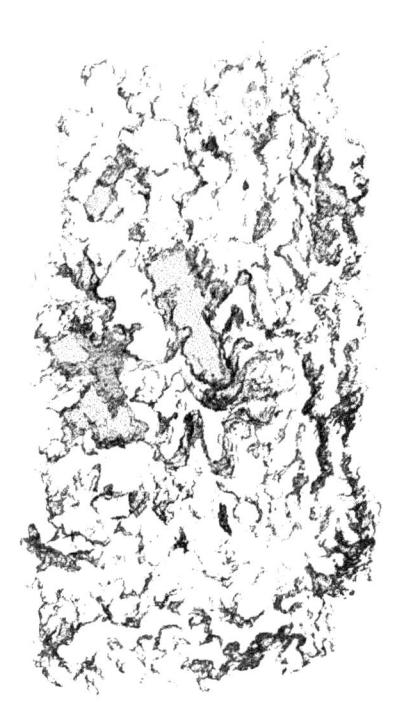

Fig. 2

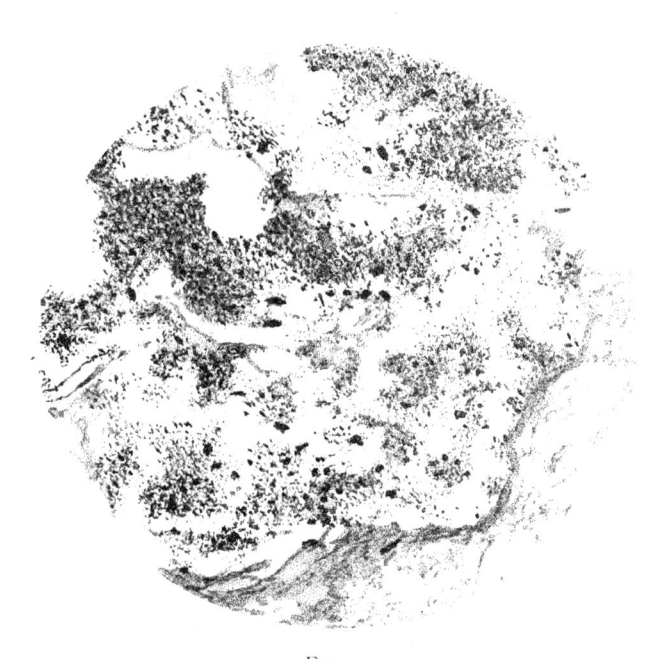

Fig. 3

PLATE XXI

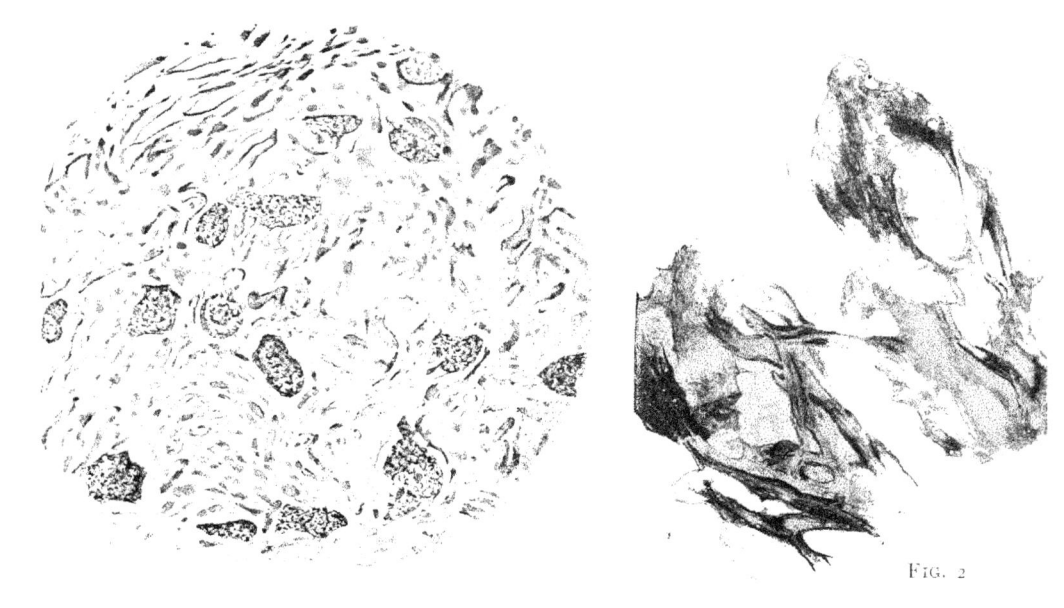

FIG. 1

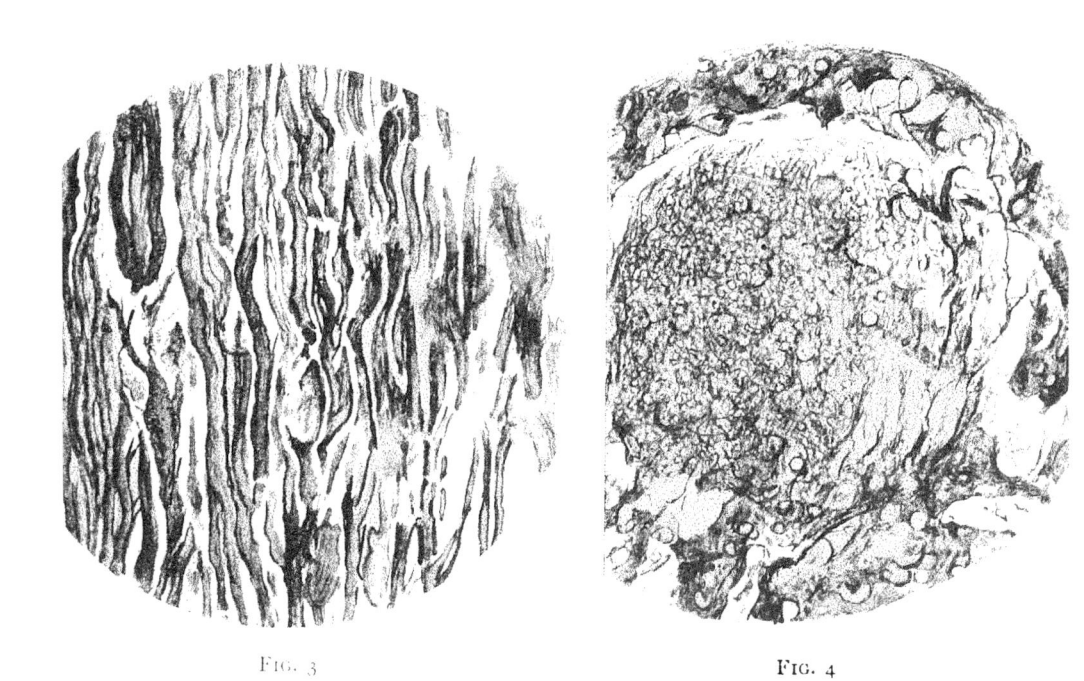

FIG. 2

FIG. 3

FIG. 4

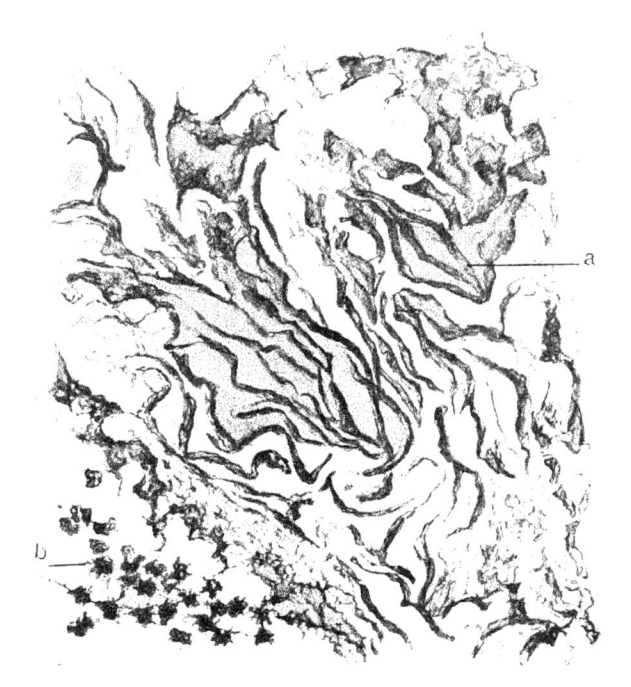

Fig. 2

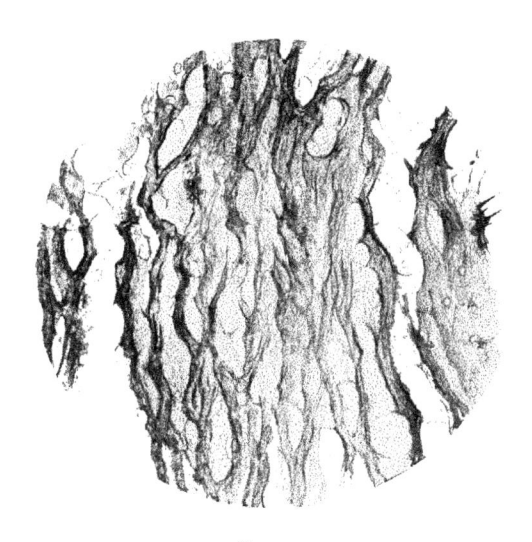

Fig.

ON OSSEOUS LESIONS IN ANCIENT EGYPTIANS[1]

(*Journal of Pathology and Bacteriology*, Vol. XVI [1912])

In 1907 the Egyptian Government decided to make an archaeological survey of that part of Nubia which would be flooded more or less permanently when the Assuan dam was raised. Dr. Elliot Smith, at first alone, afterwards in collaboration with Dr. Wood Jones and Dr. Derry, was entrusted with the anthropological side of the inquiry, and the results of the exploration were published in the *Bulletins of the Archaeological Survey of Nubia*. It is not too much to say that, quite apart from archaeological contributions, the anatomical and pathological discoveries fully justified the expenditure necessary for this work.

This, as far as we know, was the first systematic investigation regarding the diseases of old Egyptians.

As early as 1889, however, our friend Dr. Fouquet published several observations on pathological specimens found in Egyptian tombs.[2] Although we are very far from invariably agreeing with this observer's diagnoses and conclusions, yet he has the undoubtedly great merit of having been a pioneer in this branch of science.

Lastly, a new department of pathological research was opened up when one of us (M. A. R.) studied the histology of Egyptian mummies and shortly described the pathological alterations seen under the microscope.

Before entering into the main part of our paper, we should like to add that surely the time has come when a check should be put on the wholesale destruction of the pathological specimens of the past, which has been going on for over one thousand years.[3] Hundreds of mummies and dried human corpses have been removed

---

[1] This paper was written with A. Rietti as junior author.

[2] *Mémoires publiés par les membres de la Société Archéologique Française au Caire sous la direction de M. Maspéro*, 1881–84, fasc. 4. Also, De Morgan, *Recherches sur les origines de l'Égypte*.

[3] Mummies were exported from Egypt right through the Middle Ages.

from Egyptian tombs, and, with the exception of the facts enumerated in the papers above mentioned, there exist only a few very imperfect records of the state of these bodies. We hope and urge that the authorities will prohibit the exportation of skeletons, dried remains, or mummies until these have been examined by experts. Unless this is done soon, the present waste of scientific material will continue, only to be bitterly regretted before long.

Sir Gaston Maspero, Professor Flinders Petrie, Dr. Keatinge, and Professor Breccia have placed at our disposal a number of mummies and skeletons, dating from various periods of ancient Egypt. These we have examined macroscopically, and, whenever possible, microscopically. The best pathological specimens will be deposited in the Museum of the Medical School at Cairo, but a large number of diseased bones will remain over, which will be sent to any recognised pathological institute, for study and comparison with examples of the same disease occurring at the present time.

Our material came partly from Upper Egypt and partly from Alexandria. A few words about the latter are necessary.

At Chatby, near Alexandria, about two minutes' walk from the sea, lie the tombs of the Macedonian soldiers of Alexander the Great and Ptolemy I. In view of the constant growth of the town, which will soon extend over the whole of this region, the Municipal Commission ordered an archaeological survey of this site. The work was entrusted to Professor E. Breccia,[1] the curator of the Alexandria Museum, who gave us permission to examine most of the bones found in the necropolis and to be present during some of the excavations. Owing to a lawsuit, the work has been suspended for a time, and this delay is specially unfortunate because the names on the tombs to be yet opened indicate that the crypts contain the skeletons of the prostitutes who accompanied the Greek army. Here, if anywhere, evidences of syphilis and gonorrhoea should be found, provided always venereal disease existed at that period.

The bodies had been placed in rock-hewn graves. The first grave was an *ossarium* measuring about 2 c.m., and filled with sand and bones, and closed with a stone slab which had been hermetically sealed with mortar. The bones, after the bodies had undergone decomposition elsewhere, had been thrown into the ossarium *pêle-mêle*, and little care had been taken, as among the human bones the femur of a horse was found.

[1] This eminent archaeologist will soon publish a full account of his researches, which will throw much light on the habits of the Greek immigrants in Egypt.

The other sepulchres were horizontal shafts, 3.5 feet high, 6 feet deep, and about 3.5 feet wide, cut in the solid rock and closed in the same manner as the ossarium. Very rarely such a tomb contained but one body lying on a layer of sand about 6 inches deep; as a rule, several skeletons, five, six, or even more, were present. The small size of the shafts proved that the bodies were not put in together, but that the first had been allowed to putrefy and fall to pieces before the second was introduced.

Funereal urns filled with ashes or half-carbonised bones were discovered also. The Greeks of that period, therefore, were eclectic in their customs, some families burning, others burying their dead.

Unfortunately, the level of the land has sunk several feet since the last body was consigned to the grave. Hence some tombs were partially filled, others merely infiltrated, with sea water, and the bones were often found lying in water or thick, wet mud. Such skeletons were in very bad condition, and most of the smaller and some of the larger bones could not be found, even when the slush was removed carefully by hand.

Although, as might be expected, the bones were rather better preserved in dry than in wet graves, yet this was by no means the rule. The skeleton of a female, for instance, lying on a bed of dry sand was so fragile that some bones were broken when their removal was attempted; on the other hand, bones lying in liquid mud were sometimes very hard, whereas others, in the same grave, broke as soon as touched.

Sometimes the soldiers had been buried with their wives and children. Nothing could be learned from the skeletons of the latter, as hardly a single bone was preserved sufficiently well for examination.

We shall not enter into anthropometric details, as the skeletons have been handed over to an anthropologist for examination. We may say, however, that a superficial examination sufficed to show that various races were represented. Of the thirty-two skulls examined, some had high-bridged noses, others remarkably flat ones. Some were brachycephalic, others markedly dolichocephalic; two skulls were evidently negroid. The variations in stature were great also, some men being very tall, others short. These differences are not to be wondered at, considering that, from the start, Alexander's army was distinctly a "mixed crew." It is stated, for instance, in Smith's *Classical Dictionary* that of the 30,000 foot soldiers who left Greece with Alexander, only 12,000 were Greeks; the others were foreigners, Thracians chiefly.

The inscriptions on the tombs are in Greek, but it is highly probable that the soldiers settled in Egypt had intercourse with and often married native women, just as their successors have done in modern times. The present Berberine, for instance, especially when coming from Korosko, often boasts that he is a descendant of a Turkish soldier and a native woman. The term Turk, as used by him, includes Greek, Herzegovinian, Bosnian, Bulgarian, and Servian.

Part of our material is derived from the catacombs of Kom el Shougafa, which are situated close to Pompey's Pillar at Alexandria, and, according to Professor Breccia, the bodies date from the second century after Christ. The tombs contain hundreds of skeletons, most of which, owing to the gradual infiltration of water, are in such a bad condition that they cannot be examined. The few seen by us were in two tombs in which the damp had not penetrated.

It has been supposed that these catacombs contained the skeletons of the Alexandria youths who were massacred by order of Caracalla. A simple examination of the skeletons showed this supposition to be wrong, as the bones are those of men, women, and children.

On the whole, the mode of burial was almost identical with that seen at Chatby. The first body had been placed on a layer of sand about 4 inches high, and later on the skeleton had been pushed aside to make room for the second occupant. The size of the tombs precluded all possibilities of more than two or three bodies having been buried at one time. So far we have not come across any sign of cremation whatever.

We have also examined five Coptic bodies coming from Upper Egypt and dating from the fifth century A.D.

OLD EGYPTIAN SKELETONS

I. SPONDYLITIS DEFORMANS, FRACTURE OF THE LEFT FIRST RIB, SLIGHT ARTHRITIS, IN A SKELETON OF THE THIRD DYNASTY (2980–2900 B.C.)

This skeleton, that of a man called Nefêrmaat, was found by Mr. G. Wainwright.[1] We are greatly obliged to Professor W. M. Flinders Petrie for allowing us to describe the pathological lesions.[2]

The bones are extremely fragile, and were covered in many places with thick incrustations of salt. At some time or other they had been buried in, or at any rate been in intimate contact with, earth, as many of the spinal foramina were still filled with mud.

The spinal column from the fourth cervical to the coccyx, and possibly through its whole length, had been converted by disease into one rigid block. This had been broken into several pieces after death (Plate XXIII, Figs. 2–5).

Atlas, axis, and third cervical vertebra absent. Fourth to sixth cervical and first dorsal vertebrae form a rigid pillar, being firmly ankylosed anteriorly by solid new bone (Plate XXIII, Fig. 2), evidently formed in anterior spinous

[1] Gerald Wainwright, "The Mastaba of Nefêrmaat," in *Meydoum and Memphis* (3), by W. M. Flinders Petrie, Ernest Mackay, and Gerald Wainwright, 1910, p. 18.

[2] This skeleton will now be placed in the Cairo collection.

ligament. Distinct bulging of this osseous bridge opposite each space for intervertebral disc. Through gaps one can see that intervertebral discs were not ossified, as surfaces of vertebrae are perfectly smooth. Space for intervertebral discs, though empty, are not narrowed.

Posterior spinous ligament completely ossified. New bone, however, does not bulge into spinal canal, which therefore was not narrowed by bone.

Superior surface of fourth cervical vertebra had suffered much injury post mortem. Inferior border of body of first dorsal shows numerous osteophytes, forming a bridge with like prolongations on superior border of second dorsal below.

Whole dorsal region displays similar lesions (Plate XXIII, Fig. 4), both anterior and posterior borders of vertebral bodies being firmly ankylosed. Articulating surfaces with few exceptions united solidly. Spinous processes, when present, normal, save eleventh and twelfth, which are united by strong bony bridge.

Similar alterations in lumbar region, where, however, posterior spinous ligament is not ossified. The right vertebral groove opposite the twelfth dorsal, first and second lumbar vertebrae filled with mass of somewhat spongy bone about 3 cm. broad, extending laterally over articulating surfaces (Plate XXIII, Fig. 5) which are everywhere covered with thick new bone. Similar but smaller mass occupies the same situation on left side (Plate XXIII, Fig. 1).

Fifth lumbar vertebra is firmly ankylosed with the sacrum, which is completely ossified and otherwise normal.

Acetabula normal, except for some small osteophytes at junction of articular and non-articular parts.

Left femur.—Head broken off post mortem. Slight deposit of new bone at junction of head and neck.

Right femur.—Slight thickening on anterior border of articulating surface of knee-joint.

Scapulae.—Very slight roughening round scapulo-humeral articulations.

Manubrium sterni shows curious lesions. On right side there is a prolongation of bone, evidently part of the first rib firmly ankylosed with manubrium sterni (Plate XXIV, Fig. 6). This ends in a smooth, rounded surface which evidently was an articulating surface. We suggest that at some time or other there had been a fracture of the first rib, which had healed badly, and that a false joint had formed.

That the *costal cartilages* had been extensively ossified is shown by Plate XXIV, Fig. 7, representing the rest of the sternum.

In the bones of the *skull* which were left, nothing particular was found except that the internal surface of both condyles were rough and showed distinct signs of inflammation.

Left parietal bone extensively gnawed by insects.

II. SPONDYLITIS DEFORMANS AND OSTEO-ARTHRITIC LESIONS OF THE HAND IN A SKELETON OF THE THIRD DYNASTY (2980–2900 B.C.)

These bones, found by Professor W. M. Flinders Petrie in a tomb of the IIIrd Dynasty near the Fayoum pyramid, belonged to an adult of small size, whose age and sex cannot be estimated. Although few in number, they are worth describing owing to the intensity of the pathological changes in them.

Atlas.—Some osseous overgrowth at point of attachment of transverse ligament, specially on left side, where new bone forms a kind of cushion about 7 mm. long and 1 mm. thick. On left side a spear-shaped osteophyte about 4 mm. long, 3 mm. broad, and 3 mm. thick projects upwards from anterior arch (Plate XXIV, Fig. 13). Tubercle on the anterior arch greatly thickened. Superior articular surfaces smooth.

Axis.—Odontoid process very irregular and capped by an osteophyte quite 5 mm. long. Inferior anterior border prolonged into thick spear-shaped point (Plate XXIV, Fig. 16). Articulating surfaces smooth.

Cervical vertebra (fourth?).—Great thickening, round body, especially anteriorly (Plate XXIV, Fig. 10). Inferior anterior border sends off thick prolongation downwards. Judging from the worm-eaten and rough appearance of the body, it would appear that the disease possibly extended to the intervertebral discs (?).

Two cervical vertebrae firmly joined by ossified anterior and posterior spinous ligaments (Plate XXIV, Fig. 12). The disease has not extended to transverse processes.

Two separate dorsal vertebrae.—Both show much thickening on anterior and lateral borders, where new bone measures as much as 4 mm. thickness (Plate XXIV, Figs. 8 and 11).

First lumbar vertebra.—Mass of new bone 8 mm. thick, on left superior lateral border (Plate XXIV, Fig. 9).

One *metatarsal bone* shows distinct thickening at both ends (Plate XXIV, Fig. 14).

Second and terminal phalanges of one finger.—These are firmly ankylosed in a flexed position (Plate XXIV, Fig. 15).

The diagnosis, therefore, is that of spondylitis deformans, and, judging from the one metatarsal bone and the only two digital phalanges left, it is clear that other joints of the body had also suffered severely.

III. SPONDYLITIS DEFORMANS IN A SKELETON OF THE TWELFTH DYNASTY (2000-1788 B.C.)

Skeleton of a woman given us by Sir Gaston Maspero. The sarcophagus in which the body was contained had a large hole through which insects had entered and devoured almost everything save the skeleton. The only exception was a piece of organ (a muscle?), thickly covered with the pupae of insects, a piece of aorta (2.5 inches in length) at its bifurcation, and small pieces of ligament which were still attached to the spine.[1]

Skull.—All sutures except squamous ossified. Teeth much worn. Alveoli of left first premolar and all three molars, right second and third molars obliterated. Left canine carious.

Spinal column.—First four cervical vertebrae normal; fifth, distinct projection of new bone along anterior inferior border of body; sixth, normal; seventh, strong projection of new bone on left anterior inferior border.

- Dorsal vertebrae, normal, except ninth and tenth.

The lower border of the ninth dorsal in middle line and corresponding part of the upper border of the tenth united by a thick osteophyte about 1.5 cm. long (Plate XXV, Fig. 17a), the base of which is almost 0.5 cm. broad.

Second and third lumbar vertebrae show some overlipping.

Spinous processes of the tenth, eleventh, twelfth dorsal, first and second lumbar vertebrae joined together by a strong bridge of new bone.

The *other bones* showed no naked-eye lesions whatever.

The case is interesting because the disease is almost localised in front to the bodies of the ninth and tenth dorsal vertebrae, and posteriorly to the spinous processes of a few vertebrae.

[1] With regard to these insects and similar ones found in this and Ptolemaic mummies, Mr. Ad. Andres, whose knowledge of Egyptian insects is unrivalled, has kindly given us the following note:

"The fragments of insects which I have just received and which were found by Dr. M. Armand Ruffer in a mummy of the Ptolemaic epoch belong, without doubt, to Coleoptera of the Cleridae family, the scientific name of which is *Necrobia rufipes* (Geer). This species is cosmopolitan and is met with even to-day in the valley of the Nile and in Upper Egypt. Hope described it under the name of *Necrobia mumiarum*, but there can be no doubt that it belongs to the species mentioned above. (See *Coleopterum Catalogus*, par. 23, S. Schenkling, p. 143; et Charles Alluaud, *Bull. Soc. Ent. d'Égypte*, p. 31.) This is also the case with the *Necrobia glabra* (Champollion), which is identical with the *Necrobia rufipes* (Geer).

"In a communication on the subject made in October last before the Natural History Society of Alexandria, I had already drawn attention to this beetle, found together with a very large quantity of fragments of pupae of Diptera of the genus *Lucilia* and *Sarcophaga* in a mummy of the XIIth Dynasty by Dr. M. Armand Ruffer."

IV. DISEASE OF LEFT SACRO-ILIAC ARTICULATION AND BOTH HIP-JOINTS IN A MUMMY OF THE TWENTY-FIRST DYNASTY (1090–945 B.C.)

This mummy has already been partly described by Professor Elliot Smith, who wrote as follows:

In the case of an extremely emaciated old woman called Nesi-Tet-Nab-Taris, a curious state of affairs was revealed. Large open ante-mortem wounds—possibly bed-sores—were found on the back, between the shoulders and on each buttock. These had been made use of for the purpose of packing the back, and then two square sheets of fine leather (?gazelle skin) had been applied to cover the upper wound and the whole buttock respectively. These sheets had been sewn to the healthy skin beyond the sores and the edges hidden by straps of linen which were smeared with a resinous paste. A large opening—probably an abscess or sinus—extended transversely from the left pudendal labium outward into the buttock; this had been sewn up with string.

A long ulcer on the back of the leg had been covered up by a sheet of linen soaked in a solution of resin.

Evidently this old woman had been long bedridden. Professor Elliot Smith obligingly gave us the pelvis and lower limbs, in the hope that histological investigation might throw light on the nature of the chronic disease she had suffered from. The histological examination threw no light on the etiology of these sinuses, though we discovered that the peroneal arteries were completely ossified.

The remains of the pelvis and lower limbs having been macerated, the following pathological alterations were discovered:

Right femur.—Thick deposit of new bone round head of femur (Plate XXV, Figs. 18 and 19). Surface of great trochanter very rough, owing to deposits of whitish, spongy-looking bone, specially thick at upper extremity of spiral line. Depression for the ligamentum teres irregular, and deeply pitted at bottom.

Left femur (Plate XXV, Figs. 20–21).—Neck about 1 cm. shorter than that of right femur, owing to absorption, and this process having taken place more rapidly at the back, the neck has partly collapsed and the head of the bone looks almost directly backwards. All round the head, especially anteriorly, new bone has been deposited. Great trochanter roughened by deposit of new, whitish, spongy bone, thicker superiorly and anteriorly. Fossa for the ligamentum teres deeply pitted and much enlarged.

Pelvis.—Complete ankylosis between sacrum and right pelvic bone (Plate XXV, Fig. 22). In right acetabulum, separation between articular and non-articular parts is almost worn away by friction.

On the left side no trace of inflammation, expect on the ischial tuberosity, which is rougher than usual. In the acetabulum, a layer of new bone exists at the junction of the articular and non-articular parts. The latter has been so much worn away by friction that it is of transparent thinness.

The *bones of the leg* were normal.

We examined no complete skeleton of the XXIst Dynasty, but only the upper and lower limbs of various broken-up mummies. Among these we found several metatarsal bones, the heads of which showed evident signs of osteo-arthritis. Such a bone is photographed in Plate XXV, Fig. 23.

One radius also (Plate XXVII, Fig. 36) showed slight signs of osteo-arthritis.

V. SKELETON OF THE TWENTY-SECOND DYNASTY (945–745 B.C.)

This and the skeleton next in order were given us by Professor Flinders Petrie.

VERTEBRAL COLUMN

Atlas.—Flat projection of bone, almost 1 cm. long, surrounding nearly half outer border of right condyle. Small projection of bone, posterior border of left condyle.

Axis.—Normal, except that the left extremity of the bifid spinous process is much thickened, longer and broader than on the other side.

Foramen for the left vertebral artery is not completely closed.

Fifth cervical.—Distinct, rough new bone along lower posterior border of body extending laterally as far as the foramina for vertebral arteries.

Sixth cervical.—Some new bone all round upper and lower borders of body. Each vertebral foramen is divided into two unequal parts by very thin spiculum of new bone.

Seventh cervical.—New bone round upper border of body, more marked on the right side. Right foramen for vertebral artery narrowed by osseous growth to one-fourth of the left.

First dorsal.—Rough new bone along superior anterior border extending for about 0.3 cm. down the body of the vertebra. Upper left costal articulation very rough and irregular, especially at its outer border, where there is a slight bony projection.

Tenth dorsal.—Left costal articulation is very rough and irregular.

Eleventh dorsal.—Both costal articulating surfaces very rough, with new bone round them.

First lumbar.—Distinct thinning of body on left side.

Second lumbar.—Distinct roughening and bony formation round articulating surfaces on two upper and right lower articulating processes.

Third lumbar.—New bone round anterior part of superior border. A thin ridge of bone extends just on left of middle line along anterior part to a thick osseous excresence which almost surrounds the lower border. This is especially marked on the left side. Right superior articulating surface very rough and surrounded by osseous growth.

Fourth lumbar.—Very thick layer of new bone round anterior border, especially on left side and middle. This extends for some distance down the body of the vertebra and reaches the left lower border. Much new bone at base, and behind left superior and inferior articulating processes.

Fifth lumbar.—New bone right round superior border extending downwards along body for 1 cm. nearly (see Plate XXVI, Fig. 26).

Left calcaneum.—The antero-internal facet (Plate XXVI, Fig. 24) is divided into two secondary facets by new bone. The internal tuberosity sends out a spur of new bone for 1 cm. This is very irregular and is really formed by three small tuberosities, the largest of these being in front and below, the second somewhat smaller lies in front and above, and the smallest behind and above.

Fifth metatarsal bone.—Just in front (Plate XXVI, Fig. 25) of the articular facet for the fourth metatarsal bone, and at the proximal extremity of the internal surface, there is a large osseous tuberosity looking upwards and backwards. Another similar tubercle on the superior aspect and external margin, about 1 cm. from the anterior articulation, but separated from this by a deep groove.

Sacrum.—Small exostoses on right superior border.

First right metacarpal bone.—Small multiple exostoses on phalangeal articulation.

Femurs.—The fossae for the ligamentum rotundum are irregular owing to the presence of numerous small exostoses.

VI. SKELETON DATING FROM THE PERSIAN OCCUPATION OF EGYPT (ABOUT 500 B.C.)

VERTEBRAL COLUMN

All vertebrae present, except axis and the seventh cervical vertebra, which could not be found.

Atlas.—Cavity for odontoid process surrounded above and laterally by a strong layer of rough new bone. From the shape of the cavity it is evident that the odontoid process, instead of looking upwards, was bent slightly backwards. Right tubercle for attachment of transverse ligament slightly roughened, and so is bone just below right condylar process. Foramen in the right transverse process not entirely closed.

Third cervical.—Upper and lower surfaces deeply hollowed, especially on upper surface, where hollow is nearly 1 cm. in depth. Upper surface very rough. Some formation of new bone along anterior lower border, new bone being about 0.2 cm. thick. Whole body of vertebra very thin, measuring just

0.5 cm. in thickness. On side of lower surface there has been a good deal of absorption of the bone.

Fourth cervical.—This shows same lesions, but projection of new bone along anterior inferior border is more marked and irregular. Distinct atrophy of body, less than 0.5 cm. thick.

Fifth cervical.—Marked hollowing out of upper surface of body. Distinct formation of new bone along upper anterior, and slightly also along upper posterior border. Lower surface practically normal. Thickness of vertebra, 0.6 cm.

Sixth cervical.—No new bone; body about 1.2 cm. thick.

Seventh cervical.—Missing.

Sixth dorsal.—Left lower articulating facet very irregular in shape, rough, and nearly double the size of its fellow on account of formation of new bone round it.

Seventh dorsal.—Right lower articulating facet very irregular in shape and double the size of its fellow. The same is the case with right anterior articular facet. Bodies of both these vertebrae slightly thinner on the right side.

Eighth dorsal.—Left lower articular facet greatly enlarged, very irregular, with some thick new bone around it. Superior border of the body somewhat rough. Lower border of the body rough, with a projection of new bone 0.3 cm. thick and about 1 cm. long on right side (Plate XXVI, Fig. 27). Both upper articular facets very irregular and rough, owing to new bone, especially on left side. Right side of body distinctly atrophied.

Ninth dorsal.—Lower articulating surface very rough and irregular, especially on the left side. Upper articulating processes fairly smooth, but very irregular in shape. Upper surface of body shows large projection of new bone 2.5 cm. long and 1 cm. broad, fitting the similar projection on vertebra above (Plate XXVI, Fig. 27). There is distinct atrophy of right side of body of vertebra. Lower surface of body shows bony projection similar to that above, the two being joined by a strong pillar of new bone. The upper facet for the left rib side is enlarged, rough, surrounded by new bone, and almost unrecognisable.

Tenth dorsal.—On right upper border, a strong excrescence of new bone fitting in with the one above (Plate XXVI, Figs. 27, 28, and 29). Upper articular processes irregular, but otherwise almost normal. Distinct atrophy of right side of body. Some slight formation of new bone along right lower border of body.

Eleventh and twelfth dorsals.—Practically normal.

First lumbar.—Normal, except for some thickening round left posterior articular surface.

Fourth and fifth lumbars.—Some thickening around upper border of body.

N.B.—This skeleton belonged to a man less than twenty-five years of age, as the wisdom teeth had not yet cut through.

Bouchard's nodosities.—The hands of one mummy of the time of the Persian occupation showed enlargement of the heads of the first phalanges (Plate XXVI, Figs. 30 and 31); a malformation to which special attention has been drawn by Ch. Bouchard, and which this observer has shown to be caused by chronic dilatation of the stomach.

VII. SPONDYLITIS DEFORMANS AND OTHER ARTHRITIC LESIONS IN BODIES FROM THE TOMBS OF THE SOLDIERS OF ALEXANDER THE GREAT AND PTOLEMY I, AT CHATBY (ABOUT 300 B.C.)

This disease was very common among the people buried at Chatby. Accurate statistics as to the frequency of the disease, cannot be given, because, as has been mentioned before, the exact number of people in the graves examined can only be guessed at. Altogether, thirty-two skulls were found, but it is quite possible that the fragments found belonged to many more bodies, as the number of skulls does not agree with the number of inferior maxillae nor with that of the right femurs. Judging from the number of the latter, it is certain that at least forty adults or fragments of adult bodies were interred at Chatby in the graves we examined.

In only one grave did we find a skeleton in which no bones were missing. The body was that of a young woman whose third molars had not quite emerged. It was in a very bad state of preservation, the skull and smaller bones crumbling to bits when an attempt was made to remove them. Nevertheless, it was ascertained that the whole spinal column from end to end showed the early lesions of spondylitis deformans, namely, overlipping of the superior and inferior borders of the bodies of the vertebrae together with enlargement, eburnation, and ankylosis of the articulating surfaces. The odontoid process of the axis was capped by a layer of thick new bone.

The other bones of the body showed slight alterations only. In the lower limbs the tuberosities of the femurs were very rough, there was much thickening along the linea aspera of the shaft of the femur and the insertions of both quadriceps extensor femoris in the patellae were ossified. In the upper limbs, the only alteration observed was some thickening and pitting round the outer border and tuberosities of the olecranon. The bones of the hands and feet which could be found showed no special alterations.

In several other graves vertebrae were found ankylosed, or else in such a position that it was clear that they belonged to the same body. Typical examples of the lesions found may now be given.

CERVICAL REGION

No. 1.—Ankylosis of axis and third cervical articular surfaces joined by strong new bone, extending backwards on right side almost to spinous process. Posterior borders of bodies firmly ankylosed by new bone which has evidently developed in the posterior ligaments. Odontoid process very rough, especially at lower borders of groove for transverse ligament. Tip of·process rough, irregular, and capped with newly formed bone. Inferior articular process of third vertebra greatly enlarged and surrounded by osseous outgrowth. Long spur projects from inferior anterior border of third vertebra.

No. 2.—Ankylosis of third, fourth, and fifth cervical vertebrae. The upper and lower borders of the bodies, especially those of the sixth, are rather thickened; otherwise the bodies are practically normal. The disease is chiefly confined to the articular surfaces, which, with two exceptions, are enormously thickened, flattened, and bound together by thick new bone.

The atlas vertebra often shows osseous overgrowth on the upper lateral borders of the notch for the odontoid process, together with thickening and roughening of the tubercles for the attachment of the transverse ligament. As a rule, however, the articulating surfaces are healthy.

In the axis vertebra, the disease chiefly affects the inferior articulating surfaces which are flattened, irregular in shape, eburnated, at the same time worm-eaten and considerably enlarged, sometimes measuring as much as 2.5 cm. in their widest part. In such cases, the whole articulating surface is surrounded with strong new bone.

The anterior surface of the odontoid is sometimes eburnated, and a prolongation of eburnated bone may extend for 2 or 3 mm. above the tip of the process and for a similar distance laterally. This condition must have caused considerable limitation of movement during life.

Similar lesions occur frequently in the cervical vertebrae (Plate XXVII, Fig. 37), and are not seldom limited to the articular surfaces. The spinous processes always escape apparently. In one vertebra, the lower border was greatly enlarged owing to a V-shaped prolongation of new bone. Whereas the upper and lower surfaces of the bodies of the dorsal vertebrae are almost always normal, the same surfaces in the cervical vertebrae are often very rough and deeply pitted. The anterior part of the body is frequently greatly worn away, so that the vertebrae of the neck must have fallen together to some extent in front, with extensive deformation of the neck as the result.

In one specimen the skull and the three first cervical vertebrae (Plate XXVII, Fig. 40) were firmly ankylosed together as the result of osteo-arthritis, and the deformity during life was doubtless very great. The spinal canal formed an obtuse angle with the foramen magnum, so that the man's chin almost touched his chest.

DORSAL REGION

The dorsal vertebrae show changes very similar to those found in the cervical vertebrae. Very often three or more vertebrae are firmly ankylosed (Plate XXVII, Fig. 34). The following may serve as a typical example:

Bony mass consisting of three dorsal vertebrae. In first vertebra upper border of body considerably thickened, especially anteriorly where new bone measures at least 0.5 cm. Lower border on right of middle line throws out a flat osteophyte measuring 1 by 2 cm. This exactly fits with a similar osteophyte growing from the vertebra below. Upper and lower articulating surfaces very rough, irregular, and enlarged. Next vertebra shows changes similar to the one above. The top of the transverse process is rough and thickened. The costal articulating surfaces are very rough. Anterior border of last vertebra very rough, throws out a strong osteophyte fitting with similar projection from bone above. Lower border of body somewhat thickened. Superior articulating surfaces very rough, irregular, enlarged, and partly surrounded by new bone, especially thick, on right inferior border. Lower articulating surfaces somewhat rough, enlarged, and irregular, though alterations less marked than in vertebra above. Tip of left transverse process enlarged, rough, and costal articulating surfaces almost worn away.

Such ankylosed masses are of common occurrence, and the large majority of the dorsal vertebrae found showed inflammatory changes more or less profound.

The early stages of the disease usually show themselves in the dorsal and lumbar regions (Plate XXVII, Fig. 33) on the anterior borders of the body on either side close to the middle line. They are characterised by the formation of a small lip which meets a similar prolongation projecting from the vertebra above or below. Occasionally this overgrowth measures as much as 2 or 3 cm. in length, the body of the vertebra remaining normal. Sometimes the new bone spreads as a thick ridge all round the anterior border of the body and forms powerful masses which may extend over the side of the vertebra; these, meeting with similar ridges on the vertebra above or below, all three vertebrae become firmly ankylosed. The anterior and lateral spinal ligaments in such cases are firmly ossified, though recognisable.

The disease seldom extends to the posterior spinal ligament, and even should the latter become completely ossified, the new bone never intrudes on the canal.

The intervertebral cartilages were apparently quite normal, as there are no signs of inflammation on the surfaces of the body. Not infrequently the disease extended to the transverse processes, and especially to the articulating surfaces, which are then firmly tied together by new bone, sometimes as much as 5 mm. thick. The articulating surfaces may measure as much as 2.5 by 1.5 cm., and are then frequently eburnated and look worm-eaten.

The costal articulating surfaces usually escape. Occasionally they are rough, uneven, with signs of inflammation round them.

The spinal processes are normal, with the exception of a few cases where small osteophytes are present.

As a rule, the bodies of the vertebrae are not atrophied at all. The deformation of the spine during life cannot have been very marked therefore, even when there must have been considerable limitation of movement.

LUMBAR REGION AND PELVIS

The lumbar vertebrae show changes identical with those seen in the dorsal region. One example will suffice:

This specimen consists of two lumbar vertebrae (Plate XXVII, Fig. 32) which are firmly bound together by a strong mass of new bone extending almost right round the adjoining bodies of both vertebrae. The strong prolongations show that the disease extended to the vertebrae both above and below.

The changes in the spinous process are often very marked, and vary from simple irregularity and roughness to complete ankylosis, so that all the spinous processes are joined together by strong bone.

The number of lumbar vertebrae showing marked changes is enormous. Indeed, the majority of lumbar vertebrae which were found exhibited lesions, more or less severe, of spondylitis deformans.

Osteo-arthritic changes in sacrum and coccyx.—The sacrum was firmly ankylosed with the right ilium in two cases (Plate XXX, Fig. 49) and with the fifth lumbar vertebra in two other specimens (Plate XXX, Fig. 52). In two others the ankylosis between the fifth lumbar and the sacrum was not complete. In another (Plate XXX, Fig. 53) a strong osteophyte extended upwards from the left anterior superior border of the sacrum to the fifth lumbar vertebra.

The coccyx was never found diseased.

On the whole, therefore, the sacrum and coccyx often escaped.

Osteo-arthritic and other changes in the pelvis.—One pelvis is not only firmly ankylosed to the sacrum, but shows other points of interest.

The ankylosis is complete anteriorly as far as the lower border of the first sacral vertebra, posteriorly the bones are united by two strong bridges of osseous tissue separated by an interval. The whole length of the ischial ramus on its external surface, and especially near the inferior border, is covered with thick, rough new bone, which though becoming less is still very prominent near the ramus of the pubes. The inner and outer borders of the obturator foramen are very rough owing to stalactite-like outgrowths of inflammatory osseous tissue. The superior ramus of the pubes and ilio-pectineal eminence are covered with small osseous excrescences on their external surface.

The left (Plate XXX, Fig. 48) side of the pelvis shows the same lesions as the right, and the stalactite formations round the obturator foramen are even more marked.

In the right acetabulum, the non-articular portion remains normal, whereas a strong ridge of new bone lines the upper border of the articular portions, especially on the outer side. Much evidence of inflammation on right ischial tuberosity, especially on its external and inferior border. The left acetabular cavity is much worn, though there are no signs of inflammation.

Pathological changes in the acetabula are fairly common. In some, friction has completely worn away the separation between the articular and non-articular portions. In others, some deposit of new bone had taken place at the upper margin of the non-articular portion of the acetabulum.

FEMUR

In contrast to the spine, the femurs showed, as a rule, but slight lesions, and even these did not occur often. Altogether only nine femurs showed any lesions, the most pronounced of which, at the upper end, were as follows:

No. 1.—On upper surface, at junction of head with neck, there is a deposit of thick new bone, which, narrowing gradually, extends almost round the head. Insertion of ligamentum teres surrounded by thick new bone measures 2 by 1.5 cm., and the floor is rough. Numerous small spiculae of bone behind greater tuberosity, as if tendons of muscles inserted there were partially ossified. Some formation of new bone just below the small tuberosity.

The following is a description of the most conspicuous example of disease at the lower extremity of the bone:

No. 2.—*Lower extremity of right femur.*—Great thickening round external and internal borders of both condyles, especially marked behind inner condyle, where new bone forms a thick ridge separated from the bone beneath by a space of about 2 mm. Conspicuous eburnation of inner condyle. Just above the eburnated part there is a small raised nodule of rough new bone, about the size of a threepenny piece.

In the other cases, the lesions were very slight, consisting only of some small deposit of bone round the head, some roughening of the great trochanter or of the intertrochanteric line. At the lower extremity of the femur the changes consisted only of some slight thickening round the borders of the condyles.

A peculiar deformity of the femur is shown in Plate XXVIII, Figs. 41, 42, and 43.

Here the great trochanter and the intertrochanteric line are capped by an enormous growth of spongy bone measuring about 5 cm. in thickness, which is reflected in a thick layer round the junction of the neck of the bone with the shaft. The neck of the bone itself is practically normal. This enormous growth consists of loose, spongy bone, which microscopically shows nothing peculiar. Anteriorly, this growth ends at the lower end of the linea aspera, which is considerably broadened and flattened.

The head of the bone shows some, but not very marked, thickening at its posterior border. The cup for the cotyloid ligament had been considerably damaged, and exhibits no special sign of disease. The lower extremity of the femur presents some slight signs of osteo-arthritis round the borders. The shaft of the femur is nowhere enlarged.

The diagnosis in this case must remain doubtful. We thought at first that we were in presence of a specimen of osteoma or osteo-sarcoma. Against this diagnosis we may point to the fact that the shaft of the femur itself appears to be quite normal, and the surface of the tumour, except over the great trochanter, is everywhere quite smooth. The interior of the growth is composed of normal loose osseous tissue.

Considering that this person had slight osteo-arthritic lesions of the lower extremity and of the head of the bone, it may be argued that the more striking lesions were also of the same nature. Assuming this to be possible, it is not a little strange that the lesions should be almost entirely limited to the posterior region round the trochanters.

Unfortunately, the other bones belonging to this skeleton could not be discovered, this femur lying loose in the ossarium before mentioned.

Another interesting femur found in the same ossarium is the one shown in Plate XXIX, Fig. 44. Here the head of the femur had been almost completely worn away, though signs of inflammation could still be seen along its upper and outer border. The great trochanter had been badly smashed. In this instance, we do not think the possibility of the lesions having been tubercular can be excluded.

TIBIA

The tibia is normal, as a rule, and in only one were severe lesions noticed. This is a left tibia in which there is marked eburnation of the upper articulating surface posteriorly.

PATELLA

This bone shows no changes, as a rule. In several cases, however, the upper surface is very rough, and upper border throws out a flat excrescence of bone formed in the tendon of the quadriceps extensor femoris. There must have been, therefore, considerable limitation in movement.

CALCANEUM

Marked osteo-arthritic lesions of the calcaneum were never found. On the other hand, the tendon of the gastrocnemius muscle was ossified in two cases for a distance of 2–2.5 inches at its insertion into the calcaneum. The insertion of the plantar fascia in the calcaneum also was converted into a spur of bone 3–5 cm. in length, in four subjects (Plate XXVII, Fig. 38).

BONES OF THE FOOT[1]

The following were the lesions noted:

1. *First metatarsal.*—Right shows well-marked osteo-arthritic lesions of head.
2. *First metatarsal.*—Left about one-third of internal part of head with a portion of internal half of shaft broken off. Osteo-arthritis distinct in remaining portion of head.
3. *First phalanx of great toe.*—Right, slight lesions of head.
4. *First phalanx of great toe.*—Left, slight lesions of head.
5. *Fifth metatarsal.*—Right, slight lesions of head.
6. *Fifth metatarsal.*—Left, slight lesions of head.
7. *Fifth metatarsal.*—Right, slight lesions of head.
8. *Fifth metatarsal.*—Right, slight lesions of head.
9. *Third metatarsal.*—Right, slight lesions of head.
10. *Second metatarsal.*—Right, slight lesions of head.
11. *Second metatarsal.*—Right, slight lesions of head.
12. *A metatarsal bone.*—Proximal end so much modified by disease that it is not possible to be certain whether it is the second, third, or fourth.
13. *D.D. phalanx of first row, second toe.*—Slight lesions of head.

BONES AND ARTICULATIONS OF THE UPPER EXTREMITY

Like the lower, the upper extremities were but seldom the seat of disease.

The scapulo-humeral articulations are always normal, as also the head of the humerus generally. In eight cases there is some slight deposit of new bone round the anatomical neck, and three times on the large and small tuberosities also.

[1] We are greatly obliged to Dr. Wahby, professor of anatomy at the Cairo Medical School, for much help in the examination of some of these bones, as also the bones of the hand.

A curious change was noted in one left humerus in which, at the junction of the head and the upper tuberosity, there is a depression about 1 cm. deep, 1 cm. broad, and 4 cm. long, with somewhat irregular borders, and perfectly smooth walls. The inferior posterior part of the head is somewhat worn away.

In only two cases did the inferior extremity of the humerus show any signs of disease. In the first, eburnation of the capitellum is a conspicuous feature, and there is also some roughening and formation of new bone in the olecranon fossa.

In another case, the ridge between the capitellum and internal condyle is almost completely worn away.

BONES OF THE FOREARM AND CARPUS

These were remarkably healthy, no lesions whatever being found. Only three metacarpal bones were found diseased:

1. *First metacarpal bone.*—Right, the digital extremity is modified in a typical manner by osteo-arthritis. The bone is thick and long, and must have belonged to a very big hand.
2. *First metacarpal bone.*—Right, slight lesions of osteo-arthritis.
3. *First metacarpal bone.*—Left, slight lesions of osteo-arthritis.

Fractures.—Lastly, among the pathological specimens may be included two fractures of the bones of the lower limbs.

The first (Plate XXIX, Fig. 45) is a consolidated fracture of the femur of one of the soldiers of Alexander the Great. The bone had been very badly set, and the result was deplorable from every point of view.

The second (Plate XXIX, Figs. 46 and 47) is a fracture of the tibia and fibula found in a mummy dating from the time of the Persian occupation (about 500 B.C.). Here the result was much better, as the tibia shows only 0.5 cm., shortening when compared with its fellow.

These are the only examples of injury that we found.

Exostosis.—One Greek rib (Plate XXXI, Fig. 55) had a curious rounded exostosis about 2 cm. long, tapering to a blunt, round extremity. This was unfortunately broken by a somewhat too muscular visitor. The exostosis was composed of dense cancellous tissue, as is well shown in the photograph.

ON OSSEOUS LESIONS IN ANCIENT EGYPTIANS   113

EXAMINATION OF DECALCIFIED BONES

In order to study the histological changes present in spondylitis deformans, some vertebrae and other bones presenting the typical lesions of the disease were decalcified in alcohol containing 3 per cent of nitric acid. After complete decalcification this fluid was replaced by strong spirit, which was changed on three consecutive days or oftener. The bone can then be easily cut through with a knife or a strong razor.

By this method it was ascertained that in the vertebrae and in the other bones the lesions never extend to the interior of the bones, and were entirely superficial. The interior of the bone, vertebra, or femur is to the naked eye absolutely normal. In the vertebrae this condition is specially evident, for in no case except in the cervical region did the surfaces in contact with the intervertebral discs show any changes whatever to the naked eye. The only exception is that the surface of the body of the vertebra near the anterior border appeared to decalcify more slowly, and to be of somewhat tougher consistence than normal.

Where eburnation has taken place, as, for instance, in the articulating surfaces of the cervical vertebrae, the change is entirely superficial, probably as a result of friction, as the bone immediately underneath the eburnated surface presents no pathological lesions.

Similarly, in sections through the thickenings round the head of the femur or round the lower condyles of the tibia, the lesions did not affect the bone at all, and were limited to the periosteum and neighbouring tissues.

The evident eburnation proved that the cartilages had atrophied and disappeared, but in no case did we find any signs which would lead us to believe that ossification had taken place in the cartilages. Even in the one case of complete ankylosis of the second and third phalanx of one finger, the cartilage had disappeared without leaving a trace.

ROMAN PERIOD (ABOUT 200 A.D.)

We have cleared only two tombs of that period, containing eight adult bodies. Of these eight skeletons no less than four showed marked lesions of arthritis deformans. One skeleton, indeed, resembled to a remarkable extent that of the IIIrd Dynasty, which has been described already, for the whole of the vertebral columns had been converted into a rigid block of bone. Two sections of the column are shown in Plate XXXI, where Fig. 60 represents the lower cervical, and Fig. 61 the lumbar, region. In the latter the disease had spread to the spinous processes, which were firmly held together by the osseous overgrowth. Plate XXXI, Fig. 58, is a photograph of two dorsal vertebrae of the same column in which the pathological changes are obvious.

The femurs also show obvious signs of disease. At the junction of the head and neck (Plate XXXI, Fig. 54) a thick layer of new bone almost surrounds the whole. The great trochanter is much roughened owing to new deposit, and small osteophytes protrude for some distance. The articulating surfaces of the knee-joint, especially laterally, are also greatly thickened from the same cause. The left ulna is diseased also, as the borders of the greater and lesser sigmoid cavity and the olecranon are very rough and show considerable osseous hypertrophy.

One of the metatarsal bones (Plate XXXI, Fig. 59) also presents the typical deformities of arthritis deformans.

The innominate bones are peculiar. The rami of the ischium and pubes, together with the tuberosity of the ischium, are very rough. Between the inferior curved line and the upper border of the acetabulum (Plate XXX, Fig. 51) the bone is extremely rough and covered with minute rounded elevations of new bone, which greatly resemble those already described in Plate XXX, Fig. 48. The sacrum was normal.

Three other skeletons showed typical deformities due to spondylitis deformans, and in them the disease appeared to be strictly limited to the spine. The lesions of the vertebrae were absolutely characteristic, and in one case the lumbar vertebra was firmly ankylosed with the sacrum.

OSSEOUS LESIONS IN COPTIC BODIES

Coptic body given us by Professor Breccia, and dating from the fifth century A.D. It had been enclosed in a coffin which had been buried in sand, and had never been artificially mummified.

The external surfaces of the ramus of the pubes and part of the body were covered with a layer of new bone. The new bone was fairly smooth, though with a worm-eaten appearance in places. It measured 4 by 4.5 cm., and was in places about 0.75 cm. thick. Superiorly the new bone was sharply limited by a ridge and a deep groove (Plate XXX, Fig. 50). There was some evidence of periostitis along the lower border of the ramus of the pubes as far as the junction with the ramus of the ischium.

The internal surface of the bone was quite healthy.

The articulating surfaces of the symphysis pubis were smooth. On the internal surface on each side of the joint there was a layer of new spongy bone 0.5 cm. broad and about 2.5 mm. thick on the right, and a layer quite 1 mm. thick on the left side. Otherwise the left innominate bone was quite healthy.

We found no trace of an abscess round the pubes.

An interesting point was that both the dorsal and the lumbar vertebrae showed a small amount of overlipping owing to the development of new bone along the upper and lower anterior borders of the body. The disease here had evidently begun in the bone, for the intervertebral discs and the ligaments showed no signs of ossification.

It is certain that this woman had been long bedridden, possibly owing to the pelvic disease, as there was a huge bedsore in the lumbar region, in which micro-organisms were found in enormous numbers.

The Coptic sacrum (Plate XXXI, Fig. 57) showed a curious malformation. The first sacral foramen was not closed by bone internally, and a deep spoon-shaped fissure extended right away to the sacral canal. There were no signs of inflammation along the fissure, and we may suppose that it was due to congenital deformation.

SUMMARY AND GENERAL CONSIDERATIONS

The majority of the lesions discovered in the skeletons of old Egyptians, coming from a period extending over more than three thousand years, were typical of chronic arthritis. The spinal column was most often the seat of the disease, the alterations varying from slight overlipping to complete ankylosis, sometimes accompanied by lesions of the sacro-iliac articulation and of the long bones of the lower, more seldom by changes in the long bones of the upper, extremities.

The frequency with which the bones of the hand and the foot are affected could unfortunately not be estimated, as, in the majority of cases, it was not possible to say with certainty to what skeleton the bones belonged. Although the number of diseased smaller bones was certainly small, yet it is a peculiar fact that, in almost every case where the whole or the larger part of the skeleton was found, the phalanges were also altered by osteo-arthritis, though the lesions were slight as a rule. On the whole, it would appear that the foot was more often affected than the hand.

Lesions of the carpal bones were never seen, and those of the tarsus were very rare.

In many cases the fasciae, the insertions of muscles, or the muscles themselves were certainly invaded by the ossifying process. This is well shown in a skeleton of the IIIrd Dynasty, where a bony mass, which had evidently developed in the muscles and tendons, occupied the vertebral groove. Slighter pathological changes, such as small osteophytes at the insertion of muscles and fasciae (e.g., insertion of the plantar fascia, great trochanter, etc.), though less demonstrative, point to the same conclusion. It is certain also that the lesions were present far oftener than our examination showed, as all the smaller osteophytes, etc., must have been broken off and could not be discovered in the sand of the graves.

The complete or partial ankyloses of the sacro-iliac articulations may be assumed to have been caused by the same disease as the spondylitis deformans. In our opinion it is very doubtful whether lesions such as are shown in Plate XXX, Figs. 48, 50, and 51, should not be classed in a separate category. In these cases the pathological process is conspicuous, not so much in the joint as on the flat surfaces of the bones.

Nowadays the tendency is to think that the lesions of chronic arthritis are due either to a chronic infectious process or follow on an acute infectious disease. Assuming this theory to be true, we cannot say, nevertheless, to what infectious disease the osteo-arthritic lesions of old Egyptians were due. That the old Egyptians suffered from bacterial diseases, identical with those seen now, has been shown by the investigations of Elliot Smith,[1] Ruffer,[2] and Ferguson,[3] but we do not know what was the incidence of such diseases in Egypt. Until that is ascertained, the etiology of the osteo-arthritic lesions of old Egyptians cannot be even guessed at.

Undoubtedly, however, the manner in which the disease spreads along the spine points to its having been due to a chronic infectious process occasionally giving rise to metastases in other articulations.

We could not get any definite evidence as to whether the disease was more common in man than in woman.

Certainly the malady was one occurring more frequently in old than in young people. The "determinative" of old age, for instance, in hieroglyphic writing is the picture of a man deformed from chronic arthritis. That it occurred among people in early adult life is shown by the fact that typical lesions were discovered in two young people who had not yet cut their wisdom teeth.

Dr. Elliot Smith and Dr. Wood Jones had already drawn attention to the frequency with which arthritis deformans, and especially spondylitis deformans, occurred in Old Egypt. Dr. Wood Jones[4] in his monograph on the subject expresses himself as follows:

The causal factor of the disease is essentially one of environment and not of race; it is the conditions of life in the Nile Valley at all those periods from which the remains of man have been studied, which have produced the development of such a common disease.

The foreign Christians who came to Philae in the early centuries of the Christian era, and left their remains in such quantities in the cemeteries on the islands of Biga and Hera, were subject to the disease, although it was not so universal in them as in the indigenous population of the older cemeteries.

The present inhabitants of Nubia are also afflicted with the disease. . . . . Among the modern Egyptians also the signs of the osteo-arthritic changes do occur. . . . . It is probable, therefore, that the disease is associated with the

[1] Grafton Elliot Smith and Marc Armand Ruffer, "Pott'sche Krankheit an einer ägyptischen Mumie," *Zur historischen Biologie der Krankheitserreger*, Heft 3.

[2] Marc Armand Ruffer, "Remarks on the Histology and Pathological Anatomy of Egyptian Mummies," *Cairo Scientific Journal*, Vol. IV (January, 1910), No. 40.

[3] Marc Armand Ruffer and A. R. Ferguson, "Note on an Eruption Resembling That of Variola in the Skin of a Mummy of the Twentieth Dynasty (1200–1100 B.C.)," *Journal of Pathology and Bacteriology*, Cambridge, XV, 1.

[4] *The Archaeological Survey of Nubia, Report for 1907–8*, II, 273.

country of the Nile Valley and the mode of life of its population. Although the people whose remains have been examined vary in their racial characters, the Egyptians, Negroes, and a foreign element from the Eastern Mediterranean are all represented, still it is probable that the habits and mode of life of these races, when once they had become inhabitants of the Nile Valley, did not greatly differ.

At all periods the Nile was the chief factor in their lives; it gave them their livelihood and supplied their wants, and it probably gave them then, as it gives them now, the bulk of their diseases.[1]

Every member of the riverside population has it as his birthright that a great part of his whole life shall be spent dabbling in the water of the Nile, even at those times of cold which are not at all uncommon during the Nubian winter. The men, for their ablutions, their fishing, and their many processes of irrigation, are forced to spend much of their time in and out of the water; and the women of a Nubian household are never free from the constant duty of filling their waterpots at the river.

It may be this exposure, with the alternate wetting and drying in a climate which may be of severe cold or intense heat, that has produced, and is producing this remarkable frequency of osteo-arthritic changes in these people.

The theory propounded by Dr. Wood Jones is practically the once fashionable theory that osteo-arthritis is due to wet and cold. He argues that the men and women in Nubia having been exposed to heat, cold, and wet in their occupations, therefore the osteo-arthritic changes were due to these conditions.

As far as temperature is concerned, extremes of heat and cold are met with in every country, and not in Nubia only. It is true that the differences between the night and day temperature are very great, but they are hardly felt by human beings who spend their nights in houses or caves. Moreover, the exposure to wet owing to their occupations is the rule among all agricultural, fishing, or hunting people, and could not therefore account for the apparently greater frequency of osteo-arthritis in Nubia. The exposure of the agricultural population of Egypt to wet is almost limited to the hands and feet, which are quickly dried as soon as the work is finished. It is not to be compared as an etiological factor with the thorough drenching that a European labourer gets several times a year, and who often cannot change his clothes for some time.

[1] This statement we cannot allow to pass without pointing out that the evidence in favour of it is by no means conclusive.

Our observations at Alexandria show that the race cannot have had anything to do with the etiology of the disease, and there are also evidences that climate as such has no part in it.

It would indeed be difficult to find a greater contrast between the temperate, moist, marine climate of Alexandria, with its constant sea breezes, heavy winter rainfalls, mild summer, warm nights, with the Nubian desert climate, characterised by scorching days, cold nights, and excessive dryness.

Further, our observations show that occupation does not appear to have had anything to do with the causation of the disease. The Nubians were for the most part agriculturists, the Alexandria people soldiers or townspeople, and there is no reason why the latter at any rate should have dabbled in water. The Nile did not flow at Alexandria, and the enormous Roman cisterns even now in existence show that water was a precious article, and that there was none to waste, as in Nubia. Even allowing, therefore, that the Greek soldiers might have contracted this disease owing to exposure to wet and cold during their campaigns, this theory cannot account for the frequency of this disease in townspeople.

A further argument against the theory that osteo-arthritis in the past was due to exposure is that pet animals, carefully kept in temples, suffered a great deal from the same or a similar disease. Lortet and Galliard, for instance,[1] have described like lesions in monkeys at Thebes, perhaps one of the driest spots in the world, and situated miles away from the Nile.[2]

We cannot agree with Poncet that these lesions are due to tubercle, for they present none of the appearances of that disease.

Indeed, except for one very doubtful case, we have not come across one single bone showing the typical lesions of tubercle. Strange to say, lesions indicating the presence of rickets or syphilis were completely absent.

Lastly, we must not forget that it is quite possible that further investigations may show that during that period which we have

[1] See *La faune momifiée de l'Égypte*, Série II, p. 26.

[2] One of us (M. A. R.) has seen a gazelle, born in captivity in Egypt, and which had never been exposed to wet and cold, which presented the typical symptoms of arthritis deformans.

studied, osteo-arthritis was as common in other countries as it was in Egypt.

TEETH OF GREEK PERIOD

A difficulty presented itself in estimating the percentage of dental disease owing to the fact that many teeth dropped out after death and could not be found. As a rule, therefore, we were obliged to consider as diseased only such teeth the alveoli of which showed partial or complete absorption. Far from overstating the number of diseased teeth, we have therefore certainly done the reverse, for the majority of teeth showing only slight signs of decay perforce escaped our notice.

The following tables give the number of diseased teeth in the upper and lower jaws:

UPPER MAXILLA

N.B.: + indicates that a tooth was present but decayed.

No.	Register	Incisors R.	Incisors L.	Canines R.	Canines L.	Premolars R.	Premolars L.	Molars R.	Molars L.	Remarks
1	Ch. G	....	....	....	....	....	....	....	....	Young person; twelve teeth only cut through.
2	Ch. A. I	....	....	....	....	....	....	....	....	Young adult; all teeth perfect.
3	Ch. A	....	....	....	....	....	....	....	....	Adult; skull partly calcined.
4	Ch. G. II	....	....	....	....	....	....	....	1st	Young adult.
5	Ch. L	....	....	....	....	....	....	....	....	Young adult; teeth white and perfect.
6	Ch. B	....	....	....	....	....	....	....	....	Young adult; teeth good, slightly worn.
7	Ch. Y	....	....	....	....	....	....	....	....	All teeth present; slightly worn.
8	Ch. Y. II	....	....	....	....	....	....	....	....	All teeth white, somewhat worn.
9	Ch. III	....	1st	....	....	....	....	....	....	Young adult; basilar suture united, but not the others. In connection with the missing tooth there had been an abscess, which had perforated through the palate.
10	Ch. G. III	....	....	....	....	....	....	1st 2d 3d	1st	Old man; remaining teeth worn, but not carious.
11	Ch IV	1st 2d	1st 2d	1	1	1st 2d	2d	1st 2d 3d	1st 2d 3d	Old man; all alveoli completely obliterated, except first left premolar.
12	Ch. V	....	....	....	....	....	....	....	....	Young man; only twelve very white teeth present.
13	Ch. VI	1st 2d	....	1	....	1st 2d	1st 2d	1st 2d 3d	1st 2d 3d	Adult, but not old; basilar and frontal sutures ossified, but not the others.
14	Ch. VII	....	....	....	....	....	....	....	1st + 2d 3d +	Adult; frontal suture obliterated, but not the others.
15	Ch. VIII	....	....	....	....	1st + 2d	....	2d 3d	2d 3d	Old man; the first molar was deeply carious, and pushed forwards by periostal inflammation behind the fangs.

UPPER MAXILLA—*Continued*

N.B.: + indicates that a tooth was present but decayed.

No.	Register	Incisors R.	Incisors L.	Canines R.	Canines L.	Premolars R.	Premolars L.	Molars R.	Molars L.	Remarks
16	Ch. IX	....	....	....	....	....	....	1st 2d	1st	Adult; frontal suture ossified, others only partially so.
17	Ch. X	....	....	....	....	....	....	....	....	Young person; fourteen teeth only, already much worn.
18	Ch. XI	....	....	....	....	....	....	1st +	....	Young woman; basilar suture ossified, all others open.
19	Ch. XII	....	....	....	1	2d	2d	1st 2d 3d	1st 2d 3d	Young woman; basilar suture not quite ossified.
20	Ch. XIII	....	....	....	....	....	....	....	....	Teeth perfect; no tartar; basilar suture not ossified; all others not.
21	Ch. XIV	....	....	....	....	2d	1st	....	1st 3d	Woman, probably negress; suture except basilar unclosed.
22	Ch. XV	....	....	....	....	....	....	....	....	Young woman; basilar suture not closed; teeth beautifully white.
23	Ch. XVI	....	....	....	....	....	....	....	....	Young woman; fourteen teeth only, beautifully kept.
24	Ch. XVIII	....	....	1+	....	....	2d	2d+	....	

SUMMARY

Number of right 1st incisors missing...................... 2
Number of left 1st incisors missing....................... 2
Number of right 2nd incisors missing..................... 2
Number of left 2nd incisors missing...................... 1
Number of right canines missing.......................... 3
Number of left canines missing........................... 2
Number of right 1st premolars missing................... 3
Number of left 1st premolars missing.................... 3
Number of right 2nd premolars missing.................. 5
Number of left 2nd premolars missing................... 5
Number of right 1st molars missing...................... 6
Number of left 1st molars missing....................... 6
Number of right 2nd molars missing..................... 6
Number of left 2nd molars missing...................... 5
Number of right 3rd molars missing..................... 5
Number of left 3rd molars missing...................... 6

Our tables are of comparative value only; nevertheless, the results of our observations are so definite that they may find a place here.

Out of twenty-four, twelve had good teeth, but it must be remembered that many were young people.

The table shows that in those times, as now, the molars suffered most, and especially the third molar. Of twenty cases in which the molars had been cut, no less than seven had lost one or both wisdom teeth.

In the lower jaw the same deficiencies in the teeth are observed, namely, the molars have disappeared more often than any other teeth. The third molar especially has suffered a great deal, no less than six people having lost one or both wisdom teeth.

MANDIBLE

N.B.: + indicates that a tooth was present but decayed.

No.	Register	Incisors R.	Incisors L.	Canines R.	Canines L.	Premolars R.	Premolars L.	Molars R.	Molars L.	Remarks
1	Ch. x							1st		Teeth beautifully white.
2	Ch. B								1st, 2d, 3d	Teeth white, not worn.
3	Ch. G									Perfect; teeth but little worn.
4	Ch. A. II					1st				Two molars much worn; left ramus only present.
5	Ch. g									Part of right ramus only; teeth clear and white.
6	Ch. a. III				1			1st		Deep abscess in connection with left canine.
7	Ch. d									Left ramus only; teeth not worn.
8	Ch. A. I								2d, 3d+	Deep abscess in connection with outer fang of right second molar. Alveolus filled with bone.
9	Ch. E									Normal teeth; not worn.
10	Ch. G. I									Wisdom teeth not out yet; perfect.
11	Ch. I									Partially calcined; no visible lesions.
12	Ch. n									Very young person; second molars just erupting; teeth good, not worn.
13	Ch. D						2d		1st	
14	Ch. D. I								2d+	Left ramus only.
15	Ch. O							1st+		Right ramus only.
16	Ch. D. II									Wisdom teeth not out yet.
17	Ch. Y									Left ramus, teeth not worn.
18	Ch. B									Left ramus, teeth not worn.
19	Ch. C			1						Right incisor congenitally absent.
20	Ch. VII						2d	2d, 3d	1st, 2d	Much tartar; teeth yellow, not worn.
21	Ch. X								3d	No wisdom teeth on right side.
22	Ch. A. IV					2d	2d	1st	1st, 3d	An impacted tooth behind left second molar; distinct swelling of ramus in that position.
23	Ch. D. III		1st, 2d		1st	1st, 2d	1st, 2d	1st, 2d, 3d	1st, 2d, 3d	Very powerful jaw; evidently male.

SUMMARY

Number of right central incisors missing............... 0
Number of left central incisors missing................ 1
Number of right lateral incisors missing............... 0
Number of left lateral incisors missing................ 1
Number of right canines missing....................... 1
Number of left canines missing........................ 2
Number of right 1st premolars missing................. 2
Number of left 1st premolars missing.................. 1
Number of right 2nd premolars missing................. 2
Number of left 2nd premolars missing.................. 4
Number of right 1st molars missing.................... 5
Number of left 1st molars missing..................... 5
Number of right 2nd molars missing.................... 2
Number of left 2nd molars missing..................... 5
Number of right 3rd molars missing.................... 2
Number of left 3rd molars missing..................... 5

There are several other points of interest, which are revealed by the examination of the teeth.

In a few cases an abscess in connection with one of the teeth had formed. These abscesses in every case had penetrated deeply into the bone or had perforated into the palate, and yet in severe cases apparently nothing had been done to relieve the patient of the pain, which must have been agonising. In two cases the offending tooth, although loose, was still present in the alveolus.

In almost every book on ancient Egyptian medicine one reads of the Egyptians being learned in dentistry, yet judging from these and other observations they often did not pull out a painful tooth, an operation of all surgical operations certainly the most obvious.

We have never found the slightest evidence that the Egyptians knew anything about filling teeth, though in more than one treatise it is stated that they were skilled in this science. Lastly, we have never seen artificial teeth except in one instance, which was shown us by our friend, Professor Breccia. A number of teeth were bound together by gold wire, and were found in a *Roman* tomb in Egypt. It is evident, however, that this apparatus was for show and not for use, as it could not possibly have been used for mastication.

The examination of the teeth shows that the quality of the food was different from what it was in Upper Egypt in early times. The teeth are, with few exceptions, not worn down by the coarse vegetable food of the fellah, but the crowns are, as a rule, perfect save in very old people. The food was therefore soft, and consisted probably chiefly of meat.

Many of the people used the tooth-brush or some similar instrument freely. Deposits of tartar are rare, and as a rule the teeth are beautifully white and clean.

We have also often been struck with the small size of the wisdom teeth. In this connection we may refer to Darwin's remarks[1] on the subject of the third molar teeth. "It appears as if the posterior molar or wisdom tooth were tending to become rudimentary in the more civilised races of man. These teeth are rather smaller than the molars, ... and they have only two separate fangs."[2]

He also refers to a letter from Professor Mantegazza in which this observer states that "in the higher or civilised races they are on the road towards atrophy or elimination."

Morton Small and J. F. Colyer[3] express themselves as follows:

At the present time the first permanent molars are more prone to caries than other teeth, and the mandibular more than the maxillary. The second molars probably follow the first molars in liability to caries, the mandibular being attacked with more frequency than the maxillary. It is extremely difficult without reliable statistics to place the incisors and premolars as regards their liability to caries. Judging from experience, there seems little to choose between the first and second maxillary premolars in this respect, but with regard to the mandibular premolars the liability to caries is much more marked in the second than in the first. The mandibular incisors are comparatively immune to caries. . . . . The liability of the third molars to caries, in mouths where all the teeth are present, is attributable to difficulty in keeping them free from food débris.

[1] *Descent of Man*, p. 20.

[2] Darwin appears to have been under a misapprehension in this respect. Quain's *Anatomy*, II (1882), 549, states: "In the wisdom teeth of both jaws the fangs are often collected into a single irregular conical mass, which is either directed backwards in the substance of the jaw or curved irregularly; this composite fang sometimes shows traces of subdivision, and there are occasionally two fangs in the lower tooth and three in the upper."

[3] *Diseases and Injuries of the Teeth*.

Our observations, as far as they go, show that the liability of particular teeth to disease in Greek times was much the same as it is now, except that the third molar was perhaps more often affected than it is at the present day.

Without entering into the question as to whether these facts do or do not favour the idea advanced by Darwin, we would point out that all these characteristics existed more than two thousand years ago.

DESCRIPTION OF PLATES XXIII–XXXI
(For particulars see text)

PLATE XXIII

FIGS. 1–5.—From skeleton of IIIrd Dynasty.

PLATE XXIV

FIGS. 6, 7.—From same skeleton as Figs. 1–5.
FIGS. 8–16.—From another skeleton of the IIIrd Dynasty.

PLATE XXV

FIG. 17.—From a skeleton of the XIIth Dynasty. (*a*) Points to osteophyte growing between ninth and tenth dorsal vertebrae.
FIGS. 18–22.—From a mummy of the XXIst Dynasty.
FIG. 23.—Metatarsal bone from a mummy of the XXIst Dynasty.

PLATE XXVI

FIGS. 24–26.—From a skeleton of the XXIInd Dynasty.
FIGS. 27–29.—From a skeleton dating from the Persian occupation of Egypt.
FIGS. 30 and 31.—Bouchard's nodosities. From a skeleton dating from the Persian occupation of Egypt.

PLATES XXVII–XXIX

FIGS. 32–35.—From skeletons of soldiers of Alexander the Great.
FIG. 36.—Radius of skeleton of XXIst Dynasty.
FIGS. 37–45.—From skeletons of soldiers of Alexander the Great.
FIGS. 46 and 47.—Fracture of both bones of the leg. From a mummy of the time of the Persian occupation.

PLATE XXX

FIGS. 48 and 49.—From skeletons of soldiers of Alexander the Great.
FIG. 50.—From a Coptic skeleton. (*a*) Points to a deep groove between the old and newly formed bone.

Fig. 51.—From a skeleton of Roman times. (*a*) Points to bony excrescences.

Figs. 52 and 53.—From skeletons of soldiers of Alexander the Great.

PLATE XXXI

Fig. 54.—From a skeleton of Roman times.
Fig. 55.—Exostosis on rib of a soldier of Alexander the Great.
Fig. 56.—Lower jaw with alveolar abscess of a soldier of Alexander the Great.
Fig. 57.—From a Coptic skeleton.
Figs. 58–61.—From a skeleton of Roman times.

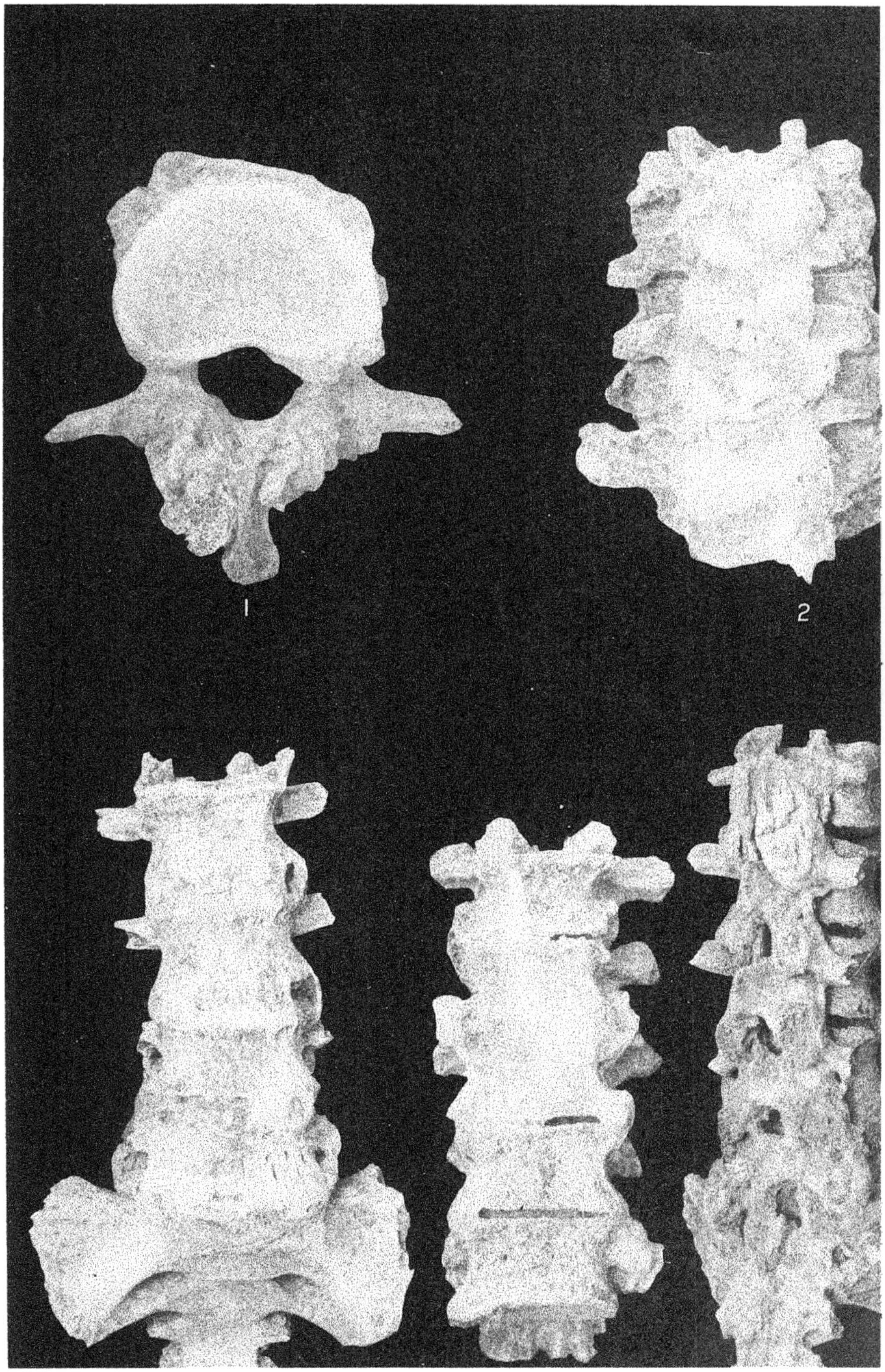
1
2

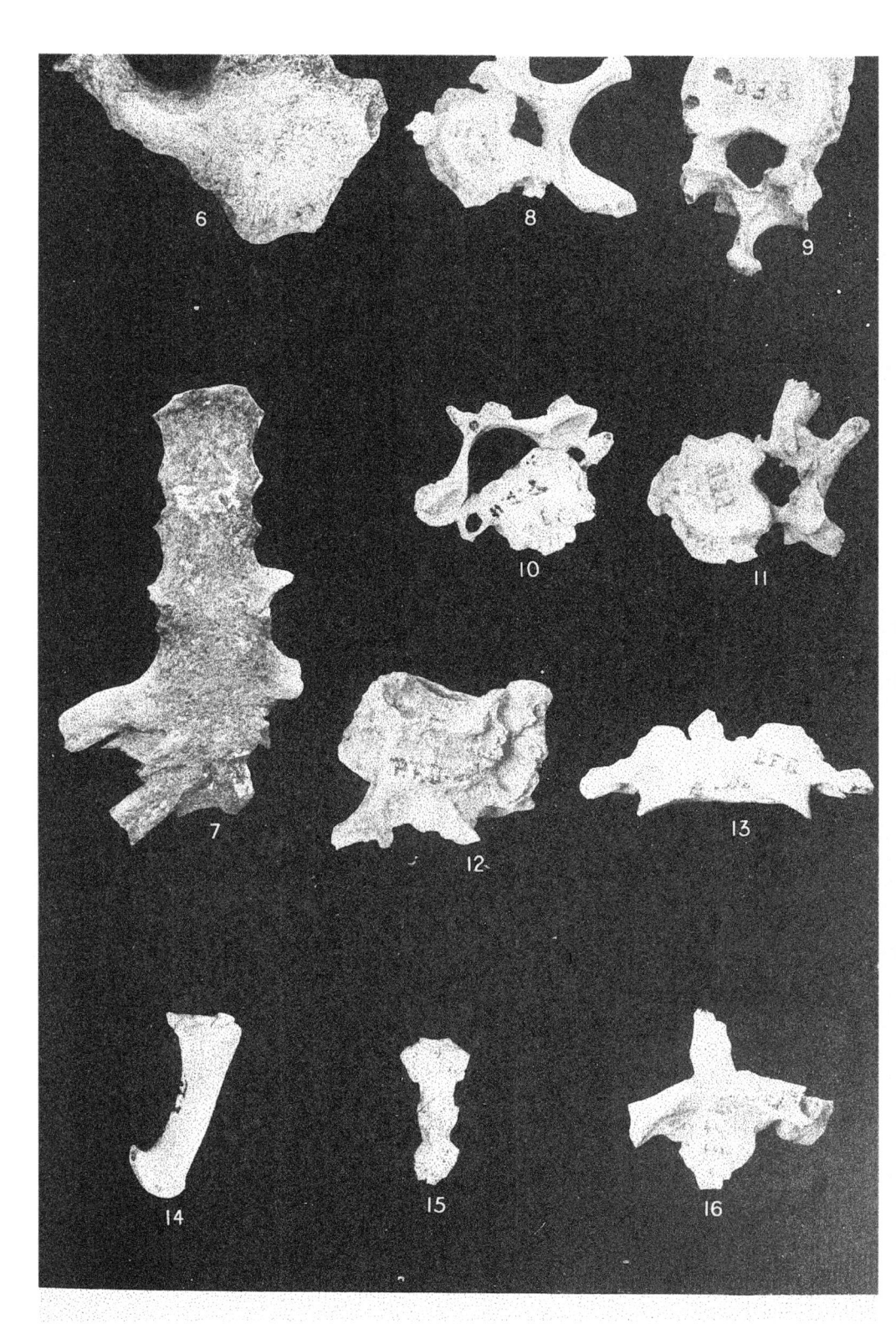

6
8
9
7
10
11
12
13
14
15
16

17

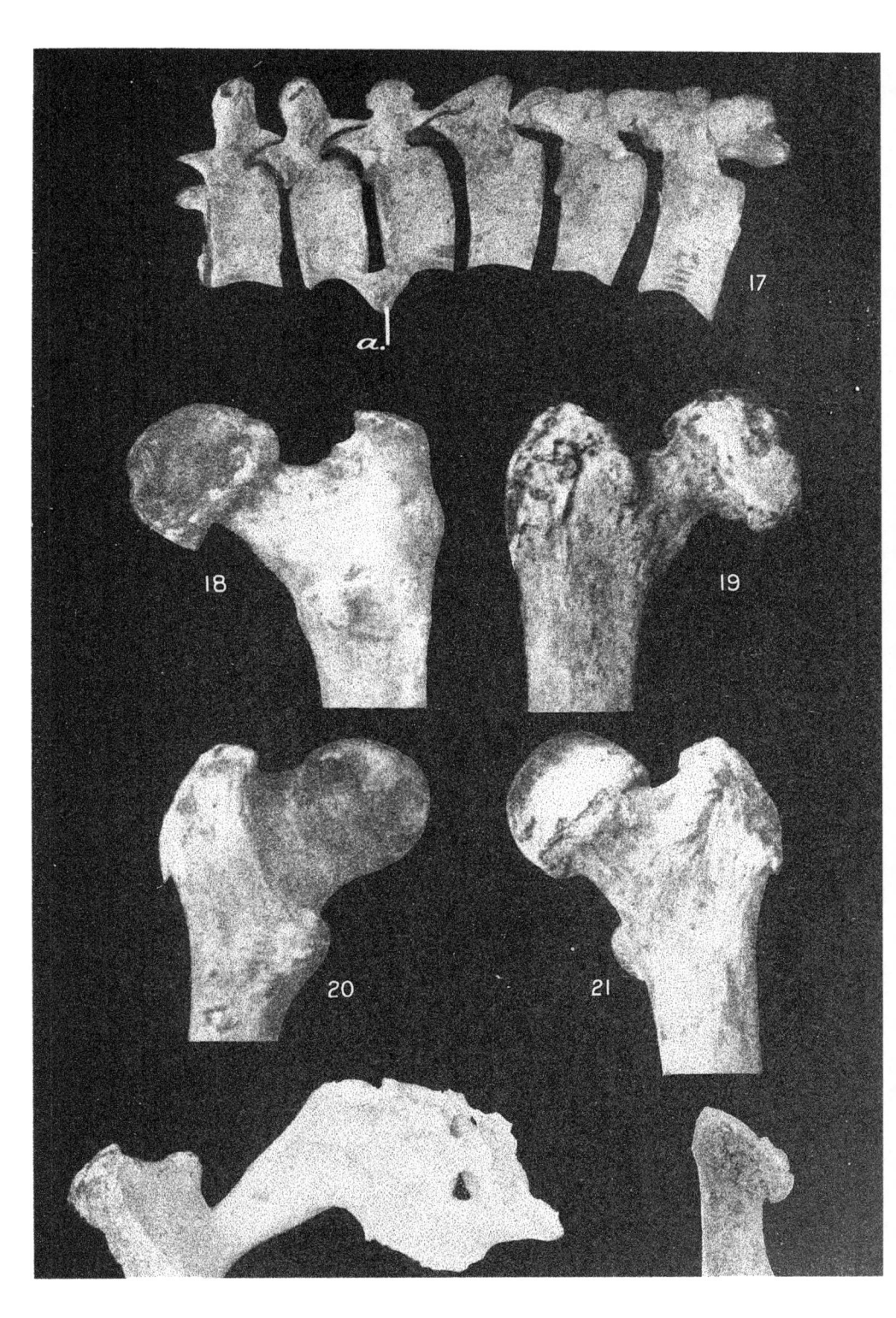

18   19

20   21

24

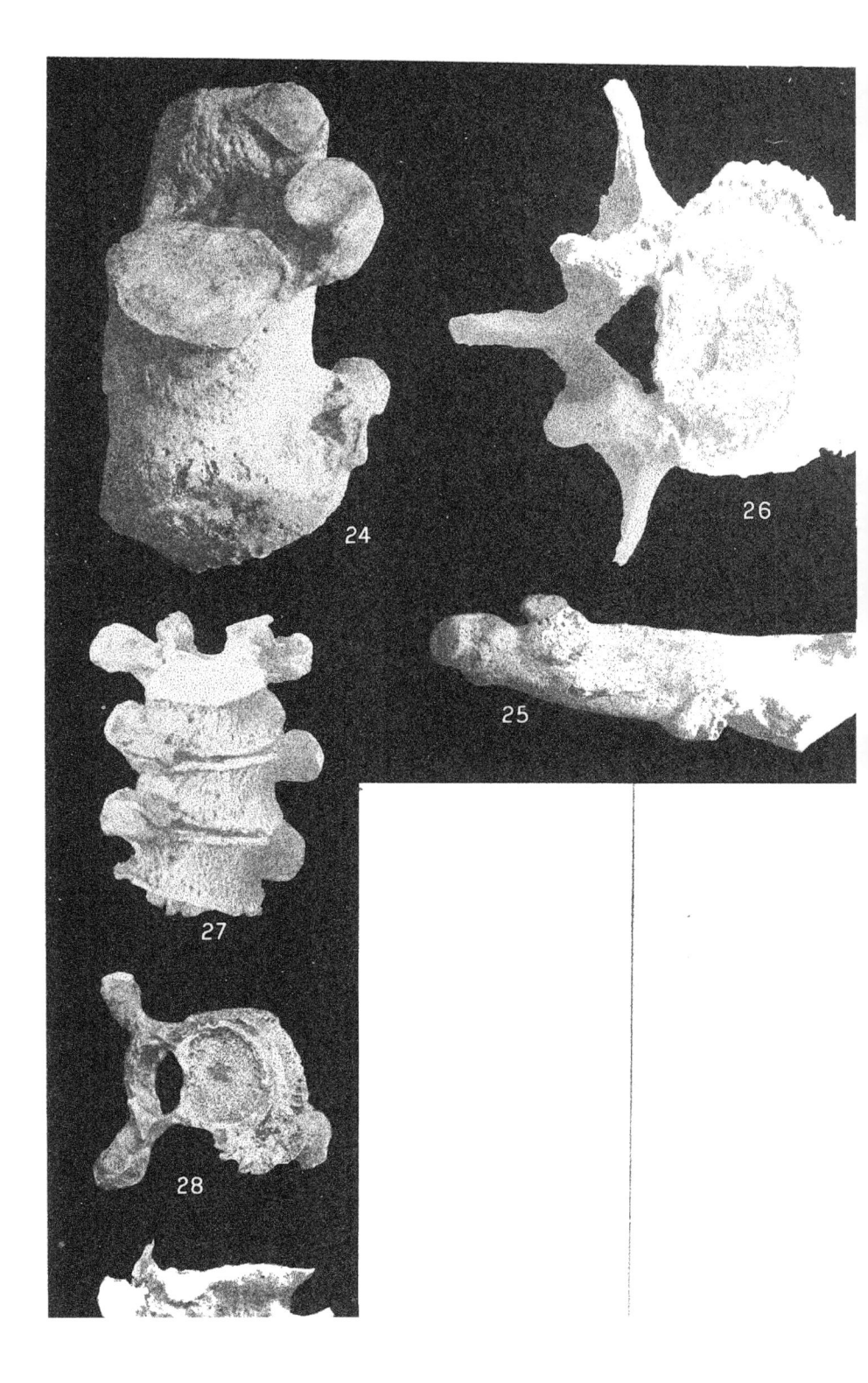

25

26

27

28

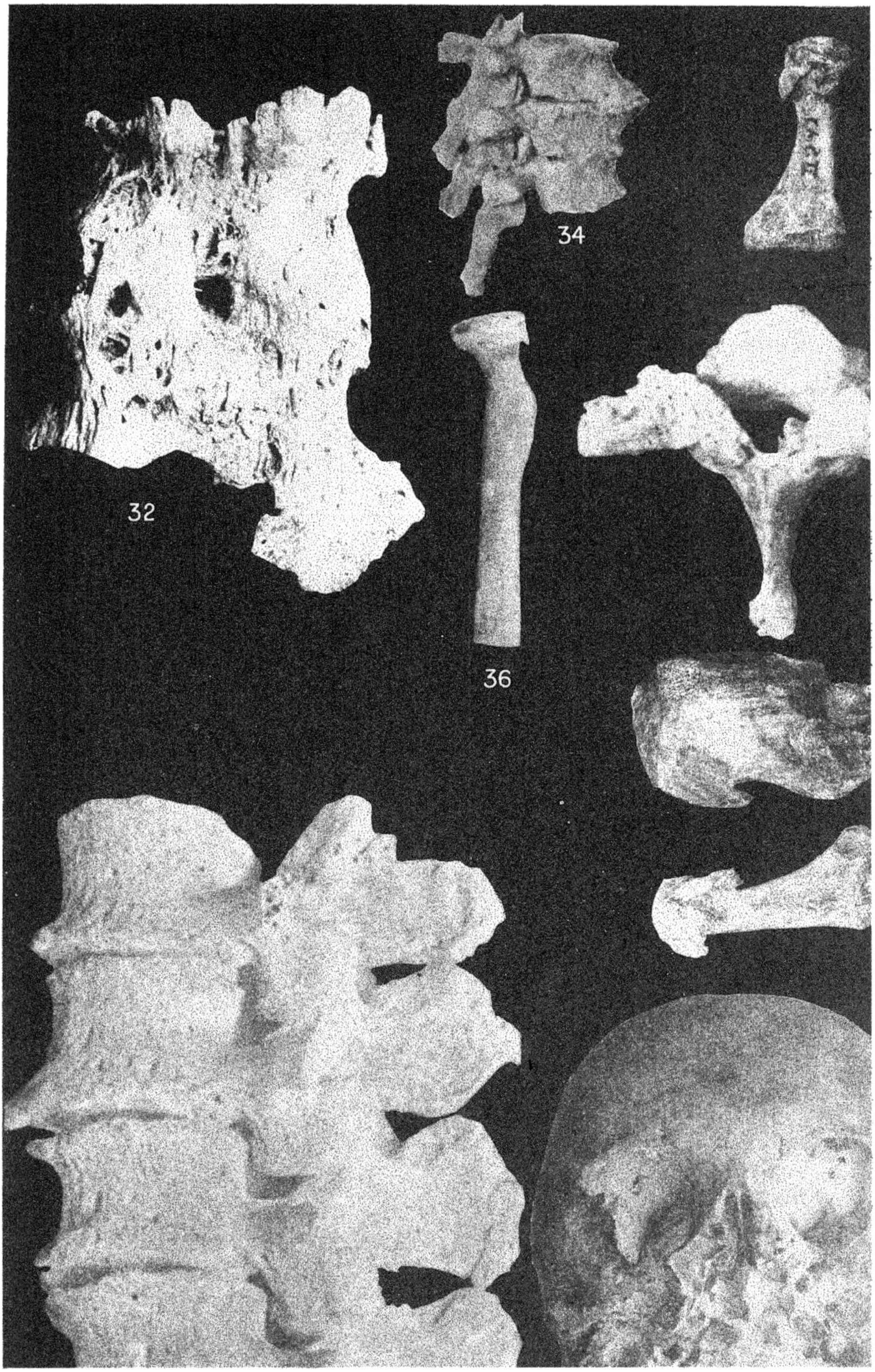
34
32
36

41

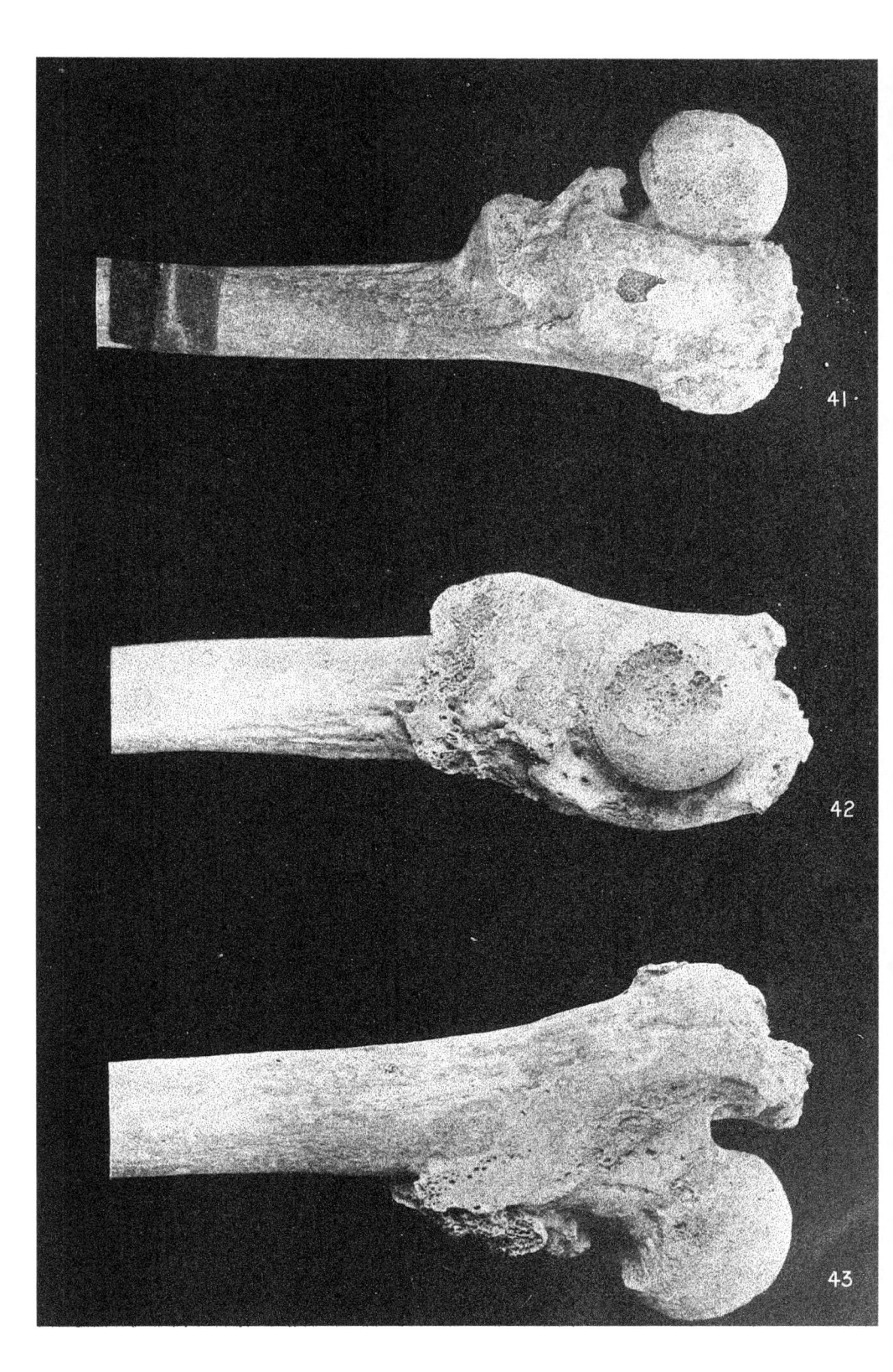

42

43

44

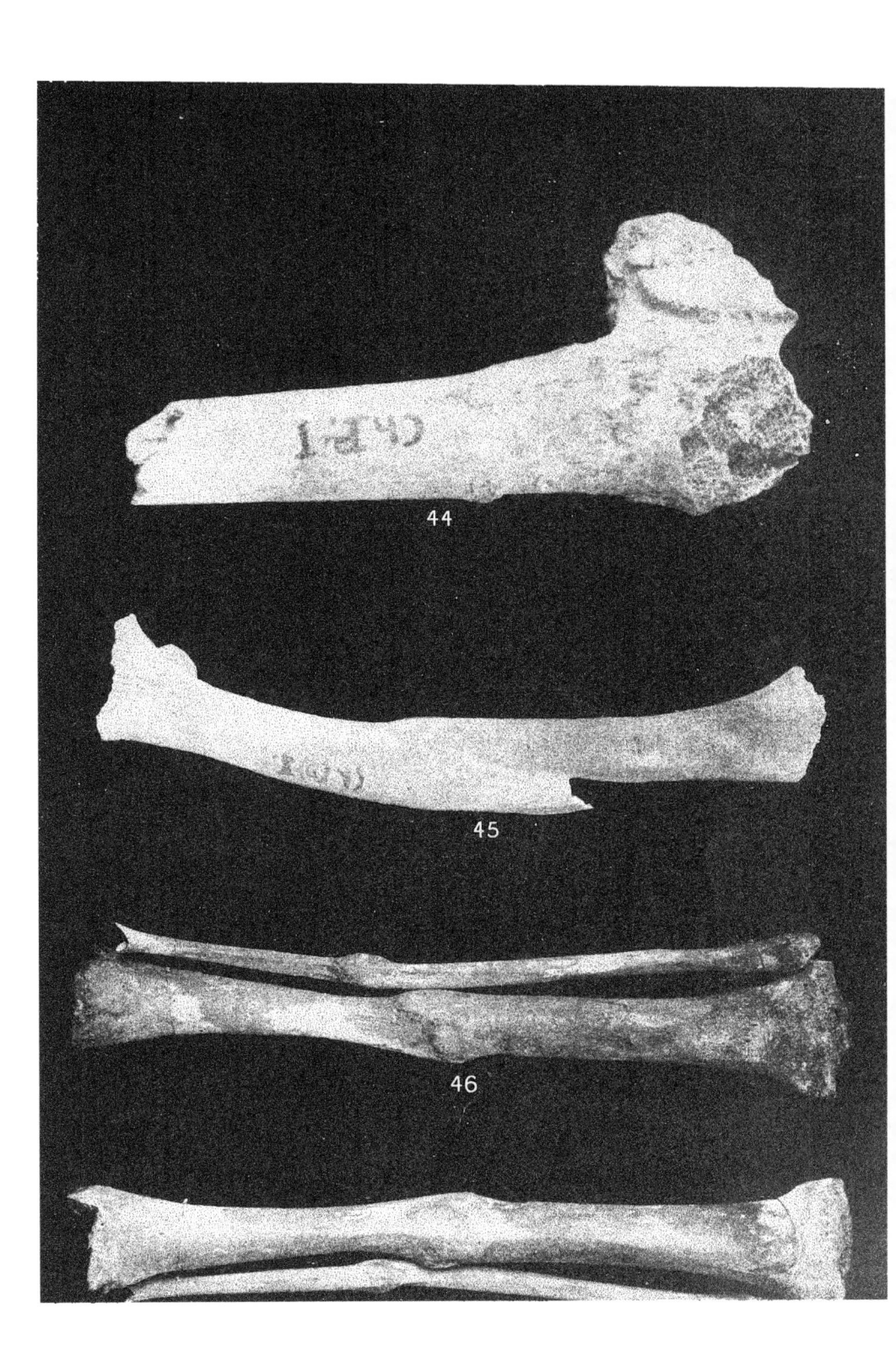

45

46

48

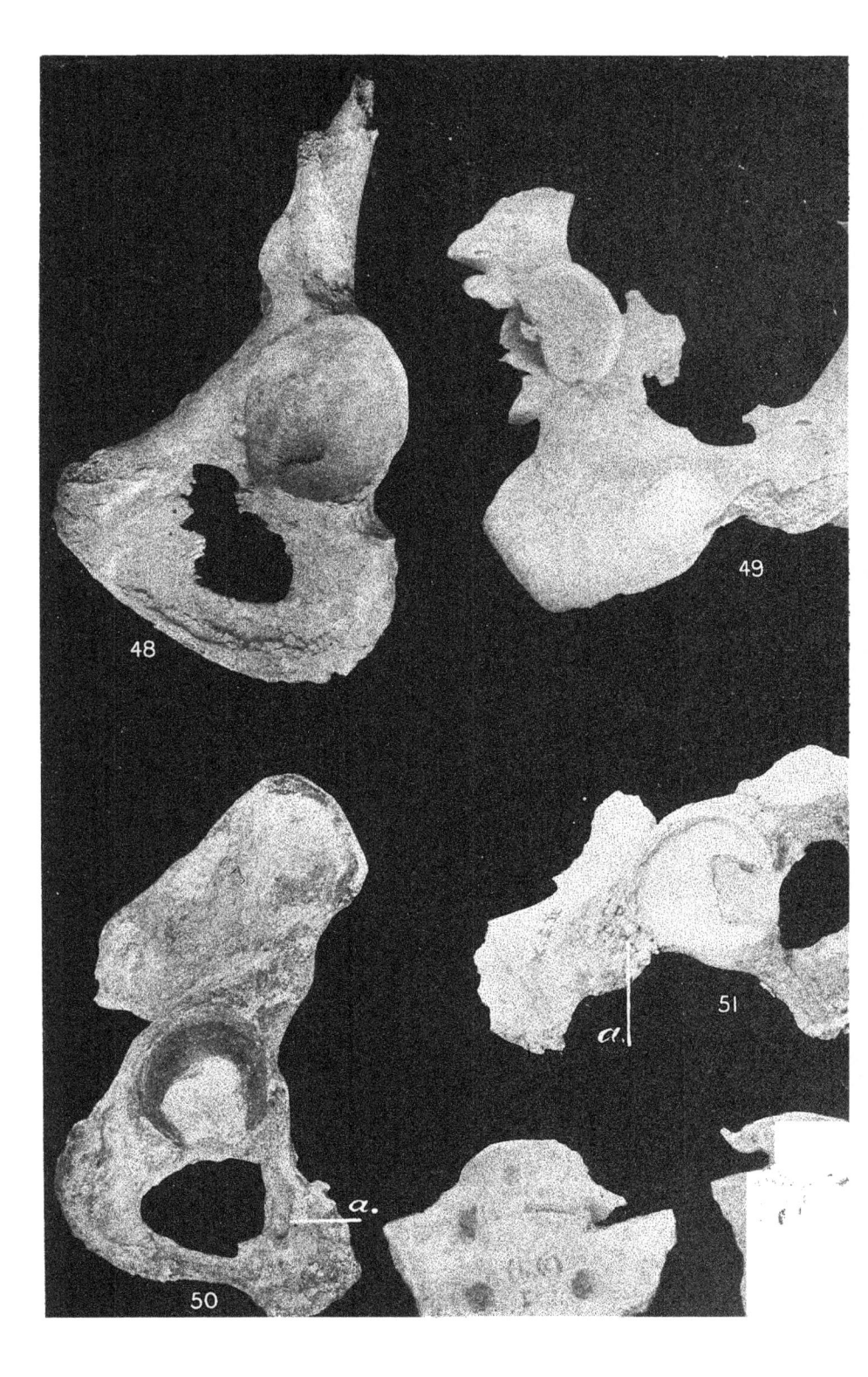

49

50

51

a.

a.

54

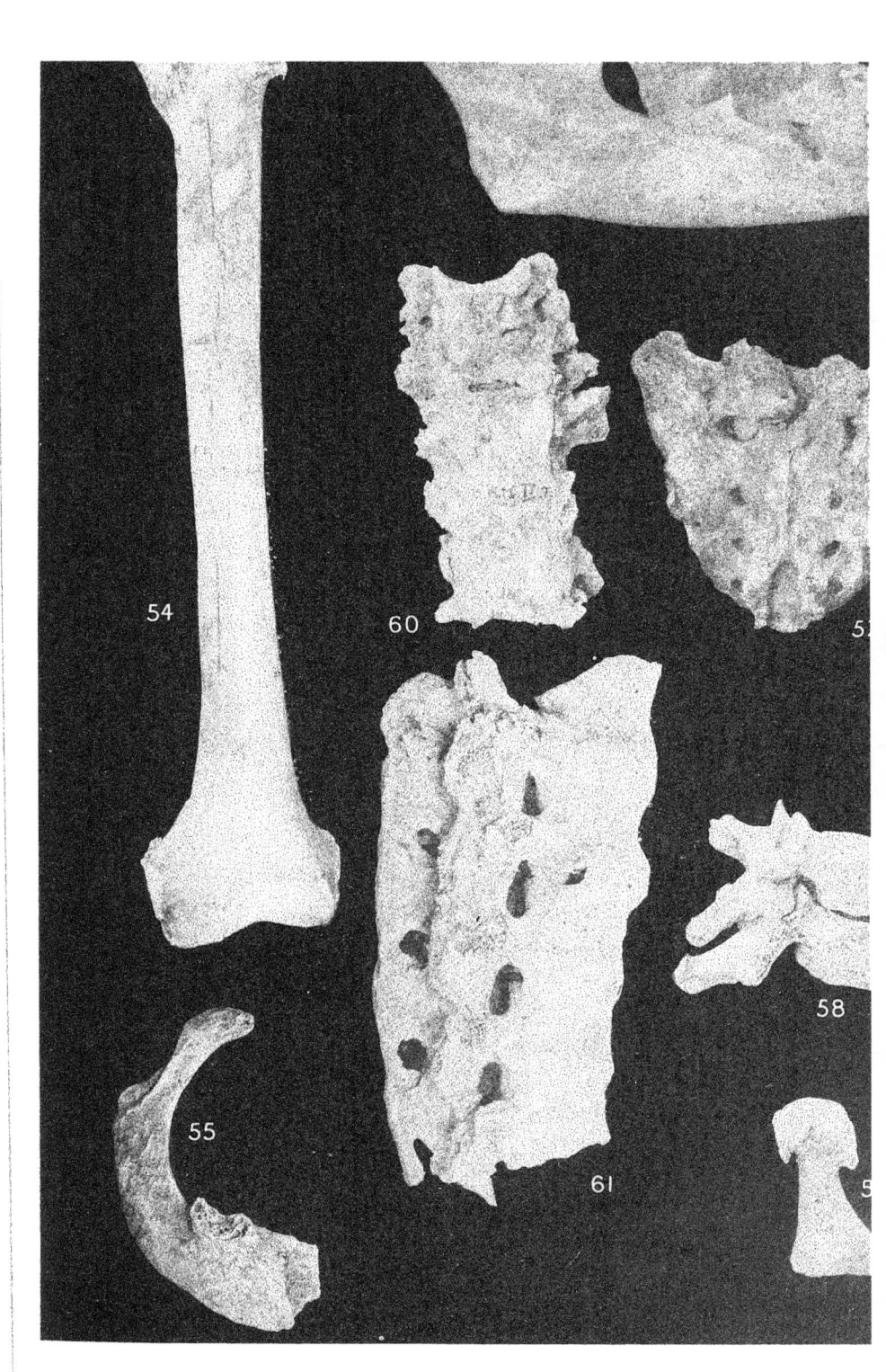

55

60

58

61

NOTES ON TWO EGYPTIAN MUMMIES DATING FROM THE PERSIAN OCCUPATION OF EGYPT[1] (525-332 B.C.)

(*Bulletin de la Société Archéologique d'Alexandrie*, No. 14 [1912])

In spite of numerous works on embalming, but few facts are known regarding this process, for with a few brillant exceptions, such as Pettigrew, Maspero, Fouquet, Elliot Smith, Derry, Wood Jones, most writers have been content to copy ancient or modern textbooks, and have added little that is new to our knowledge.

We do not intend to give here an account of methods of embalming, but merely to put on record two observations which appear to us to be of some interest.

The two mummies to be described now were given us by Professor W. M. Flinders Petrie, who informed us that they belonged to the date of the Persian occupation of Egypt.

MUMMY NO. 1

The first mummy was that of a woman, and we give here the notes taken during its examination.

NOTES OF EXAMINATION

Mummy very light. Length, when unrolled, 1 metre 50 centimetres. On unrolling, the following layers of bandages presented themselves:

1. External surface of shroud (Plate XXXII, Fig. 1), adorned with small bandages 2.8 centimetres in breadth, most of which, however, had been torn away. Remaining bandage wound twice round the neck. Some small pieces of cartonnage still left over neck and lower part of legs.

2. Broad longitudinal band passing over head to centre of back, where it was lost in a lump of gum.

---

[1] This paper was written with A. Rietti as junior author.

This band, 20 centimetres in breadth, was split into two, near the feet, each of these two pieces going round feet, and then running up over head to back, which was greatly soiled with gum.

3. Large number of linen rags (Plate XXXII, Fig. 2.), which had been forced between the legs and laid over the abdomen; also forcibly pushed between side of head and bandages passing from head to shoulder. Back also covered by a large number of similar rags greatly begrimed with gum.

4. Body lying with legs fully extended and arms crossed, right arm over left. Bandage (Plate XXXII, Fig. 3), 4 centimetres broad, passed several times round body, both arms, over legs and finally tied round feet.

5. Piece of linen forming a shroud over the legs, arms, abdomen, and chest.

6. Whole mummy, from head to feet, was now seen to be a model of beautiful bandaging.

Bandages made of rather coarse linen. One, obtained entire, measure 6 metres in length and 2.8 centimetres in breadth. Free end fringed like a scarf; the other end hemmed, showing that it had been torn off from a piece of cloth 6 metres long, the breadth of which we could not ascertain.

Head held in position by bandage passing over vertex, round one side of the neck, over the head again, and again on the other side of the neck. Finally, several turns round the forehead kept all these bandages together. Over the face, bandages looked pink and white alternately; an appearance produced by small strips of pink linen placed under each bandage, each of which overlapped the white bandages for about half a centimetre. Strips of pink linen had been neatly tied just above each wrist, elbow, ankle, and knee, forming bracelets or anklets.

Bandages ran up in figures of eight, over the chest and round the shoulders, and again from the toes, legs, round the abdomen and groins, just as surgical bandages are applied now for wounds in the same regions. No reverses anywhere.

Exact method of bandaging the abdomen and chest not ascertainable, owing to soiling of back by gum.

Fingers were not bandaged, but enclosed in a piece of linen covering the whole hand. Nails of fingers (but not of toes) (Plate

XXXIII, Fig. 4) tied on by little pieces of string, in the same manner as has been described by Professor Elliot Smith in mummies of the XXIst Dynasty.

7. After removal of bandages, the mummy was found to be covered by a long broad piece of linen, entirely encasing it (Plate XXXIV, Fig. 5).

8. Bandages running irregularly over the body and legs, holding together flat strips of linen, measuring 14 centimètres, placed in various positions as a padding, plainly in order to simulate the shape of the body. These strips most numerous on inner surface of thighs, on calves and chest, round neck and underneath chin. They were always put in perfectly flat, and from the way in which they were placed it appears probable that one person endeavoured to imitate the shape of the thighs, legs, etc., by holding these strips of linen in position, while another bandaged over them. On one hand, bandages kept in position by passing through interdigital spaces of second and third fingers.

9. Near the skin, bandages intensely black from gum, hard, and brittle. It was impossible to follow them, but one had the impression that a very fine piece of linen had been first placed all along the skin. The pieces had to be picked away bit by bit, until the skin underneath was exposed.

10. At the back, after picking away the bandages from top and bottom, one came in the centre of the back to a mass of coarse linen saturated with gum and so hard that it was impossible to remove it (Plate XXXV, Fig. 6a). Here the skin and muscles had entirely disappeared. Plainly a large hole at the back had been filled up by linen saturated with gum.

11. The body now looked extraordinarily thin. The skin was so brittle that in spite of every possible care holes were made in wall of abdomen. After a search lasting several hours, the line of the incision in the left flank was found, a piece of linen which was still sticking between the edges of the wound proving a guide to it.

12. Body jet-black, in some places almost of a slaty colour. The chest and abdomen look just as if painted with black shiny varnish (Plate XXXIV, Fig. 7).

Head was cleaned with difficulty owing to linen closely attached to skin. Strips of rag had been put behind the ears, and bandages so arranged as to press ears forward (Plate XXXVI, Fig. 8). The top of the head was clean-shaved.

Very peculiar appearance was presented by mouth, its left angle being distinctly depressed (Plate XXXVI, Fig. 8). Right angle normal apparently, but tongue protruded for about half a centimetre, and strongly indented by teeth. Mouth contained no foreign matter. Eyelids jet-black just as if they had been varnished. Eyebrows could not be recognised, but eyes themselves were easily seen, the globes not having been removed. Eyelashes perfect.

13. Front of abdominal walls and chest now cut away bit by bit with scissors. The genital organs had been removed, and a round, sacklike piece of stiff linen, filled with some vegetable powder and about 3 inches in diameter, had been rammed into the pelvic cavity through the perineum. This had plainly been put there in order to close the cavity.

14. Spine had been fractured just above the second lumbar vertebra. The first lumbar vertebra found lying almost behind the second. The sacrum looked almost horizontally backwards.

Dorsal vertebrae seen vaguely at bottom of wound, but extraordinarily black, very unlike the lumbar vertebrae below. A piece of stick (the rib of a palm leaf) had been put in vertically and was resting just below and behind Poupart's ligament on right side and on first rib above. This can only have been introduced through the perineum by the embalmer, and had evidently been put in to prevent collapse of body (Plate XXXVI, Fig. 8).

Absolutely no trace of any internal organ could be found. The whole of the abdominal cavity was lined everywhere by a black, hard, glistening substance, which posteriorly formed a layer almost 2 inches thick. There were also a few thick pieces of coarse rag crammed into right iliac fossa, and just above and behind the second lumbar vertebra.

The body was so brittle that it was useless to try to dissect it in this condition. Accordingly, after detaching the head, it was placed into the usual softening solution for twenty-four hours.

15. When the body was taken out of the solution, hardly a trace of the dorsal vertebral column could be discovered. All that remained of the vertebrae consisted of some small crumbling pieces of bone, though several intervertebral discs were found, which exhibited no sign of disease. On the other hand, cervical and lumbar vertebrae, sacrum and pelvis were normal.

At the lower end of the dorsal region, there was a hole extending from the back to the abdominal cavity. This cavity had been plugged from the abdominal cavity and from the back by linen soaked in gum. The two plugs when joined together looked like an hour-glass. There had therefore evidently been a large cavity which had been filled after death in order to prevent the embalming material from escaping. The fluid, gummy material, nevertheless, had found its way for some distance, between the muscles of the back, into the axillae and groins on both sides.

No gum whatever discovered in the limbs or in the mouth, though it had found its way into the pharynx and posterior nares.

The body had been bandaged tightly when it was still fairly soft, as the marks of the bandages could be seen on several parts of the thighs.

16. Head contained small pieces of resin and stump of a tooth, all of which had evidently fallen in after death. Skull otherwise empty, except near the foramen magnum where pieces of membrane were still adherent. Cribriform plate of ethmoid and small wing of the sphenoid had been fractured on each side by embalmers when the brain was taken out through nostrils.

Bony and cartilaginous septa of nose unhurt.

No trace of pits for Pacchionian bodies in vault of skull.

EXAMINATION OF TEETH

Grinding surface of teeth, especially of molars, much worn.

Wisdom teeth present.

Lower maxilla. Alveoli of both first molars completely obliterated.

Upper maxilla. *Left:* third molar, alveolus completely obliterated; second molar, alveolus partly obliterated; first molar, laveolus completely obliterated. *Right:* second and third molars, alveoli completely obliterated; first and second premolars, alveoli completely obliterated.

HISTOLOGICAL EXAMINATION

Only parts examined were skin of abdomen, back, and fingers, also arteries and nerves. These were placed in softening solution, where they became pliable, showing that the body had in no way been carbonised. Epidermic layers could still be made out as flattened cells, and the general structure of the corium was fairly well retained.

No sweat glands could be seen. Muscular fibres were teased out with caustic potash and showed the striation fairly well. Arteries of the limbs showed no alterations. In the nerves, epineurium and endoneurium were perfect. Medullary sheath made out in transverse sections. Axis cylinders absent.

PATHOLOGICAL EXAMINATION

The hands showed deformation described by Professor Bouchard, and which is generally called by his name (Plate XXXIII).

Attention has been drawn already to the peculiar deformity of the face, simulating left facial paralysis. Perhaps very much importance must not be attached to this nor to the protrusion of the tongue, as such an appearance may possibly have been caused by manipulations after death. Still, we must say that it is the only mummy in which we have ever observed this appearance.

A remarkable point is the almost total disappearance of the dorsal vertebrae.

Some of the dorsal vertebrae were noticed lying in the body cavity, though they looked strangely altered. We regret we did not endeavour to remove them before placing the body in the macerating solution, as it is now impossible to know why they dissolved almost completely.

As the lumbar vertebrae, the ribs, clavicles, bones of the arm, cervical vertebrae, treated exactly in the same way, did not show any signs of dissolution, we conclude that extensive pathological changes may have existed in the dorsal vertebrae and rendered them susceptible to the dissolving action of weak carbonate of soda. Whatever the pathological change may have been, it did not extend to all the intervertebral discs, for some we found were normal. Our only excuse for neglecting to remove the dorsal vertebrae is that we have never had this experience before.

The articular surface of the knee-joints was jet-black, although not a trace of foreign material could be discovered with the microscope.

Mr. A. Lucas kindly gave us the following notes on the results of the chemical examination of materials removed from the body.

Bandages near pubis.—The resinous-looking material on the bandages is not resin, but possibly gum altered by age and exposure; it contains a small amount of combined soda, also sodium chloride and sulphate, possibly *indicating the use of natron.* The results of the analysis are as follows:

	Per Cent
Soluble in petroleum ether	0.70
Soluble in absolute alcohol	2.70
Soluble in water after alcohol	40.90
Insoluble organic matter (by difference)	50.00
Mineral matter { soluble in water*	3.20
insoluble in water	2.50
	100.00

*Sodium salts.

Bandages with white spots.—The bandages contain a small amount of an aromatic, resinous substance, together with a small amount of combined soda and also sodium chloride and sulphate, possibly *indicating the use of natron.*

Gum between skin and muscles of back.—The sample is not a resin, but is possibly gum altered by age and exposure; it contains a small amount of combined soda, also sodium chloride and sulphate, *possibly indicating the use of natron.* The results of the analysis are as follows:

	Per Cent
Soluble in petroleum ether	trace
Soluble in absolute alcohol	1.60
Soluble in water after alcohol	52.30
Insoluble organic matter (by difference)	36.70
Mineral matter { soluble in water*	5.00
insoluble in water	4.40
	100.00

*Sodium salts.

REMARKS

The method of embalming in this case appears to have been as follows:

An incision having been made in the left flank, the viscera were removed, and, unfortunately, their ultimate fate is unknown. The body was then probably immersed in the pickling solution. This solution may or may not have contained natron, as the amount found was small, and in fact the only evidence we have that a pickling solution was used is that the nails were tied to the fingers.

During these manipulations it is possible that a large hole was made in the back, possibly through clumsiness or on purpose. It is more probable, however, that owing to some disease (e.g., tubercular caries, secondary cancer, bedsore, etc)., a weak point existed in that situation during life, and that a careless workman greatly extended this defect.

The back being broken, the body would have collapsed, had not a stick been introduced which acted as an artificial backbone. The cavity was plugged with coarse bandages and the body treated with thick gum, applied very hot externally and internally; the excess of hot gum being allowed to escape through the perineum, which was plugged afterwards. The gum was then allowed to set almost hard and the body bandaged in the manner described above.

Such mummies more or less artificially built up are probably by no means rare, and several such instances are on record already.

Maspero, in his classical work (*Momies royales*), tells us that the Princess Sitamon was supposed to have been buried in a small coffin bearing her name. The mummy, however, actually consisted of a thin layer of bandages containing a parcel of *djerids* topped by a child's cranium; the whole measuring about 1 metre 20 centimetres in length.

Not infrequently the mummy was robbed and broken up by robbers, who made up an artificial mummy and substituted it for the original. This was the case with the mummy of the princess Manshont-timihou and that of Prince Siamon (see Maspero, *Momies royales*, pp. 544 and 538).

The body of the princess consisted of a bit of yellow coffin with yellow varnish, the handle of a mirror and some small objects, while a parcel of rags simulated the head and another parcel the feet.

The mummy of Prince Siamon had been robbed in olden times and broken into pieces. When it was made up again, no care was taken to reconstitute the skeleton, and the bones were simply thrown together higgledy-piggledy to form an oblong parcel.

The Museum of Lyons (Lortet, *Faune momifiée*, Fasc. 2, p. 35) possesses a very interesting specimen brought back by M. Chantre, which is composed of the body of a man from the head to the waist. The pelvis is absent; the thighs are replaced by branches of acacia bearing at their extremities small female legs, of which the flexor and extensor tendons of the toes "had evidently been dissected by a long maceration in the water of the river." (?)

This process of substituting part of the body for the whole extended even to bodies of animals. Lortet (*Faune momifiée*, Fasc. 2, p. 53) states: "It is interesting to note that cats like ibis were not always embalmed whole. One has seen mummies of ibis which contained only the back and the feet, or some feathers."

In the *Archaeological Survey of Nubia* (1907-8, pp. 204-5) Wood Jones has recorded several cases where, in the Ptolemaic period, the head of the body had been connected with the trunk by means of a stick.

In the case of a child
the body was kept intact by a stick which passed through its entire length, for the child had been spiked by a stick pushed into the vagina, thence through the abdomen and thorax, into the cavity of the skull. The lower end of the stick extended down below the knees, and no attempt had been made even to trim its rough end. The outward appearance of the mummy, however, was quite normal and aroused no suspicion of these curious manipulations.

We may also draw attention to the fact that although we were quite convinced that, in the first case, the black substance used for mummification was bitumen, yet as a matter of fact not a trace of this substance was found by chemical analysis.

MUMMY NO. 2.

To all outward appearances, this mummy was exactly like the one just described. The following are the notes taken at the examination of the body.

NOTES OF EXAMINATION.

1. After few remaining narrow outer bandages there came:
2. Strips of linen arranged diagonally across, but untidily and without any definite order.
3. A broad piece of linen forming a shroud covering the whole.
4. Beneath this, band 9 centimetres in width running along one side of the body, over head, down other side and wrapped several times round feet.
5. A mass of rags very untidily arranged and greatly begrimed with gum, kept in place by several long bands 20 centimetres broad, which ran over head and feet of mummy and along whole length.
6. Another mass of rags very untidily arranged, held in position by transverse broad bands also arranged without order. In the region of the pelvis, a metacarpal bone was found lying between these rags.
7. The rags having been carefully removed, a mass of bones was found lying in a kind of crate made of ribs of palm leaves (Plate XXXVII, Figs. 9 and 10). At the bottom of the crate, six little sticks placed vertically upwards and surrounded by masses of bandages represented the feet.

The bones, being greatly begrimed with earth, had evidently been buried first and then placed inside the crate.

The two tibiae were at the lower extremity of the crate. Then came the two femurs, right one upside down and on left side. One fibula lay behind the femurs.

Most of vertebrae massed together in pelvic region, and majority of the bones of feet were in right abdominal region, and had been thrown in anyhow.

Right shoulder formed by an iliac bone, whereas other iliac bone represented the front of the chest. One scapula, placed upside down, stood for other shoulder. Lower end of the sternum was lying transversely across the chest, the manubrium near scapula on left side. Some vertebrae and sacrum occupied left abdominal region.

A long stick, consisting of a rib of palm leaf, had been passed through the atlas vertebra (which was still hanging on the stick) and the foramen magnum into the head, and had been tied by bandages to lower end of crate (Plate XXXVIII, Fig. 11).

No traces of skin or organs remained, but here and there small remnants of tendons, cartilages, and muscles were still attached to the bones.

Orbits were full of earth. Lower jaw and hyoid bone were lying together under the skull. The alveoli of the teeth, many of which had fallen out after death, were filled with earth. Some of the teeth were lying loose behind the head, but after much searching, we accounted for all of them.

Crate consisted of seven ribs of palm leaves, tied together at the top and bottom by fine palm fibres (Plate XXXVIII, Fig. 11).

The bones belonged to a young man, certainly under twenty-five years of age, for the wisdom teeth had not emerged. Nevertheless, many of the bones showed the typical lesions of chronic osteoarthritis.

REMARKS

The dismemberment of the body had been deliberately done, though not by violence, as there were no signs of cuts or injuries.

It appears to us certain that the body was first buried in soft, moist earth, until all the soft parts had disappeared, and that, afterwards, the bones were gathered together and arranged in the crate in the manner described.

We do not think that this was the work of robbers, for in order to spoil the body thieves would hardly have taken the trouble to bury it and then replace the bones in the crate. Where thieves have interfered, the work is rough and ready and evidently done in a hurry. In this case, on the other hand, some care was taken to arrange the bones so that in outward shape, at any rate, the whole should resemble a human mummy.

It appears to us far more probable that we have to deal with a cheap method of preparing bodies for burials. According to our theory, those who could not or would not afford an expensive form of embalming had the body buried, disinterred, and then rearranged in the form of a mummy.

Time will show whether this theory is correct or not.

NOTES OF EXAMINATION.

1. After few remaining narrow outer bandages there came:

2. Strips of linen arranged diagonally across, but untidily and without any definite order.

3. A broad piece of linen forming a shroud covering the whole.

4. Beneath this, band 9 centimetres in width running along one side of the body, over head, down other side and wrapped several times round feet.

5. A mass of rags very untidily arranged and greatly begrimed with gum, kept in place by several long bands 20 centimetres broad, which ran over head and feet of mummy and along whole length.

6. Another mass of rags very untidily arranged, held in position by transverse broad bands also arranged without order. In the region of the pelvis, a metacarpal bone was found lying between these rags.

7. The rags having been carefully removed, a mass of bones was found lying in a kind of crate made of ribs of palm leaves (Plate XXXVII, Figs. 9 and 10). At the bottom of the crate, six little sticks placed vertically upwards and surrounded by masses of bandages represented the feet.

The bones, being greatly begrimed with earth, had evidently been buried first and then placed inside the crate.

The two tibiae were at the lower extremity of the crate. Then came the two femurs, right one upside down and on left side. One fibula lay behind the femurs.

Most of vertebrae massed together in pelvic region, and majority of the bones of feet were in right abdominal region, and had been thrown in anyhow.

Right shoulder formed by an iliac bone, whereas other iliac bone represented the front of the chest. One scapula, placed upside down, stood for other shoulder. Lower end of the sternum was lying transversely across the chest, the manubrium near scapula on left side. Some vertebrae and sacrum occupied left abdominal region.

A long stick, consisting of a rib of palm leaf, had been passed through the atlas vertebra (which was still hanging on the stick) and the foramen magnum into the head, and had been tied by bandages to lower end of crate (Plate XXXVIII, Fig. 11).

No traces of skin or organs remained, but here and there small remnants of tendons, cartilages, and muscles were still attached to the bones.

Orbits were full of earth. Lower jaw and hyoid bone were lying together under the skull. The alveoli of the teeth, many of which had fallen out after death, were filled with earth. Some of the teeth were lying loose behind the head, but after much searching, we accounted for all of them.

Crate consisted of seven ribs of palm leaves, tied together at the top and bottom by fine palm fibres (Plate XXXVIII, Fig. 11).

The bones belonged to a young man, certainly under twenty-five years of age, for the wisdom teeth had not emerged. Nevertheless, many of the bones showed the typical lesions of chronic osteo-arthritis.

REMARKS

The dismemberment of the body had been deliberately done, though not by violence, as there were no signs of cuts or injuries.

It appears to us certain that the body was first buried in soft, moist earth, until all the soft parts had disappeared, and that, afterwards, the bones were gathered together and arranged in the crate in the manner described.

We do not think that this was the work of robbers, for in order to spoil the body thieves would hardly have taken the trouble to bury it and then replace the bones in the crate. Where thieves have interfered, the work is rough and ready and evidently done in a hurry. In this case, on the other hand, some care was taken to arrange the bones so that in outward shape, at any rate, the whole should resemble a human mummy.

It appears to us far more probable that we have to deal with a cheap method of preparing bodies for burials. According to our theory, those who could not or would not afford an expensive form of embalming had the body buried, disinterred, and then rearranged in the form of a mummy.

Time will show whether this theory is correct or not.

DESCRIPTION OF PLATES XXXII–XXXVIII[1]

(For particulars see text)

PLATE XXXII

FIG. 1.—Mummy unrolled.
FIG. 2.—Shows mass of linen rags packed under outer shroud.
FIG. 3.—Shows method of tying limbs to body.

PLATE XXXIII

FIG. 4.—Hands of mummy. The nails are fastened to fingers by string.

PLATE XXXIV

FIG. 5.—Shows long shroud covering the body.
FIG. 7.—Body after removing all bandages.

PLATE XXXV

FIG. 6.—Shows plug of bandages closing the cavity at the back.

PLATE XXXVI

FIG. 8.—Body opened, showing rib of palm leaf supporting the body.

PLATE XXXVII

FIGS. 9 and 10.—View of bones lying in crate.

PLATE XXXVIII

FIG. 11.—Crate with long stick passing through the foramen magnum into the skull. Near the skull, the atlas vertebra is seen hanging from the stick.

[1] Figs. 1–8 from first mummy, Figs. 9–11 from second body. All the photographs were taken by Dr. Arnoldo Rietti.

PLATE XXXII

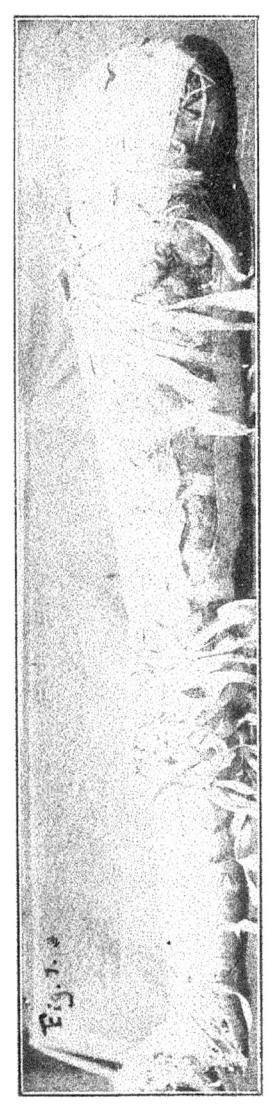

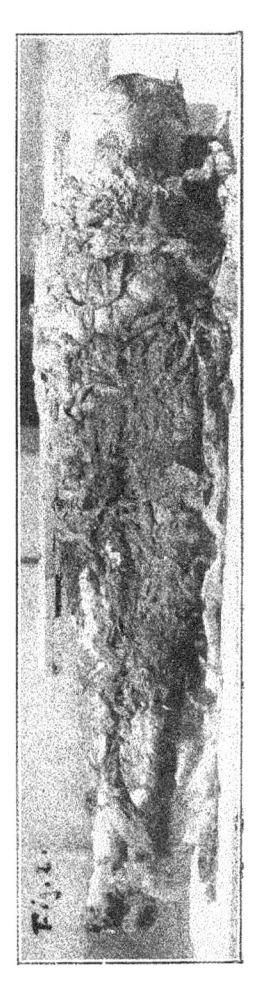

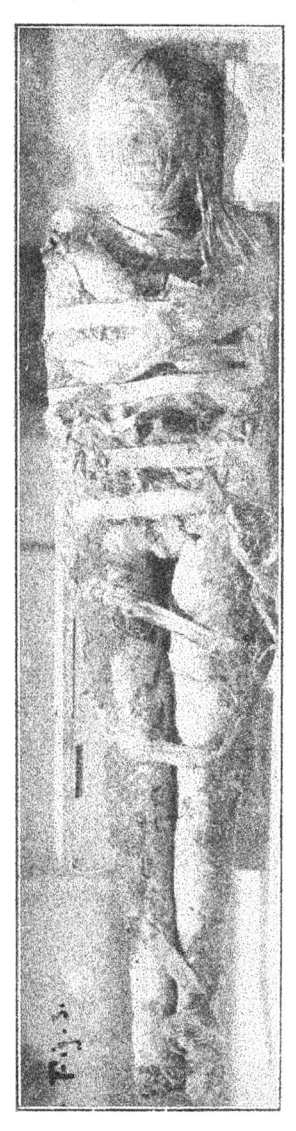

FIG. 1   FIG. 2   FIG. 3

PLATE XXXIII

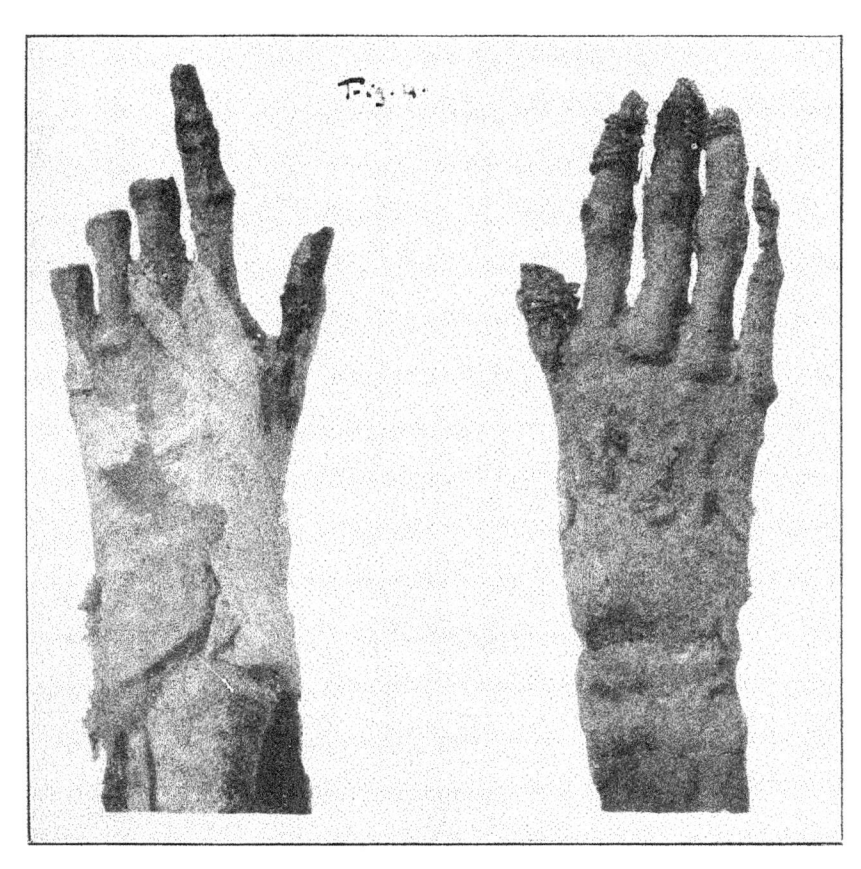

FIG. 4

PLATE XXXIV

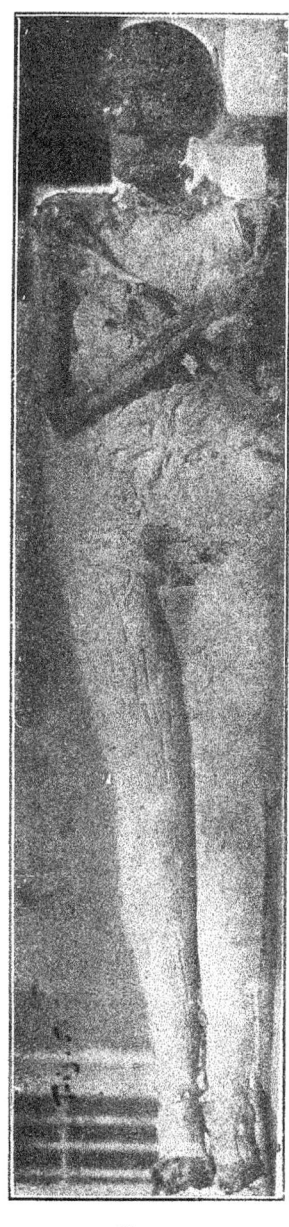

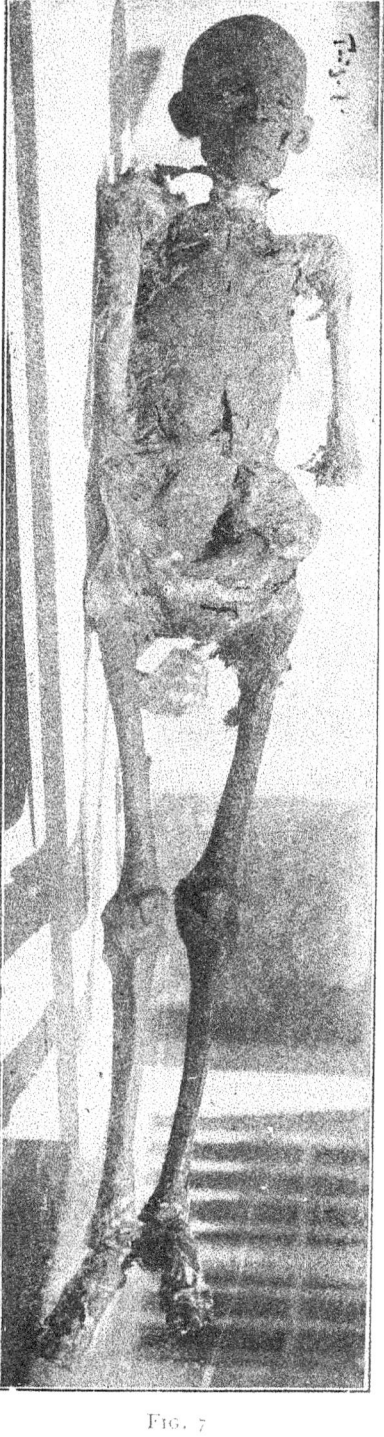

FIG. 5

FIG. 7

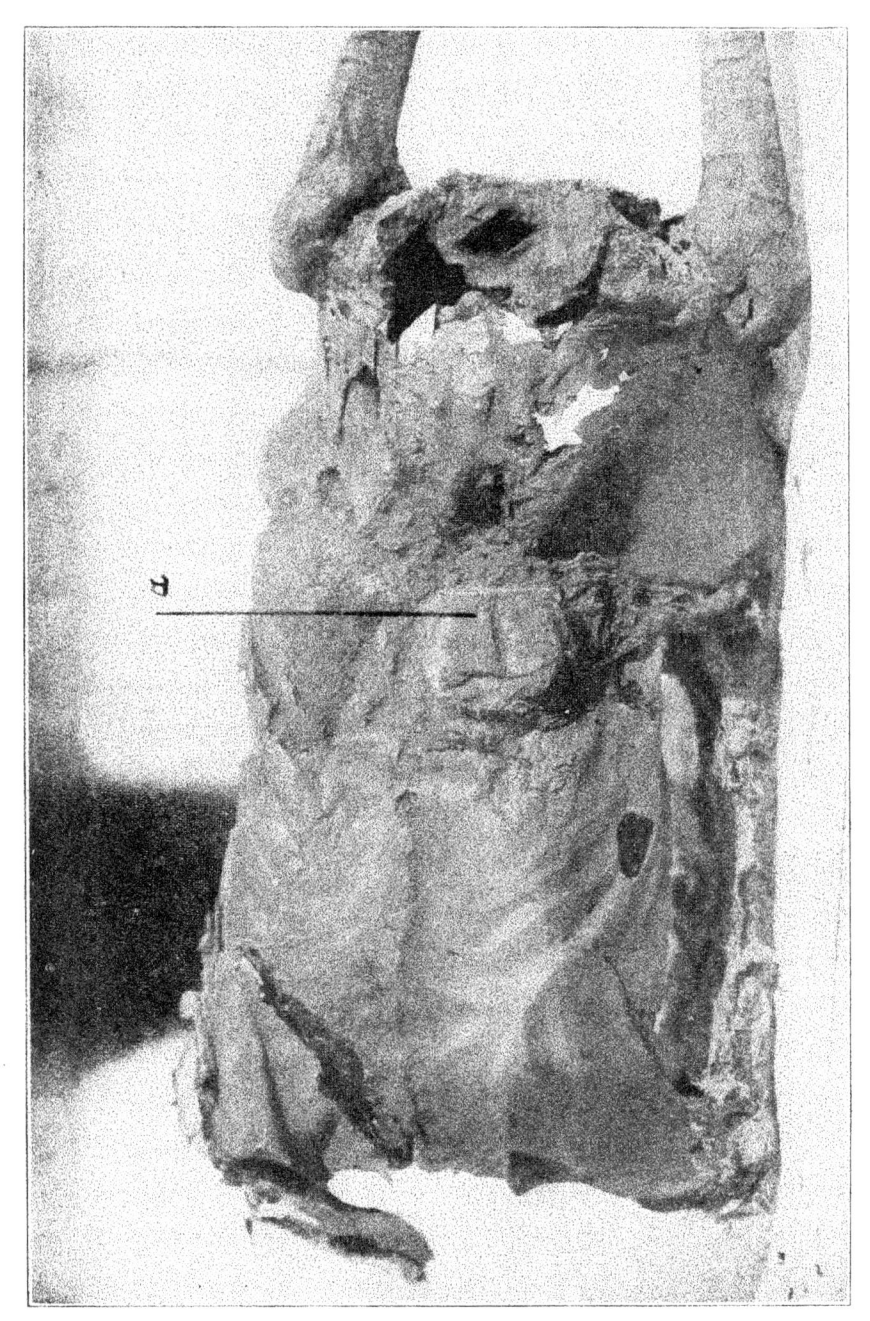

PLATE XXXV

FIG. 6

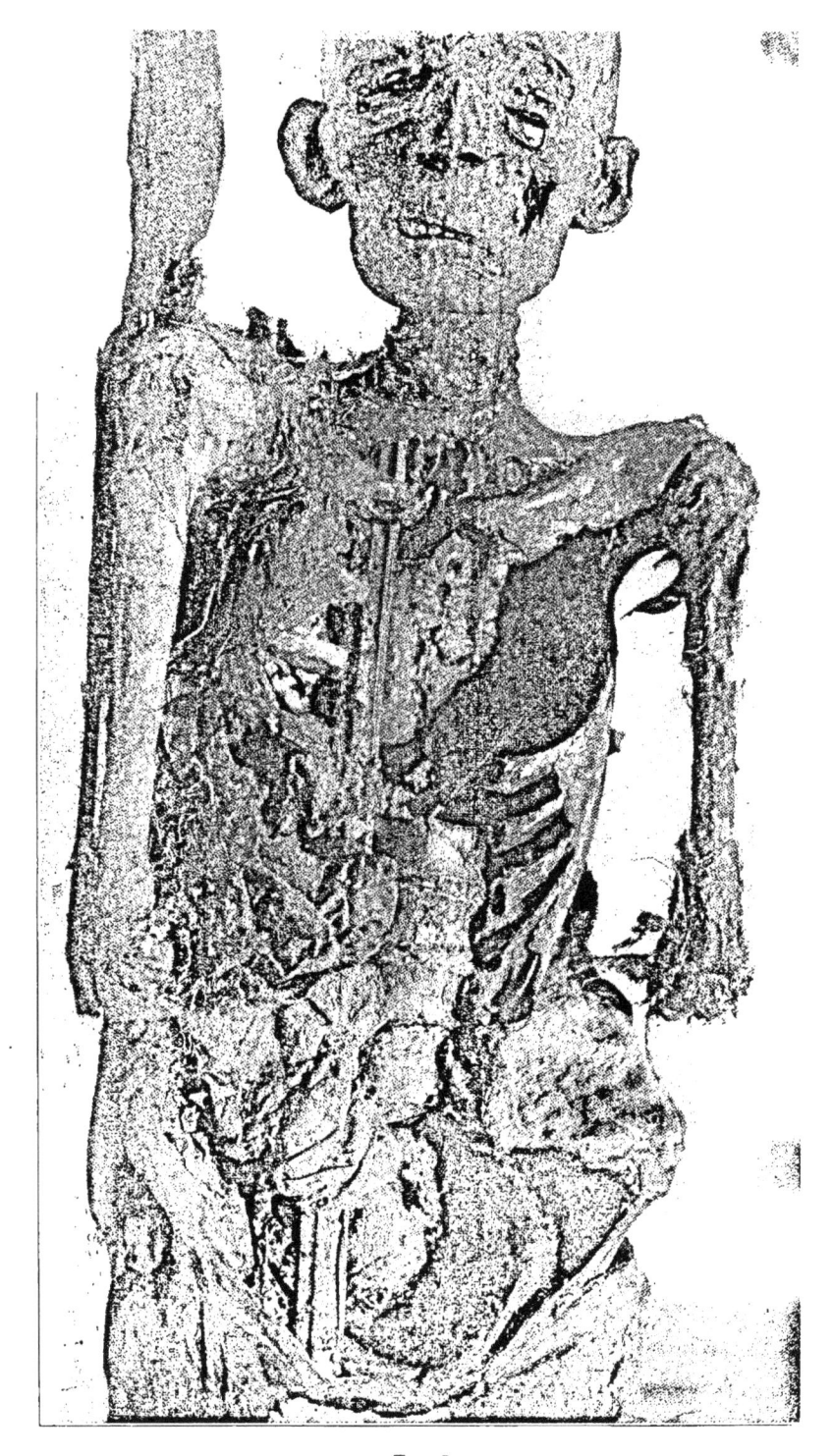

Fig. 8

FIG. 9

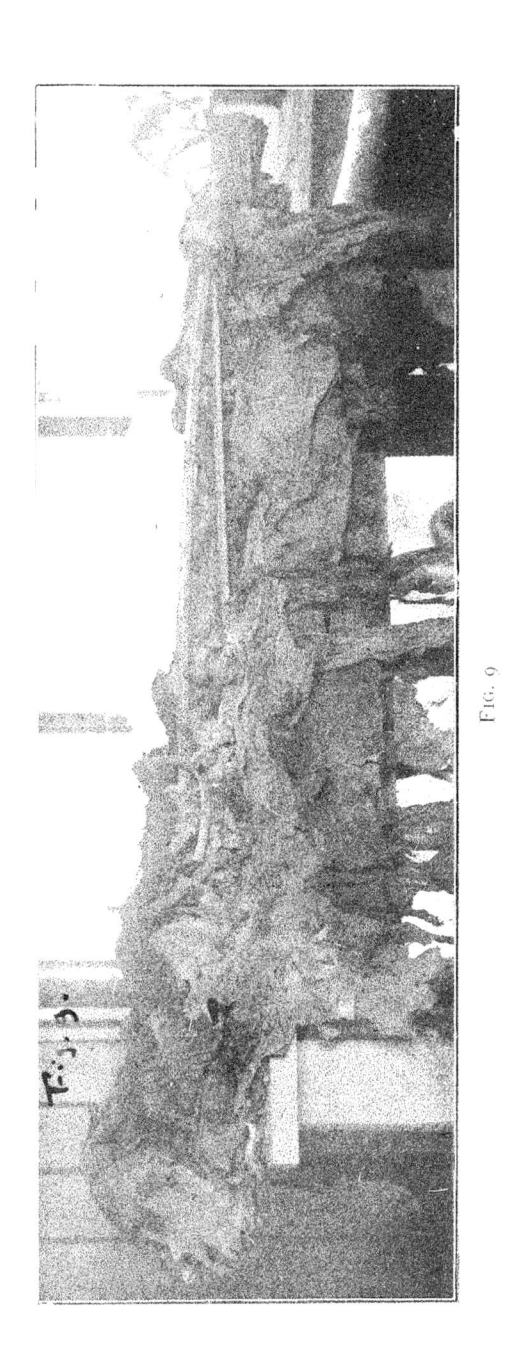

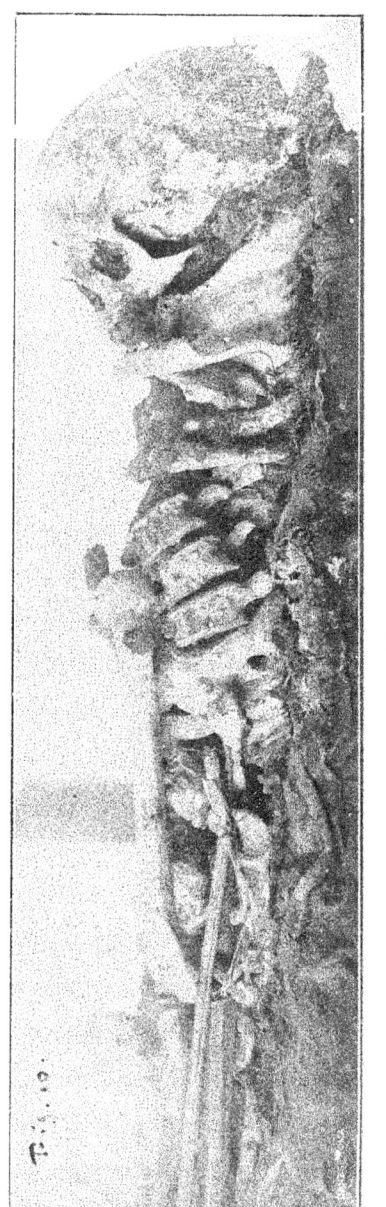

FIG. 10

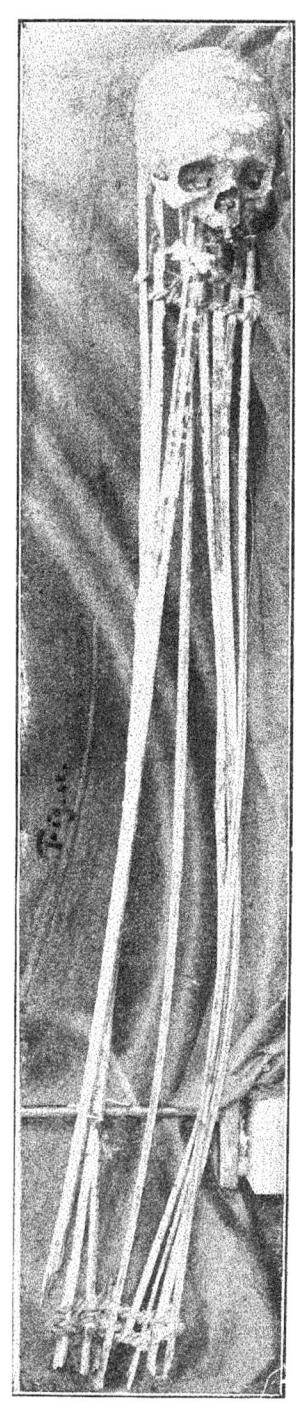

FIG. 11

ON PATHOLOGICAL LESIONS FOUND IN COPTIC BODIES (400-500 A.D.)

(*Journal of Pathology and Bacteriology*, Vol. XVIII [1913])

A word of explanation for the subject-matter of this paper is necessary.

In trying to express clearly the object of the studies which Dr. Fouquet, Dr. Elliot Smith, Dr. Wood Jones, Mr. Shattock, Dr. Ferguson, Dr. Rietti, and I have published during the last few years, I found no word exactly suitable. Hence, I coined the word "palaeopathology." Palaeontology is defined as "the science of extinct forms of life": by *palaeopathology*, however, I do not mean the science of extinct diseases, but *the science of the diseases which can be demonstrated in human and animal remains of ancient times.* I did not adopt this term without consulting several Greek friends, notably that excellent scholar, Dr. Demetriades, who assured me that the word carried the meaning which I attributed to it.

The Coptic bodies which I have studied were given to me by Professor Breccia, curator of the Alexandria Archaeological Museum, and came from Antinoë in Upper Egypt. They dated from the fifth to the sixth centuries after Christ, and were therefore about fourteen to fifteen hundred years old.

It is certain that most of these people were Christians, as the shirts in which they were dressed were decorated with embroideries typical of Christian times, and a beautiful Coptic cross was carved on one of the coffins.

The bodies had been originally enclosed in wooden coffins and buried in sand. Some years ago they were dug up and enclosed in rough deal coffins. When handed over to me for examination, they were dressed in the long linen shirts in which they had been buried. From the embroideries adorning these garments I concluded that the people had belonged to a wealthy class of the community.[1]

[1] These embroideries, now cleaned and looking almost new, are deposited in the Alexandria Museum.

Remains of strong leather boots were found on some of them. In one case the boots were well preserved and reached almost to the knee. The point is interesting, as some lesions discovered in the phalanges (Plate XLIII, Figs. 22 and 23) might be attributed, with some probability, to the wearing of tight footgear.

These bodies differed considerably from the mummies of preceding periods. Never having been opened by the embalmer, the organs were in situ, and they contained no resin, gum, or any materials (such as mud, sand, rags, sawdust, etc.) generally used in Old Egypt for packing the body, after removal of the organs. The only preservative found, and this in two cases only, was common salt. In one, a lump of salt, the size of a man's fist was lying on the abdomen, and Mr. Lucas, of the Survey Laboratory in Cairo, pronounced it to be sodium chloride. In another, small lumps of the same material had been scattered over the abdomen and chest.

There was nothing to show that the body had been macerated, for the skin, where no insects had penetrated, was untouched and the epidermis readily demonstrated. In one body, however, there was in the lumbar region a distinct swelling, and when opened a large abscess cavity was revealed. The contents to the naked eye were grey, granular, and easily removed. No cause for this abscess was discovered (Plate XXXIX, Fig. 2a).

The nails, which had evidently been cleaned and cut after death, were not tied to the fingers. The hair of the head was long (Plate XXXIX, Fig. 1), both in males and females, and all the adult men had yellowish-red beards.[1]

The penis had suffered considerable damage during the 1,400 years which had elapsed since death, so that, in most cases, I could not make sure whether it had been circumcised or not. In one case it had certainly not been circumcised.

During the process of desiccation, the hands and feet had become greatly contorted and were often typically claw-shaped. The bones of the hands and feet, however, were found normal, except for the lesions to be described further on.

The bodies, therefore, could not be called mummies in the sense in which that word is generally used. They had undergone no

[1] I could not make sure whether this red colour was due to henna or not.

artificial process except that, at one time, they had been covered, more or less extensively, with salt. The real preservative had been the dry, Egyptian sand.

Unfortunately for our purpose, the hot, moist climate of Alexandria had produced evil effects on these remains. Innumerable moulds had grown during the last two years in the acid tissues, and, occasionally, the internal organs had become converted into a sticky, glue-like, black mass with which nothing could be done; in others, however, the organs were in a very fair state of preservation. Crystals of fatty acids often covered the internal parts, especially the liver.

The *brain* was always present, not having been tampered with in ancient times. As a rule, the dura mater (Plate XLII, Fig. 9) was still adherent to the cranium; the falx cerebri (Plate XLII, Fig. 10) was perfect and the shrivelled brain lay at the back of the head (Plate XLII, Fig. 9). The lobes of the brain and some of the convolutions were recognisable, whereas the cerebellum was represented by a crumbling yellowish mass of no particular structure. The *medulla oblongata* and the *spinal cord* had completely disappeared. The *spinal dura mater* was perfect.

The *lungs* (Plate XL, Fig. 3) usually lay flat at the back of the pleural cavity. They were jet-black, not thicker than a stout piece of cardboard, and traces of adhesions were frequently found. Sometimes these organs were retracted and pressed against the side of the chest wall; they had shrunk to a length of about 6 inches and measured not more than half an inch in thickness. Nevertheless, the bronchi were recognisable with the microscope, and the alveolar structure of the organ could be made out. The alveoli, of course, were less than one-fifth the size of normal, and the whole microscopical structure had what might be described as a Lilliputian appearance. The lymphatic glands of the chest could not be found as a rule.

The *heart* (Plate XL, Fig. 3) was usually represented by a tube-like, yellow, crumbling mass. The striated fibres were easily demonstrated, and in some cases even the valves were seen. On the whole, however, this viscus was badly preserved, and its examination disappointing.

The whole mass of the *intestines*, shrivelled up to an almost incredible degree, often came away with the abdominal wall. By appropriate treatment fairly large pieces of intestine (12 inches in length) were obtained, but in spite of every possible care I seldom demonstrated greater lengths of the intestinal canal. Under the microscope the coats of the intestine were visible; and though the columnar epithelium lining of the mucous membrane had disappeared, the glands were in a remarkably fine state of preservation, except that the epithelium cells had run together. With haematoxylin the epithelium cells stained yellow, and the connective tissue was of a beautiful blue.

A remarkable fact was that in three bodies the *rectum* was enormously distended by a brown mass, consisting almost entirely of vegetable fibres, which the botanist to whom I showed them and I were unable to identify. This vegetable material was mixed with a brownish, thick substance, probably faeces, which dissolved easily in water, carbonate of soda, and alcohol. Prolapse of the rectum was seen in two cases (Plate XXXIX, Fig. 1). I have found similar masses of vegetable fibres in a dried body of the XIIth Dynasty, and in a boy of the Greek period (Plate XL, Fig. 4). In the latter, the intestine formed a large lump in the left iliac fossa, the sigmoid flexure being enormously distended. I cannot help thinking that the vegetable matter had been introduced either by mouth or anus during the last illness for some therapeutic purpose.

The *liver* (Plate XLI, Fig. 8), dried up almost into the shape of a tube, was in position in the right flank. The gall bladder was unrecognisable. The liver measured about 16–17 cm. in length, 8 cm. in thickness, and weighed 180 gm. on an average. Its substance, for the first few millimetres near the surface, was rather soft, black, and sticky, and became hard, crumbling, and of a dirty-yellow colour in the deeper regions. The cut surface was more or less granular, and when exposed to air soon became black, soft, and sticky. In an appropriate solution, small pieces, though they never swelled up to any extent, softened considerably and after a time became converted into a yellowish, sticky, gummy mass, which, when hardened in absolute alcohol, could be cut in the usual manner with the microtome.

The microscopical appearance varied considerably. In some cases long strands of homogeneous material only were seen, in which no structure could be made out. Sometimes, on the contrary, the cells were distinct. They measured about one-third of their usual size, were round or irregular in shape, and did not stain except with powerful aniline stains. Not unfrequently the nuclei were distinct in the centre of the cells and looked like vacuoles. Very often the lobular arrangement of the organ was preserved even when the connective tissue, smaller blood vessels, and bile ducts had completely disappeared. Only the larger vessels and the liver cells were left, and they, together with the thicker strands of connective tissue, stained deeply with haematoxylin.

The *spleen* (Plate XLI, Fig. 5), intensely dark in colour, was not always found, in spite of laborious searching. It measured as a rule 6 cm. in length, 4 cm. in breadth, and 2 cm. in thickness. Microscopically very little except strands of connective tissue could be recognised.

The *kidneys* (Plate XLI, Fig. 7) were flat, 1 cm. thick, 10 cm. long, 3 cm. broad, and weighed 10 gm. each. They were discovered easily. Microscopically the tubuli, connective tissue, and glomeruli were demonstrable, though of course they were greatly altered.

The *ovaries, uterus,* and *suprarenal capsules* were not seen, nor was it possible, as a rule; to separate the bladder from the surrounding connective tissue.

The *testicles* were in a very bad state of preservation, all the internal structure, except the thick connective tissue septa, having disappeared.

The *arteries, nerves,* and *muscles* were quite distinct. In two aortae well-marked calcareous plates were found.

A point to be remembered is that all the histological elements had shrunk greatly; and it is impossible to lay down a rule as to the amount of this shrinkage. Usually they were about one-third, and never more than half their natural size, so that it was necessary to work with much higher powers of the microscope than usual. The sections, in spite of numerous washings, always remained stained brownish yellow.

The *bones*, though hard and well preserved, stood maceration rather badly, and care had to be taken not to leave them in water too long. The *cartilages*, always stained intensely black, were perfect, and after maceration in dilute caustic potash could be removed whole.

Altogether sixteen Coptic bodies were examined, namely, six women and ten adult men. Of the six women, two were young girls certainly not more than sixteen years old. They showed no pathological lesions.

LESIONS OF THE TEETH

The general appearance of the teeth did not suggest that much care had been taken of them, as they were often yellow and covered with tartar. In one case, indeed, the deposit of tartar was truly enormous, being at least 2 mm. thick. Attrition was not marked, and the crowns contrasted with those of predynastic skulls of Egypt, which are often ground down to the level of the gums. In most cases, however, serious lesions of the teeth and alveoli were present, and the life of some of these people must have been one of perfect misery, owing to the state of their mouths.

DESCRIPTION OF DENTAL LESIONS FOUND

I. ADULT MAN, PROBABLY ABOUT FORTY-FIVE YEARS OLD.

Teeth missing.[1]—Maxillae: Right first molar and second premolar; left first molar. Mandible: Right second premolar and first molar; left first molar. Teeth not much worn, with exception of left third lower molar. Lower left second premolar *carious* on posterior approximate side.

II. ADULT, BUT NOT OLD.—Basilar suture ossified, other sutures still open.

Teeth missing.—Maxillae: Left first molar and probably first premolar also. Mandible: Third molar.

Other lesions of teeth.—Maxillae: First right molar extensively carious. In connection with the anterior fang (Plate XLIII, Fig. 17 A), an abscess had formed which had perforated through palate into nasal cavity. Track followed by pus evident, and opening into the nasal cavity is nearly the size of threepenny piece. No perforation into antrum. Mandible: Whole outer wall of alveolus of right first molar has been worn away, evidently by suppuration (Plate XLIII, Fig. 25). Tooth itself healthy, though crown somewhat

---

[1] As teeth often drop out after death, I consider as *missing* only those teeth the alveoli of which are completely or almost completely absorbed.

worn. Second molar has one fang only, deeply carious. Judging from size of the alveolus, I conclude that there had been some ulceration round that fang also.

The dental disease was of old standing, and the third molar had fallen out or been removed some time before death. The floor of the alveolus was partially filled up with bone. The top of it, on the other hand, was nearly 1.2 cm. wide, and in all probability there had been an abscess round that tooth also. The suppuration had extended backward along the outer side of the gums round the second and third molar teeth in the upper maxilla, as the bone in that situation is singularly smooth, and its perfectly rounded edge is in sharp contrast with the rugged edge in front. Moreover, the fangs of the teeth are exposed through their whole length owing to the absorption of the alveolar walls.

This man suffered also from chronic nasal disease, from arthritis in the glenoid fossa, from periostitis of the great trochanter of the femur, and chronic spondylitis. Racked as he must have been with dental agony, afflicted with a chronic nasal discharge, and stiff with pain in his hip and spine, his life must have been well-nigh unbearable.

III. ADULT WOMAN, PROBABLY ABOUT TWENTY-SIX YEARS OLD.—Lower third molars present, whereas upper had not emerged.

Teeth missing.—Maxillae: Normal. Mandible: Right first molar; left first and third molars.

Other lesions.—Extensive caries of posterior part of second left molar extending almost to fang. Right second and third molars extensively carious where they touch. Crowns but little worn.

IV. MAN, ADULT BUT NOT AGED, PROBABLY ABOUT THIRTY YEARS OLD.

Teeth missing.—Maxillae: All right premolars and molars. Left second premolar and third molar. Mandible: Right second molar; left molars and premolars.

Other lesions.—Maxillae: Second right incisor, carious. Region occupied by left first and second molars hollowed out into a cavity with deeply pitted floor, measuring 1.5 cm. from before backwards, and 1.2 cm. from side to side. Outer wall of the alveolus of the first molar completely gone. Evidently there had been extensive suppuration round the first and second molars, possibly beginning in the teeth themselves. These had either fallen out or been removed some time before death. It is highly probable also that there had been an abscess round right canine.

V. YOUNG WOMAN, whose third molars had not emerged yet.

Teeth missing.—Mandible: Second left premolar; first right molar, carious; right middle turbinated bone twice the size of the left.

VI. VERY OLD WOMAN.—Upper jaw completely smashed after death, probably at the time body was taken out of the grave, so no examination of it was possible. Mandible: All the teeth with exception of four incisors had disappeared long ago, and alveoli had been completely absorbed.

VII. MAN ABOUT FORTY-FIVE YEARS OLD.—Uncircumcised. All teeth perfect, slightly worn.

VIII. MAN ADVANCED IN AGE.

Teeth missing.—Maxillae (right side): All premolars, first molar, third molar, second molar present. There had been considerable inflammation round it, so that alveolus is almost completely absorbed. Left side: First premolar, second premolar, second and third molars. First molar shows the same alteration as the second molar on other side. Mandible: Left molars and premolars; right second and third molars. There is some attrition of all the teeth.

IX. OLD WOMAN.—All teeth in upper jaw missing (Plate XLIII, Fig. 15). Mandible (right): Molars, premolars, canine, and one incisor. Left: Central incisor, canine, second premolar, and all molars.

ALVEOLAR AND OTHER LESIONS

Perhaps the most striking changes are the signs of periodontitis and suppuration round the roots of the teeth, which were present in a large number of skulls.

Let us examine, for instance, Plate XLIII, Fig. 25, and Plate XLIII, Fig. 17, which come from the same body. Though the teeth are regularly planted, the fangs throughout their whole length are almost bare. This exposure is due to the absorption of the wall of the alveoli; a change generally most marked on the labial border of the teeth. In Plate XLIII, Fig. 25, for instance, it is evident that suppuration had existed round the molar teeth, which were finally contained in a smooth-walled cavity, the walls of which had been completely absorbed. Further, this process of absorption, though less complete, has proceeded along the alveolar borders of the upper maxillae and mandible, leaving the teeth bare and for the most part very loose. In my opinion, we are here in the presence of the pathological lesions produced by suppurating disease of the alveoli or pyorrhoea alveolaris.

Another mandible is very interesting from this point of view (Plate XLIII, Fig. 18). At (*a*) the alveolus has been completely absorbed, a thin bridge of bone superiorly being all that remains of it. At (*c*) the bony alveolus has almost disappeared, only the thinnest possible layer of bone remaining. The pus had evidently burrowed into the deeper parts of the mandible. The alveolus itself is of normal size, and the tooth must have dropped out either just before, or possibly after, death. In the neighbouring teeth the same process had been going on, for the fangs are partly bare, and at (*b*) a sinus has been formed. Without doubt that tooth was on the point of dropping out. It is very probable, if not absolutely certain, that the loss of the other teeth was due to this process also.

The upper jaws of the same skull are completely edentulous, and has been so for some time before death, for the alveoli have been absorbed so completely that not a trace of them is left. The suppurating process, therefore, had attacked the whole mouth, and had lasted for years before the patient finally succumbed.

In another skull one of the teeth was on the point of being shed, one fang being completely, and the other almost completely, bare, so that the tooth was fixed to the skull by one fang only and by the centre of the tooth between the fangs (Plate XLIV, Fig. 29).

As a rule, the teeth in the neighbourhood were perfectly sound, and not carious. In a few cases, however, a certain amount of odontitis had taken place and calculi had formed on the outer surface of the teeth. Sometimes, on the contrary, absorption of the tooth round the neck had taken place (Plate XLIII, Fig. 18).

The alveoli were gradually absorbed, and this absorption appears to have started from the bottom and gradually worked its way towards the neck of the tooth, so that after a time, in the molar region for instance, the fangs were laid completely bare, and the teeth were fixed not by the fangs at all, but by the centre between the fangs.

Altogether, therefore, the disease was characterised in Coptic times as it is now, by (1) loosening of the teeth; (2) absorption of the alveoli; (3) formation of fistulae.

Transverse striation of the teeth was very evident in one person (Plate XLIII, Fig. 20). The cause of it could not be ascertained.

OSSEOUS LESIONS

I. ADULT MAN, BUT NOT AGED, PROBABLY ABOUT THIRTY YEARS OLD.

Spondylitis limited to the first five cervical vertebrae.—Atlas: Slight thickening of bone on the anterior arch cavity for odontoid process. Axis: Normal, except that top of odontoid process is covered by a little cap of new bone, measuring 3×3 mm. Third cervical vertebra: Upper surface normal. Left inferior articular surface slightly enlarged; right articular surface greatly enlarged, measuring 1.5×1.3 cm. Deposit of new bone all round the edge, and surface has a worm-eaten appearance.

Right upper articulating surface and left lower articulating surface of the fourth cervical vertebra and corresponding superior articulating surface of the fifth greatly enlarged, with a worm-eaten appearance.

Lower articulating surface of the fifth cervical vertebra and rest of the vertebral column normal.

Although the characteristic lesions of spondylitis are in this case rather slight, and limited to one side of the cervical part of the vertebral column, the man must have had a very stiff neck, causing great limitation of movement.

Arthritic and other lesions in the same person.—This person is one in whom very severe dental disease was present (II). He was an adult, but by no means an old man.

Glenoid fossae: Anterior part of the glenoid fossa is much thickened and partly eburnated. On right side there is considerable thickening of bone, forming an irregular patch, measuring 2×1.2 cm., with a thickness of 0.2 cm. It extends posteriorly almost to bottom of the fossa. Condyles of mandible are normal.

Pathological changes in vertebral column merely consist in some overlapping of anterior inferior border of the second and the anterior superior border of the third cervical vertebrae. Similar changes are seen in sixth and seventh cervical vertebrae, in dorsal vertebrae from the seventh to the twelfth, and in lumbar vertebrae from first to fourth. Disease is most marked in dorsal region, where new bone forms a thick irregular festoon round anterior border. Last lumbar vertebrae, sacrum, and coccyx normal.

Pelvis shows no change, except for some distinct thickening round lower border of acetabulum.

Right nostril of the same mummy shows a curious appearance (Plate XLIII, Fig. 12). The middle turbinated bone on that side is conspicuously swollen, its free extremity being about four times as thick as that of its fellow. Swelling gradually tapers towards the attached border and occupies only anterior two-thirds of the bone, posterior third being practically normal.

This swelling had deflected the bony nasal septum very markedly to the left, and this is also perforated by numerous small holes, which, however, may have been formed post mortem.

Left middle turbinated bone had a very ragged edge, but is not noticeably swollen. Both inferior turbinated bones are practically normal.

Left femur: Thick mass of new bone fills up cavity for the ligamentum teres almost entirely, and projects over borders of cavity especially on the inner side. New bone measures 2.5×1.5 cm. (Plate XLIV, Fig. 30). Great trochanter is covered by a somewhat thick deposit of rough new bone. Lower end of femur would be normal were it not for a patch of spongy new bone about 1 mm. in thickness and the size of a threepenny bit on the lower and inner surface of the articulation, and some thickening on inner and outer borders of condyles.

The right femur (Plate XLIV, Fig. 30) shows similar changes, especially in cavity of ligamentum teres. New bone in this position measures 2 cm. in its longest and 1.5 cm. in its broadest diameter. There is some slight thickening round the edge of the lower end of the femur. A distinct rough-fitted groove separates the new bone from the old, and the whole gives the impression of a chronic process. On the other side there is a similar mass 2 cm. long, 1 cm. broad, and 4 mm. thick on the upper border near the tip, which is somewhat rough though otherwise normal.

II. VERY MUSCULAR MAN.

Spondylitis deformans (IV).—All insertions of muscles extremely prominent. The ensiform cartilage shows a curious defect in ossification (Plate XLIII, Fig. 13).

Cervical vertebrae, atlas: Formation of new bone round superior border of notch, so that top of the odontoid process is overlapped by bone growing from atlas.

Lower articular facets of third vertebra greatly enlarged, especially on right side, where they are rough and irregular, with a thin layer of new bone on inner border. Upper articular facets of fourth cervical correspondingly enlarged, especially right, which measures 2 cm., from above downwards. All other cervical vertebrae have bifid spinous processes, though otherwise normal.

Third dorsal vertebra has a strong anterior median ridge of bone projecting for about 1.2 cm., corresponding to a similar ridge on fourth.

Similar lesions on the sixth, seventh, eighth, and ninth dorsal vertebrae. Lesions specially marked on eighth and ninth dorsal vertebrae, where the corresponding ridges form a lateral prolongation, 1 cm. broad at the base, and which projects for 1.2 cm. externally.

Lesions of vertebral column, phalanges, fibula, and patellae (III).—Marked overlipping of anterior borders of bodies of twelfth vertebrae and all lumbar vertebrae.

Terminal phalanges of feet and hands (Plate XLIII, Figs. 21, 22, and 23) rough and thickened at proximal and distal ends, especially at point of insertion of great flexor muscles, and one has the impression that this person suffered from chronic synovitis. In both great toes (Plate XLIII, Figs. 22 and 23) the point of insertion of the flexor longus hallucis is greatly deepened and surrounded by a ridge of strong new bone (Plate XLIII, Figs. 22, 23 A). Moreover, the proximal ends of both halluces present marked exostoses (Plate XLIII, Figs. 22 and 23). The distal ends of all the phalanges of hands and feet are exceedingly rough, as if they had been worn away by prolonged inflammation.

Scapulae: A mass of strong new bone has formed at the tip and upper border of the right acromion (Plate XLIV, Fig. 28). This extends for a length of 3 cm. and has an irregular upper border with a maximum width of 1.3 cm.

Fibula: Ossification of lateral ligaments (Plate XLIII, Fig. 11).

Patellae: Ossification of lateral ligaments.

Lesions of phalanges and localised spondylitis deformans (XII).—Terminal phalanges of both big toes show same changes as the preceding case. Eleventh and twelfth dorsal vertebrae show prolongation of bone on anterior border = localised spondylitis deformans.

Moreover, upper articular surface for rib of twelfth dorsal (Plate XLIII, Fig. 19.1) enormously enlarged, white, ivory-like, corresponding to similar facet on rib (Plate XLIII, Fig. 16 A).

III. MALE.

Exostosis of pelvis and other lesions (VIII).—Skull: All sutures well advanced in ossification.

Pelvis: Plate XLIII, Fig. 24, and Plate XLIV, Fig. 27, give very good pictures of a remarkable exostosis of that bone. The dimensions of this exostosis are as follows: Length = 5 cm.; thickness at tip = 2.25 cm.; depth at B = 2 cm.; depth at A = 0.5 cm.; base = 4 cm. Exostosis is smooth, though deeply grooved at B and C, as if by blood vessels. There are no signs of inflammation in neighbouring bones, and symphysis is quite normal.

Last lumbar vertebra shows signs of inflammation (Plate XLIV, Fig. 26 A), and there is some slight thickening round the anatomical necks in the humeri.

On left fibula there is a sharp transverse cut, about 1 cm. long and less than 1 cm. deep. No scar of skin noticeable, but this may be due to the very bad state of the teguments.

Injuries.—The only injuries discovered were the transverse cut on the fibula, mentioned above, and a healed fractured rib shown in Plate XLIII, Fig. 14.

LESIONS OF SOFT PARTS

Hypertrophy of spleen.—In order to ascertain whether the organs were enlarged or the reverse, their average weight had to be

	Weight		Length		Breadth
	Coptic	Present Day	Coptic	Present Day	Coptic
	gm.	gm.	cm.	cm.	cm.
Liver	180	1,609	165	321	8
Spleen	12	171	6	12–13	4
Kidneys	10	140	10	10.8–11.4	3

ascertained. I give here, therefore, the weights and lengths of the spleen, liver, and kidneys of five Coptic bodies, and compare them with the average weight of the same organs in adults of the present time.

These Coptic weights correspond closely with those of the same organs of a dried body of the XIIth Dynasty. Roughly speaking, the organs weigh in Coptic bodies about one-tenth to one-fifteenth of their original weight. The length of the liver and spleen of Coptic bodies is diminished by about one-half, whereas the kidneys retain very nearly their normal length.

One spleen, however, instead of weighing 12 gm., weighed 27 gm., that is, nearly double the weight of the normal. It measured 20 mm. in length more than the normal spleen. The weight of the liver of the same person was 186 gm.—that is, a little greater than normal. In this case, therefore, we have evidence that there was during life some hypertrophy of the spleen.

The second case (XII) was still more interesting. The dimensions of the spleen (Plate XLI, Fig. 6) were: Length, 16 cm.; weight, 62 gm.; breadth, 8 cm.—that is, the spleen was at least twice as long, twice as broad, and weighed five times as much as the normal spleen of Coptic bodies. In the photograph the breadth is not seen, because the spleen was bent on itself; an appearance which, owing to the uniform blackness, could not be brought out in the photograph. The liver also was distinctly larger than normal as it weighed 280 instead of 180 gm.

Microscopical examination threw no light on the causation of the enlargement of the volume of these organs, for an enormous growth of moulds completely obscured the structure of the organ.

To speculate on the actual cause of this hypertrophy would be useless. Malaria was most probably the cause of it, and this hypothesis is supported by the fact that up to the present day it is not a rare disease in Upper Egypt where these people lived.

I may mention, in this connection, that I found a similarly enlarged spleen in a Fayoum mummy, dating from the Roman period. The Fayoum Province is, even now, infested with malaria.

SUMMARY

Already in several papers I have drawn attention to the bad state of the teeth of ancient Egyptians.

It would be difficult, however, to find anywhere so many diseased teeth as in these Coptic bodies. Practically every skull, with the exception of two,[1] had some serious dental defects. This may perhaps be accounted for by the fact that very little care of the dentition appears to have been taken. The thick incrustations of tartar are sufficient evidence that the Copts did not clean their teeth at all. In many peoples and animals the absence of the toothbrush is compensated for by the fact that the food is hard, fibrous, and raw, requiring a good deal of chewing, which mechanically cleans the teeth. In ancient Coptic times this does not appear to have been the case, for, in contrast to the predynastic bodies in which attrition is very marked, this is slight, in fact being less marked than it is in Egyptians of the present day.

It would appear, therefore, that the Copts of Antinoë lived chiefly on cooked, soft food, chewed without an effort. Caries, moreover, was extremely common, and was possibly due to the nature of the food consumed.

The fact that many of these people suffered from periodontitis and pyorrhoea alveolaris[2] may perhaps have been due to small particles of food lodging between the teeth and setting up putrefaction, inflammation, and suppuration. In Alexandria, at the present time, the poorer class of natives take very little care of the teeth, and it is perhaps owing to this fact that periodontitis and pyorrhoea alveolaris are exceedingly common among them. My friend, Mr. Webb Jones, surgeon to the Government Hospital, tells me that it occurs in almost every patient frequenting this hospital. Many Europeans suffer from it also.

Lastly, I found no certain evidence that these people knew anything about dentistry. Surely, had the practice of even simple tooth-drawing been common, such lesions as I have described, and the accompanying excruciating pain, would have been avoided by this very simple operation.

The occurrence of spondylitis deformans among ancient Copts is one more proof that the disease has existed throughout Egypt

[1] I do not give a detailed account of five skulls which were given to a foreign museum. As the mouths were not opened in order not to spoil them, I cannot say for certain how many teeth were bad, but I ascertained that all of them had diseased teeth.

[2] The disease is almost as old as the human race. At any rate, I have found evidence of it in prehistoric skulls and in Greek, Roman, Peruvian, Mexican, Merovingian, and German skulls.

from the remotest times and is independent of climate. It has been found by Dr. Rietti and myself in bodies buried close to the Mediterranean shores, in bodies from Upper Egypt and in Nubia. Quite lately I have found an example of it in a skeleton from the Meroitic kingdom (300 B.C.) and buried in the Tropics at Merawi, one of the hottest and dryest places in the world, and others in Christian skeletons at Abou Menas and Abou Sir in the comparatively damp region of Mariout. These skeletons date from about 500 A.D.

A peculiarity of the disease met with in Coptic bodies is that it was as a rule localised to few vertebrae, and in one case to two vertebrae and one rib.

The exostosis of the pelvis and the inflammatory lesions described in various parts of the skeleton call for no particular comment.

The arthritis of the tempero-maxillary condition described in this paper was a rare disease among Egyptians, for I do not possess another specimen.

Cases of hypertrophy of the middle turbinated bones in ancient peoples have not been described before, as far as I know. Since writing this paper, however, I have seen another Egyptian skull, dating from about 1000 B.C., in which the nasal passages on both sides were completely blocked by hypertrophy of the turbinated bones, and I have also found similar unilateral lesions in two Greek skulls dating from the time of Alexander the Great.

Pathological changes of the soft parts, recognisable macroscopically, were not common. Judging from the two cases of hypertrophied spleen which were found, it appears probable that these people suffered from malaria, but nothing definite can be said until a large number of bodies coming from the same locality have been examined.

DESCRIPTION OF PLATES XXXIX–XLIV[1]
(For particulars see text)

PLATE XXXIX

FIG. 1.—Coptic body with prolapse of rectum. The body, with the exception of the head and feet, was dressed in a long linen shirt. Notice that the parts not covered by the sheet have remained white.

FIG. 2.—Body with (a) deep abscess in back.

[1] Most of the photographs by Dr. Rietti.

PLATE XL
Fig. 3.—Lungs and heart stained intensely black.
Fig. 4.—Distended rectum and sigmoid flexure.

PLATE XLI
Fig. 5.—Normal spleen.
Fig. 6.—Hypertrophied spleen.
Fig. 7.—Kidney.
Fig. 8.—Liver.

PLATE XLII
Fig. 9.—Skull with cap removed. D.M.=dura mater. Part of the brain visible in situ.
Fig. 10.—Skull showing falx cerebri in situ.

PLATE XLIII
Fig. 11.—Fibula. Ossification of lateral ligament.
Fig. 12.—Hypertrophied middle turbinated bone.
Fig. 13.—Defect of ossification in sternum.
Fig. 14.—Fractured rib.
Fig. 15.—Edentulous upper jaw. The loss of teeth was probably due to pyorrhoea alveolaris, as the corresponding mandible showed all the lesions of that disease.
Fig. 16.—Rib with articular facet (*A*) greatly enlarged and eburnated.
Fig. 17.—From the same skull as Fig. 25. The first molar (*A*) is extensively decayed and a sinus leads from it into the nasal cavity.
Fig. 18.—Pyorrhoea alveolaris. At (*a*) the tooth has fallen out, and the alveolus has been completely absorbed, except for a thin ridge of bone at the superior border. At (*c*) the alveolus has been almost completely absorbed. The alveolus of the neighbouring outer tooth has been almost completely absorbed, so that the fang is nearly bare, and at (*b*) a sinus has formed. There has been absorption round the neck of that tooth also.
Fig. 19.—Dorsal vertebra with (*a*) an eburnated, enlarged facet for articulation with rib. The lower anterior border of body presents a marked exostosis (*f*).
Fig. 20.—Teeth with marked transverse striation.
Fig. 21.—Terminal phalanx. There is considerable formation of new bone round insertion of flexor digitorum profundus. The ungual extremity is very rough.
Fig. 22.—Hallux with exostosis due to chronic inflammation. At *A* an osseous ridge round insertion of long flexor (tight boots?). The ungual end is greatly roughened and has a worm-eaten appearance.
Fig. 23.—Similar to Fig. 22.

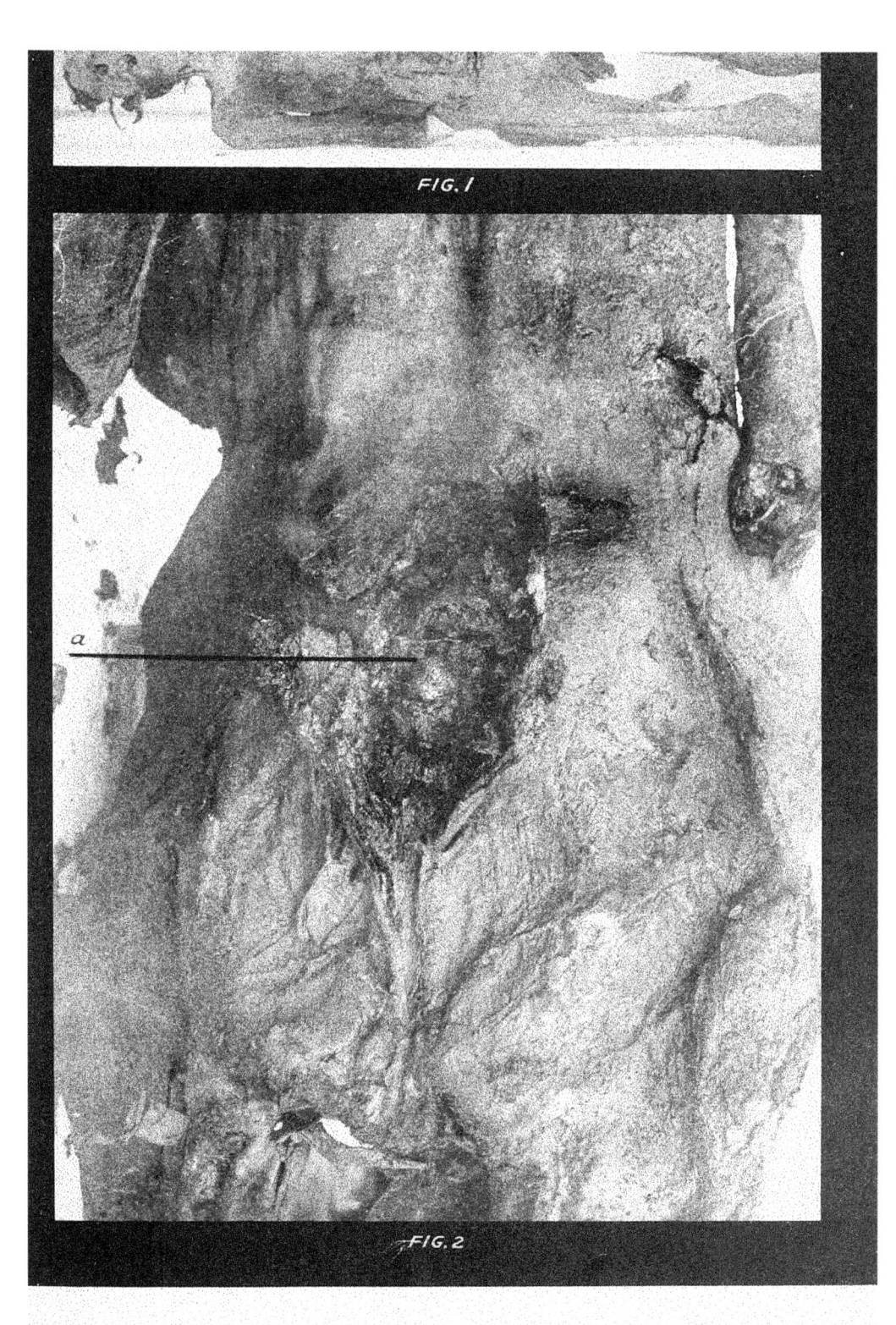

FIG. 1

FIG. 2

PLATE XL

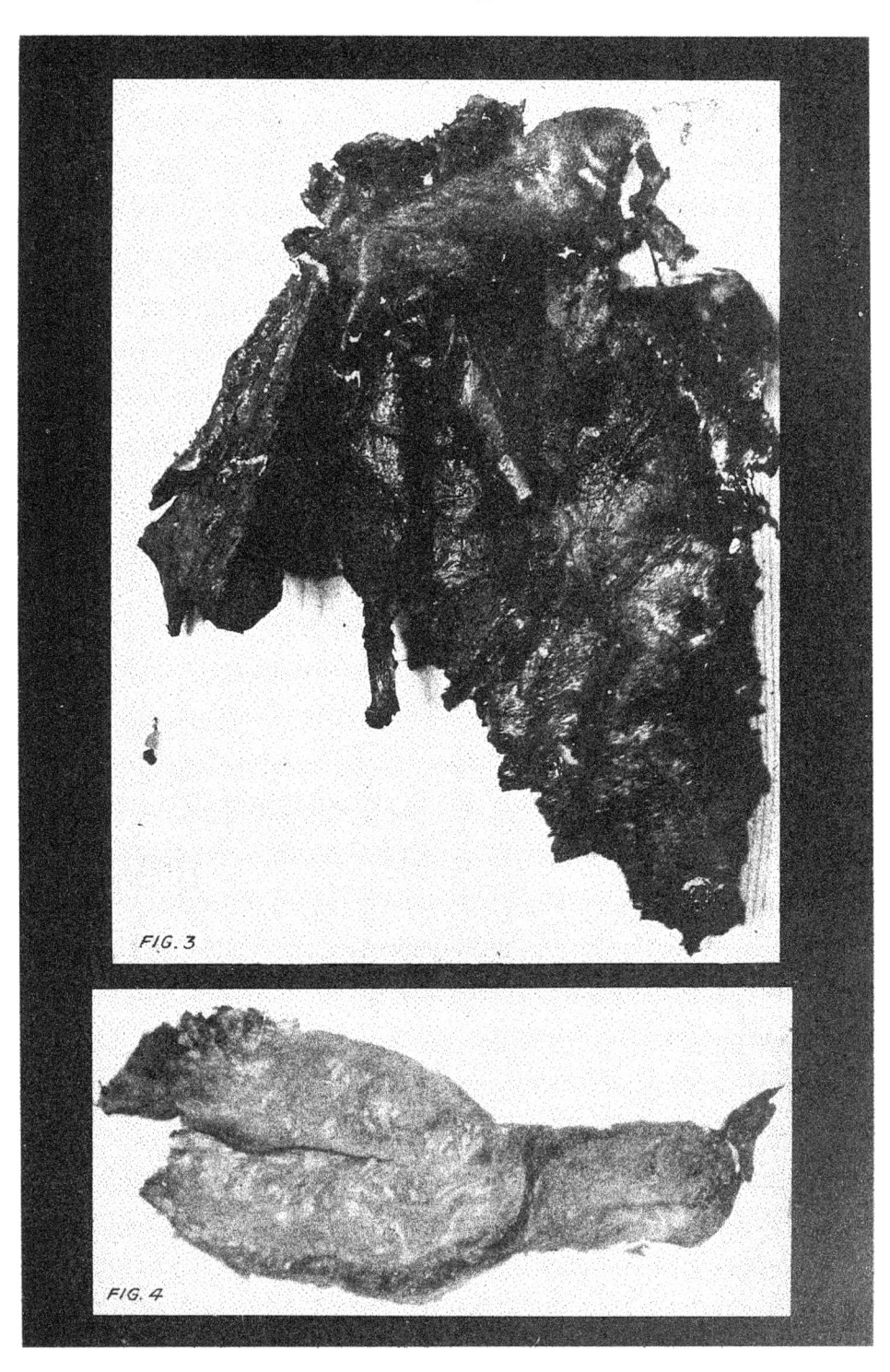

FIG. 3

FIG. 4

PLATE XLI

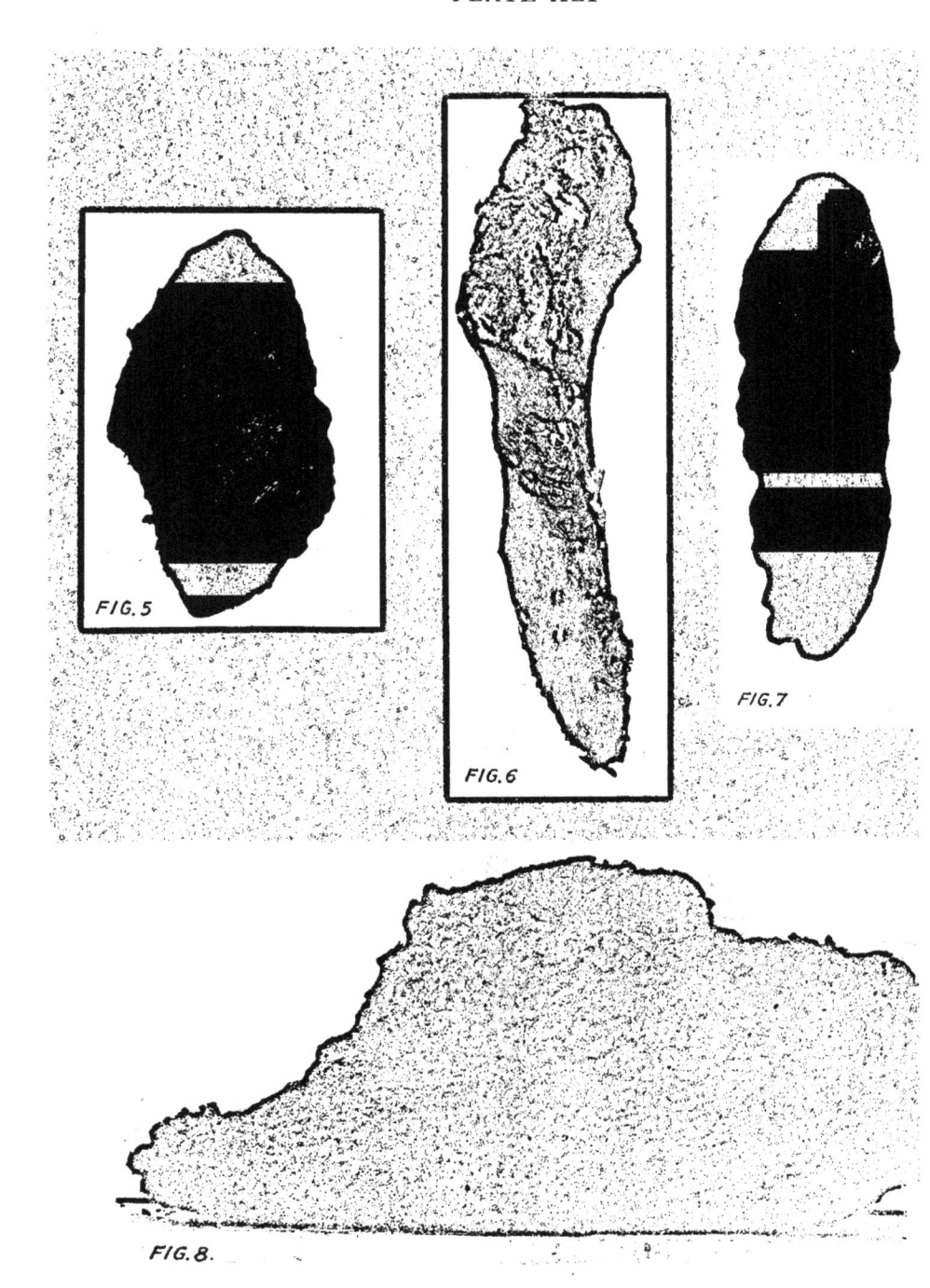

FIG. 5

FIG. 6

FIG. 7

FIG. 8.

FIG. 9

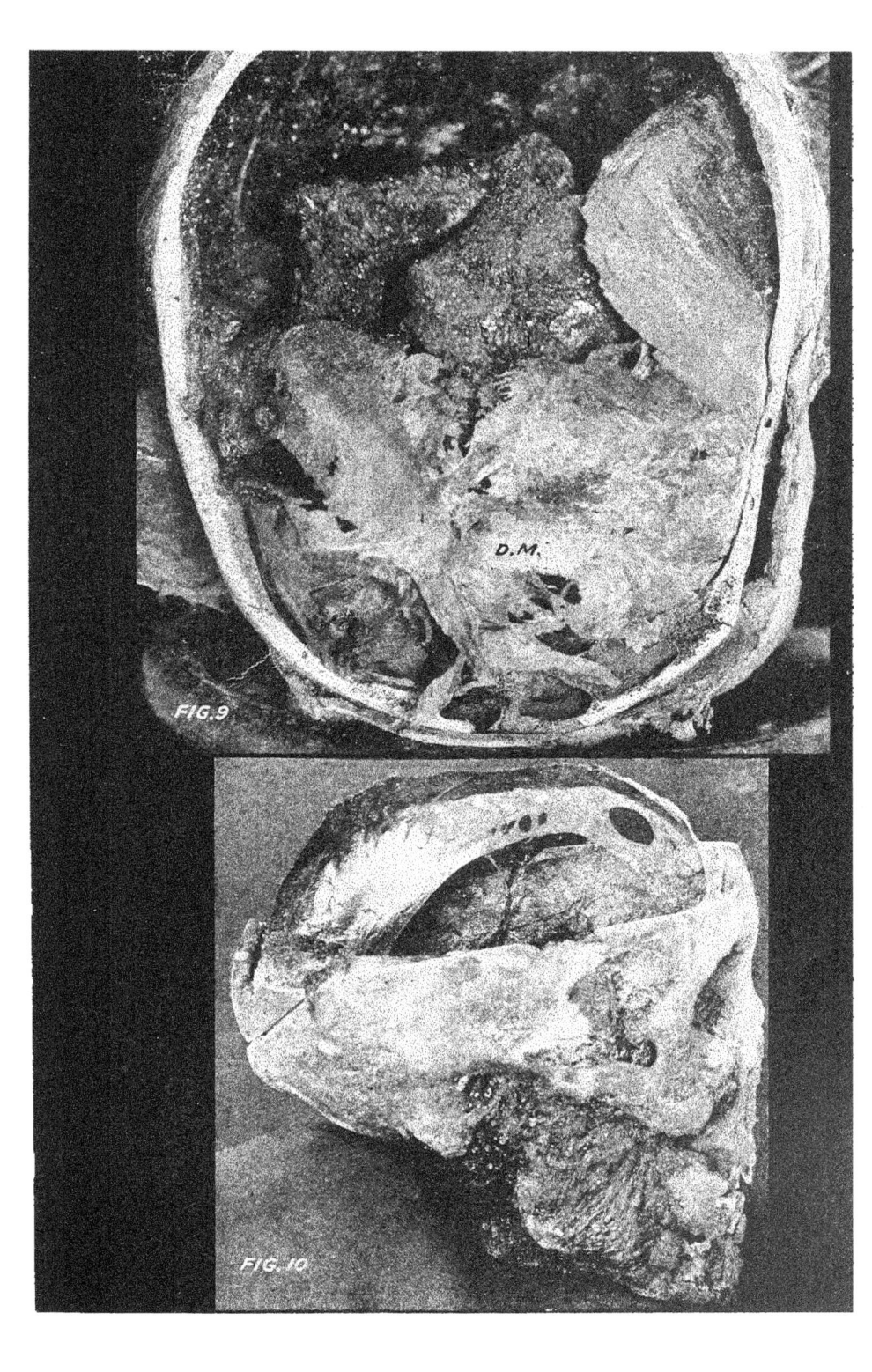

FIG. 10

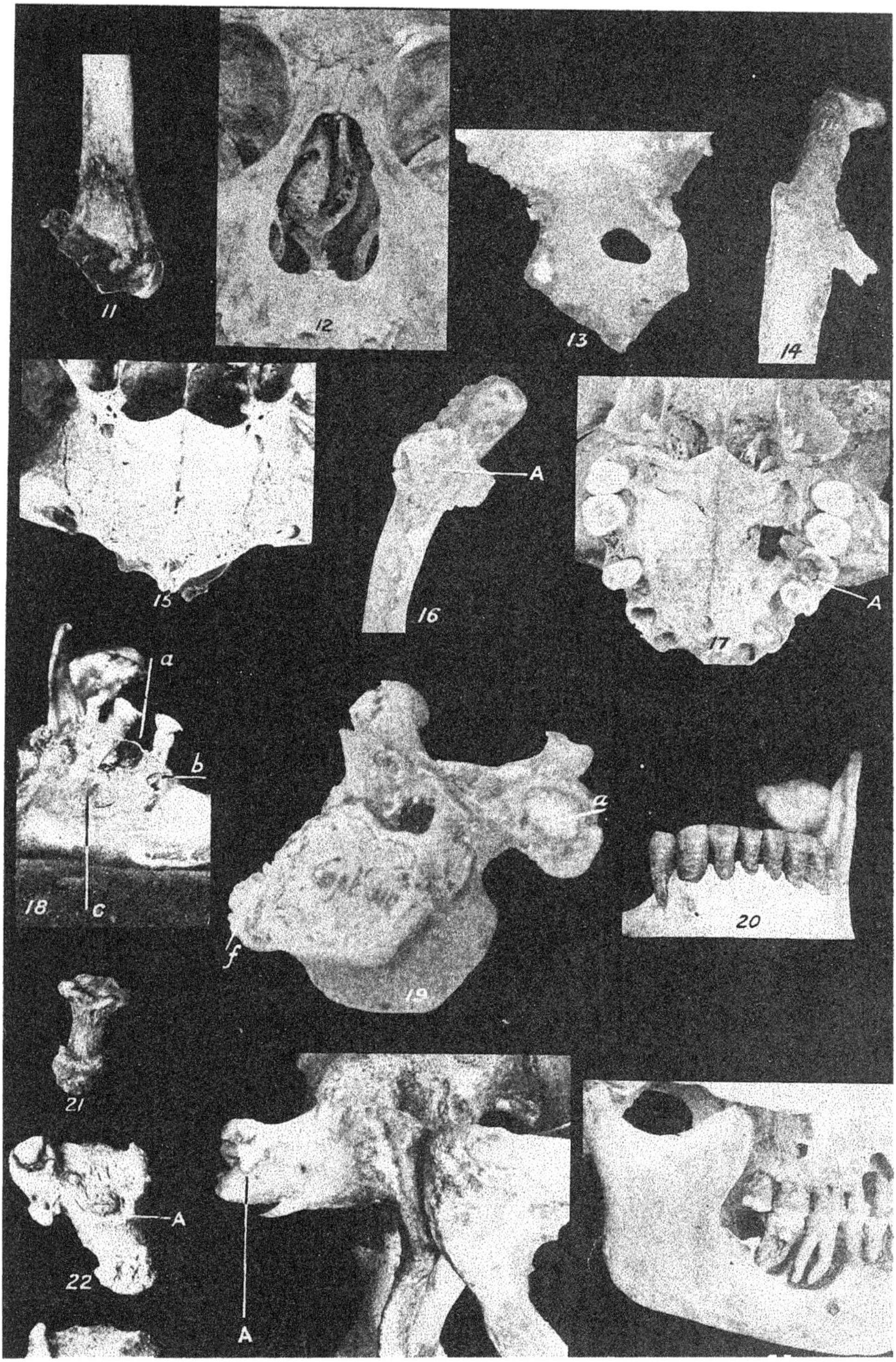
11
12
13
14
15
16
A
17
A
a
b
18
c
a
f
19
20
21
A
22
A

PLATE XLIV

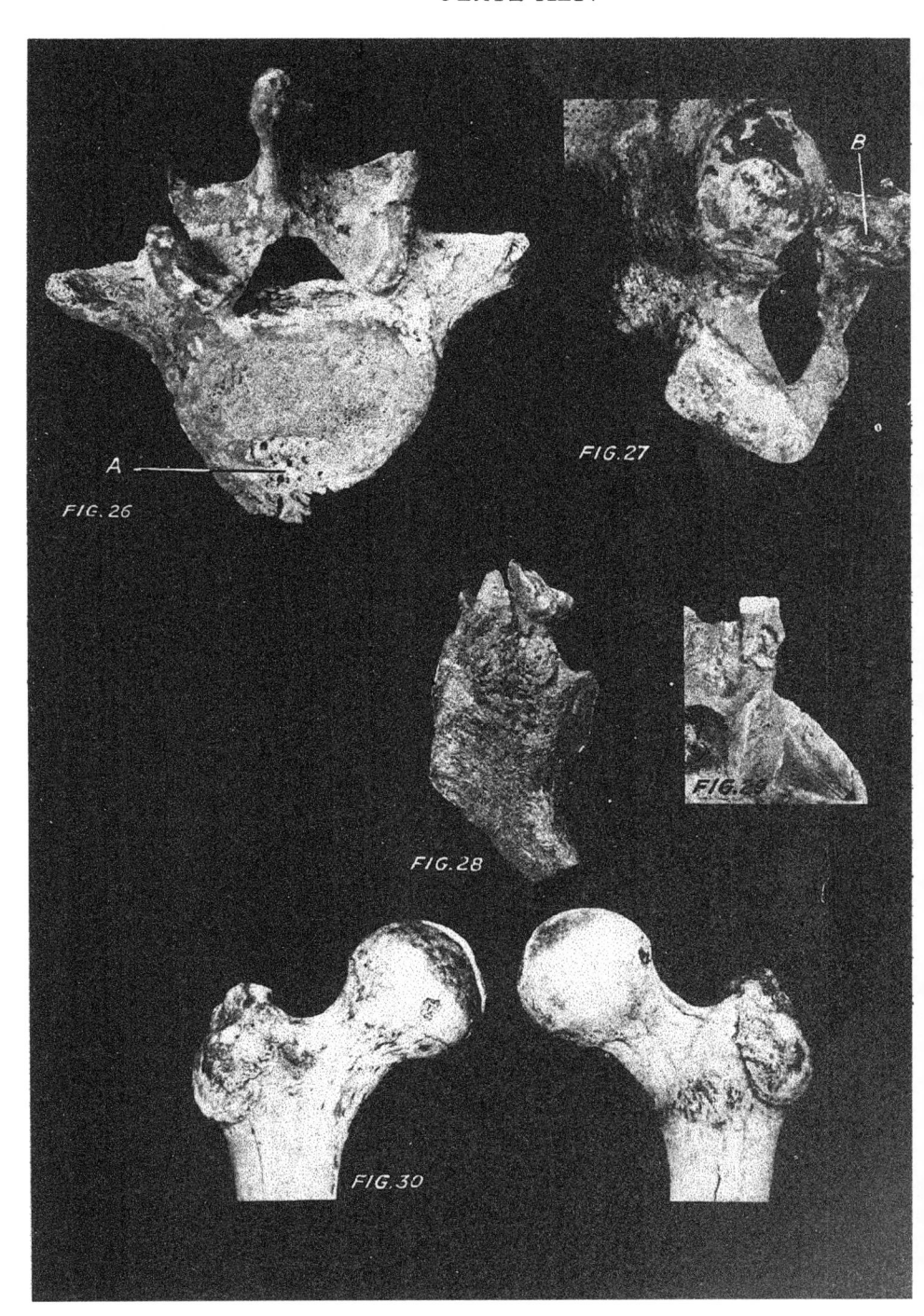

FIG. 26

A

FIG. 27

B

FIG. 28

FIG. 29

FIG. 30

Fig. 24.—Exostosis of pelvis. *A* points to groove in exostosis.

Fig. 25.—Pyorrhoea alveolaris. The second lower molar is extensively decayed. (See also Plate XLIII, Fig. 17.)

PLATE XLIV

Fig. 26.—Last lumbar vertebra. Thickening of anterior border of body with marked absorption of bone at *A*.

Fig. 27.—Exostosis of pelvis. (See also Plate XLIII, Fig. 24.) *A, B,* and *C* point to deep grooves in exostosis.

Fig. 28.—Exostosis at tip of acromion.

Fig. 29.—Pyorrhoea alveolaris. The alveoli of the third molar have been completely absorbed, the tooth being attached by its centre only.

Fig. 30.—Marked periostitis over great trochanter.

ON THE DISEASES OF THE SUDAN AND NUBIA IN ANCIENT TIMES

(*Mitteilungen zur Geschichte der Medizin u. der Naturwissenschaften*, No. 58, Vol. XIII [1914], No. 4)

During the winter of 1913, I had an opportunity of witnessing, for a few days, the excavations then in progress at Merawi (Sudan). Professor Griffith,[1] of Oxford, who was directing the work, gave me every facility for studying the skeletons still in the graves and the few skulls and bones which he had collected. He also allowed me to examine the specimens which he had dug up at Faras in 1912.

I am informed by Professor Griffith that the skeletons at Merawi dated roughly from the time of the XXVth–XXVIth Dynasties (i.e., about 750–500 B.C.), and that those from Faras were of the Meroïtic age (i.e., about 100 B.C.—300 A.D.).

Merawi[2] is situated on the Nile (18° N.), and Faras lies a few miles north of Wady Halfa, near the second cataract of the Nile.

I made no attempt to measure the skeletons, as this will be done by a competent anthropologist. I ascertained, however, that the people buried at Merawi and Faras were of two distinct races, the first probably Egyptian and the other unmistakably negroid.

At Merawi, most of the skeletons which I saw were still in their graves, and sadly altered by the action of the sand. At Faras, on the other hand, the bones had been removed from the graves the year before, duly labelled, and placed in a closed room of a mud-hut.

---

[1] To Professor and Mrs. Griffith, I may be allowed to express here my warmest thanks for their kindness to my wife and myself on this and several other occasions. To His Excellency, the Sirdar and Governor General of the Sudan, General Sir Reginald Wingate, and His Excellency Jackson Pasha, Governor of Merawi Province, I am under great obligation for all the facilities they gave me. Sir Reginald Wingate and the Government of the Sudan have lately issued an order according to which all ancient human remains discovered during excavations are to be examined by a competent anatomist, either at the time of excavation or afterwards. When will the enlightened governments of Europe follow suit?

[2] Merawi (or Meroë, or Merowe) is close to the ancient Napata. It must not be mistaken for another Meroë or Merowe which is situated further south.

DISEASES OF THE SUDAN IN ANCIENT TIMES 157

These specimens were in better condition, as the dryness of the atmosphere had rendered them resistant. Fragments from about seventy different bodies were left, and there was hardly a single perfect bone; a few débris of vertebrae, a sacrum, or a piece of an ulna, a radius, a femur, a mandible perhaps represented all that was left of one body. All the pathological specimens were set aside and sent off to Alexandria, where they were examined at leisure.

The first difficulty was to distinguish between the changes caused by the method of burial and true pathological alterations. Had this cause of error been really appreciated in the past, such a diagnosis as syphilitic ulceration would not have been made, only to be contradicted afterwards.

At Merawi, the bodies were buried in brick-lined graves filled with sand, and the effects of pressure on the long bones and the skulls were very marked. The former, for instance, were generally found broken in several places, and, through the cleanly cut fracture, the sand had penetrated into the medullary canals, which it filled from end to end, the fine, spongy tissue being completely destroyed in some skeletons. These fractures were very common, especially in the long bones of the lower limbs, the femurs suffering most. The neck of the femurs and the iliac bones were not infrequently smashed or completely destroyed by the same agency. The sand also worked its way into the heads of the bones, especially into the head of the femur, and eroding the superficial bony layer exposed and destroyed the cancellous tissue below.

The sand had occasionally shifted some of the bones out of their places, even in intact burials. A sternum, for instance, had slipped into the pelvis, or a radius was lying at right angles to the ulna.

The most remarkable changes due to sand erosion were seen in the skull. The sand penetrating into the sutures, especially of young people, separated the bones of the skull from one another almost as neatly as an anatomist might have done it. Through the sutures the sand infiltrated between the inner and outer tables of the skull, and then the former often gave way in places. Curious erosions were thus formed, which were distinguishable from pathological processes by the absence of newly formed bone and of other signs of inflammation at the edge of the eroded patch. The losses of substance so produced exactly resembled the syphilitic lesions (?) described by Fouquet in old Egyptian skulls.

Similar losses of substance caused by the action of sand occurred on the external table of the skull also, and occasionally it was extremely difficult to know whether such defects were due to a pathological process or not. In one case, indeed, even now, after prolonged examination, I am unable to decide to what agency the loss of substance was due. The lesion in question consists of a hole in the lower third of the frontal bone which measures 0.7 cm. in its longest and 0.3 cm. in its widest diameter. Its walls are quite smooth, somewhat rounded off on the inner, but not on the outer side, and there are no other signs of inflammation in the neighbourhood. At the upper edge, a smooth groove implicates the upper layer of the external table only. There are no signs of inflammation round this, but the groove is so smooth and even that it is difficult to believe that it has been caused by gritty sand. On the whole, I feel inclined to think that we are here in the presence of an injury, possibly an old and healed perforating wound of the skull.

No other case of disease of the roof of the skull nor of the nose was discovered, but as the turbinated bones were usually completely smashed the detection of pathological changes in the nose was often impossible.

Wormian bones.—These bones were not very numerous, a few, including a very large one, occurring in the lambdoid sutures and some on the coronal and sagittal sutures. I did not discover a single one in the face. Three typical specimens of os epactal and one specimen of a double os epactal were found.

Lesions and diseases of the teeth.—Malpositions were rare, and the teeth were beautifully and regularly planted as a rule. In one cranium the alveoli were not in their normal position, but as the teeth had fallen out it was impossible to be certain as to the exact malposition; in another skull, the second right upper molar was displaced to the inner side. There were also several good examples of impacted teeth.

Two malformations were observed in the fangs of the grinding teeth. In the first, two fangs were so bent that their tips met, and in the other the three fangs were joined together into one mass.

DISEASES OF THE SUDAN IN ANCIENT TIMES 159

When the sand had been removed the teeth nearly always looked very clean and white; a few were stained yellow, and deposits of tartar were occasionally present. As a rule, however, the enamel, except on the grinding surface or cutting edge, was in very good condition, and at first I had the impression that the teeth of these people were very fine. This impression was dissipated on more careful examination.

Almost all the teeth showed signs of considerable attrition. This phenomenon has been observed already in predynastic bodies, in old Egyptian mummies, and in Greek and Coptic bodies, by Flinders Petrie, Fouquet, De Morgan, Elliot Smith, Wood Jones, Derry, and also Rietti and myself.

Nevertheless, it is worthy of being carefully studied, as from this and other conditions of the teeth one may form an opinion as to the food of these people. At Merawi and Faras this alteration began quite early in life, as in some young skulls the deciduous, grinding teeth showed marked attrition. The molars were worn down irregularly, the often crescented and sharply cut cavity being generally more marked on the lingual side of the upper and on the labial side of the lower teeth. This, indeed, appears to be the rule in deciduous and in permanent teeth also.

The rapidity with which this wearing down of the crown progresses was estimated by the amount of attrition in the teeth, the age of which could be known with some accuracy. The first mandibular permanent molar, for instance, erupts at the age of seven years and three months (according to others, at six years and nine months), and the canine at ten years and seven months, i.e., about three years afterwards. Now in several mandibles, in which the canines were just pushing through the bone, the first molars showed very considerable attrition already. In three years, therefore, most of the mischief had been done.

Similarly, during the interval between the eruption of the second and third molars, the crown of the former had sometimes become much worn; though, perhaps, the degree of attrition was generally less marked than in the first case.

Attrition affected all the teeth, though to a different degree. The first molars were most worn, then the second premolars, the second molars, and to a less extent the first premolars, the canines, the incisors, and lastly the third molars.

The cavities formed by long attrition differed exceedingly according to the position of the teeth. In the incisors, canines, and often the first premolars, a bow-like cavity was formed. In the molars and second premolars, the grinding generally gave rise at first to smooth, more or less crescented cavities, and these, as has been explained before, were usually deeper on the lingual side of the upper and on the labial side of the lower teeth. Later on, the teeth were ground down evenly; the smooth surface so produced being inclined to the labial side in the upper jaw, and to the lingual side in the mandible.

Although most teeth were ground down, and although the change evidently progressed rapidly in early youth, yet it was never as marked as in predynastic skulls or modern Egyptians. It progressed in old people at a much slower rate than in young, sometimes stopping altogether in the old.

In many cases the pulp cavity was opened by the attrition, yet this lesion was not frequently followed either by caries or abscesses. The latter were often connected with carious teeth, or with perialveolar disease.

A cursory examination of the skulls made on the spot showed that about 12 per cent of the skulls had carious teeth. This, however, gives a very erroneous idea of the real state of things, for being pressed for time, my examination was somewhat superficial. Moreover, the crowns of a large number of teeth had been broken off; many teeth had dropped out and could not be found, some of which may have been carious.

Of the thirty-six skulls and fragments of mandibles from Faras and Merawi which I took home to examine, all but two showed carious teeth. As a rule, the crown of the tooth was not affected, and the carious hole was situated on the proximal or the distal surfaces, or on the labial or lingual sides.

Occasionally the results following on caries were exceedingly severe and must have caused agony during life. Let us examine some of them more carefully.

The first case was the left maxilla of a very young person, which had also an impacted tooth, just behind the first and second upper incisors. The two incisors, canines, and first premolars had either fallen out or their crowns had been broken off, after death.

The second premolar was carious on its inner, proximal side, and had evidently been infected by the first molar, which, together with the second molar, was extensively carious. In connection with the first molar there was an abscess as large as a pea, opening into the mouth.

In another mandible there was extensive caries on the lingual side of the second premolar. The first molar had probably been carious also, and, at any rate, there had been considerable inflammation round it, which was shown by the rough state of the alveolus. An abscess had formed round one of these teeth, probably of the first molar, and the pus had found its way from one alveolus to the other, through a sinus which admitted a large probe. It had then worked through the bone on the labial side of the second premolar, and lastly into the mouth.

In another case an abscess as large as a pea existed at the root of the left mandibular canine. All the teeth showed great attrition, and the pulp canal of the canine had thus been opened. The pus in this case had welled up on the inner side of the canine, where its track was easily followed.

An abscess similar to the last was found in another mandible, in which the track of the pus at the base of one incisor opened into the alveoli of both neighbouring incisors.

Among the most important and frequent lesions were those secondary to periodontal disease. Many teeth were not in position and looked as if pushed forward; the whole or part of the fangs were exposed, owing to the absorption of the alveoli by a chronic inflammatory process or periodontitis.

In early cases the alveoli were partly absorbed, so that in each tooth part of the fang was exposed. Later on, the alveoli disappeared on one side, and, in consequence, the fangs were bare along their whole length. In some skulls the alveoli had gone almost completely, most of the teeth had dropped out, and the few remaining were attached to the skull only by the tip of the fangs.

We are here, I think, in the presence of cases of rarefying periodontitis, and pyorrhoea alveolaris, with consequent loosening and final shedding of the teeth. It is most probably due to this cause that some of the skulls were absolutely toothless, the alveolar borders having been completely absorbed.

This disease rages now at Faras as it did two thousand years ago, for during my short stay there I was consulted by several men, who in consequence of pyorrhoea had lost nearly all their teeth and were in a fair way of shedding the remaining few. It is spread all over Egypt, and when in the desert of Sinai near Akaba, I was visited by the garrison of seven men who held a small fort there. All seven showed the typical symptoms of this disease and were in a wretched state of health in consequence.

Two perfectly toothless mandibles and maxillae are worthy of notice, for judging from the state of the cranial sutures, it is extremely probable that their owners were still middle-aged at the time of death. Yet, they had lost their teeth some considerable time before death.

To resume: The lesions of the teeth found at Marawi and Faras may be tabulated as follows: (1) impaction; (2) attrition; (3) caries; (4) abscesses and fistulae; (5) periodontitis and pyorrhoea alveolaris. On the whole, therefore, the state of the dentition in those times was remarkably bad.

Injuries of bones.—Injuries of bones in the shape of fractures appear to have been fairly common, as I came across four of them in a very short time.

The first, discovered at Merawi, was an oblique, simple fracture at the junction of the lower and middle thirds of the humerus. There was a good deal of callus, and the fracture had been very badly set, so that a marked deformity existed.

In the case of a fractured ulna, it is doubtful whether the lesion was due to disease or to injury. At the junction of the lower and middle thirds of the bone, there was an oblong, osseous swelling which entirely surrounded the bone. The specimen had been waxed before I saw it, and its condition could not be satisfactorily ascertained. I believe, however, that the lesion was due to disease and not to injury, for there were two holes with smooth, rounded walls, evidently two sinuses, opening over the swelling and probably caused by some disease of the shaft of the ulna, e.g., osteomyelitis, which led to formation of a sinus, fracture of the bone, and incomplete formation of callus round the fracture. That osteomyelitis existed in Old Egypt is shown by a typical ancient specimen of this disease, now in the Cairo Pathological Museum.

A third specimen is a fracture of the lower end of the fibula. The fracture had not been well set, and there was considerable twisting of the bone. It did not extend into the joint, the lower end of the bone being normal.

At Faras, I found a healed, impacted fracture of the upper part of the femur. Only part of the bone was present, but although the fracture was completely healed, there had been considerable shortening. Further, the numerous osteophytes round the fracture showed that the healing process had taken a very long time, and that, probably, there had been some suppuration also.

Such a fracture is very difficult to treat, and even now the results obtained are often very unsatisfactory. We cannot wonder, therefore, that the old Meroites were not more successful.

The two specimens of uncomplicated fractures, however, namely of the humerus and fibula, do not give one a very high opinion of the surgery of those days, as the final results of the treatment can only be considered as bad. This observation agrees very well with what I have seen in Egypt of other fractures dating from a similar period.

Arthritic lesions. Spondylitis deformans.—The investigations of Elliot Smith, Wood Jones and Derry in Nubia, and of Armand Ruffer and Rietti in Egypt have shown that this disease was common in predynastic, dynastic, Greek, Roman, and Coptic times. At the Pathological Museum of the Medical School in Cario, I have arranged specimens of Egyptian vertebrae exhibiting the characteristic signs of this disease, dating from 4000 B.C. to 300 A.D.

I was naturally anxious, therefore, to see whether this disease existed at Merawi and Faras. At the first site, owing to the very bad state of the bones, I was for a long time unsuccessful. Finally I discovered in one grave three lumbar vertebrae with marked overlipping of the anterior borders of the bodies. In another grave were two lumbar vertebrae, which showed some overlipping of their borders and were joined together on one side by a strong bridge of new bone measuring about 1.5 cm. in width and about 0.5 cm. in thickness.

At Faras, the vertebrae which had been saved were very few and badly preserved. Three sacra, however, showed marked signs of spondylitis deformans. This disease, therefore, existed at Merawi as well as at Faras; that is, in two of the dryest and hottest places of the world, so that it is difficult to believe that it is due to cold and damp.

Other cases of arthritis.—The only two other cases of arthritis were found at Faras. The first was a humerus in which there was a border of new bone, more marked on the anterior side, round the anatomical neck. The bone was smooth, white, and had evidently been formed some time before death.

The other was the lower end of a femur which showed two remarkable osteophytes; the largest measuring about 2.5 by 2 cm. and more than 0.5 cm. in its thickest part. This must have caused considerable limitation of movement during life.

Considering the few bones I had occasion to examine, it is not a little remarkable that not less than six fragments, belonging to different bodies, should have exhibited signs of chronic arthritis. It is very probable, therefore, that this disease was very common.

Other lesions of bones.—Neither tubercular nor syphilitic lesions were discovered.

Two bones showed deformities which may possibly have been caused by rickets. The first was a femur in which the antero-posterior curve was greatly exaggerated. Unfortunately the lower end was missing.

The other case was more instructive. It was a sacrum in which the last two vertebrae were bent forward sharply, almost at right angles to the others. The whole sacrum was remarkably light and brittle, and, except for the deformation just described, exhibited no other pathological changes. It appeared to me most probable that this deformity was due to rickets.

A word remains to be said about the age of these people at the time of death. Were they in fact a short-lived or a long-lived race? As we have seen, the skeletons were generally those of adults, and it is often extremely difficult to determine accurately the age of an adult person from the state of the skull, and the other parts of the skeletons were of no use for that purpose. In both places the state of the teeth was of little assistance in estimating the age of these people, as attrition was present even in the young, and the thickness of the parietal bones and the weight of the skull were no guides, owing to the bad state of preservation of the specimens.

In most skeletons the sutures with the exception of the basilar were still wide open and there was no sign of obliteration, nor did I find a single case of complete synostosis of the cranium.

My impression, therefore was that the majority of these people died before they were fifty years old.

PATHOLOGICAL NOTES ON THE ROYAL MUMMIES OF THE CAIRO MUSEUM[1]

(*Mitteilungen zur Geschichte der Medizin u. der Naturwissenschaften*, No. 56, Vol. XIII [1914], No. 2)

In 1889, Sir Gaston Maspero, the eminent Director General of the Antiquities' Department of Egypt, published his great monograph, *Les Momies royales de Deir el Bahri*, in which he gave a full account of the appearances presented by these mummies at the time they were unrolled. Since that time the royal mummies have rested in the Cairo Museum.

Maspero's account, although supplemented by the notes of Fouquet, was that of the pure Egyptologist, and gave little consideration to anatomy and pathology. Nearly twenty years afterwards, Maspero requested Elliot Smith to re-examine the mummies and to report on their anatomical and pathological characteristics, and I feel sure everyone will agree that no one could have done the work better. In the course of this enquiry, however, it soon became obvious that little could be done from an anatomical or pathological point of view without dissection. This, of course, was out of the question, as these mummies rank as archaeological documents of the first importance and must remain intact. Fortunately, however, Elliot Smith examined a large number of mummies less exalted in rank than the royal mummies, and on these he based his researches published some years ago.[1] W. A. Schmidt, A. Lucas, W. M. Colles discussed the subject from the chemical point of view. Marc Armand Ruffer gave a full account of the histology of mummies, or in collaboration with W. R. Ferguson also described some of the pathological lesions which can be detected with the microscope.

The paper contains a full account of the process of embalming, but, considering that this has been fully discussed elsewhere and reported at its proper time, I may pass it over to-day. Many valu-

[1] Service des Antiquités de l'Égypte, *Catalogue général des Antiquités égyptiennes du Musée du Caire*, Nos. 61051–100. G. Elliot Smith, F.R.S., *The Royal Mummies*, Le Caire, 1912.

able pathological observations, however, are scattered in this memoir, and it is of these only that I wish to speak in this review.

The appearance of mummies is very deceptive. At first sight, a casual observer might conclude that ancient Egyptians were a singularly thin people, and a glance at the photographs reproduced in this volume would confirm him in this manner of thinking. More careful examination shows that this conclusion would be entirely wrong, and that not only were most of these people well nourished, but some suffered from marked obesity.

The mummy of Ramses III (1198–1167 B.C.),[1] for instance, looks like the body of a very thin man. Examination shows that the wrinkled skin forms behind the neck under the chin, round the thighs and joints, enormous folds imbricated one over the other. The king, therefore, was very corpulent at the time of his death. King Merneptah (1225–1215 B.C.) also was a singularly fat man, for, although the body is now reduced to little more than skin and bone, the redundancy of the skin of the abdomen, thighs, and cheeks leaves no doubt on that point. The same remark applies to King Thutmose II (about 1501 B.C.), to Zabdptahefônkhou, a priest of Amon, and to others. The skin of the priest of Amon, for instance, is thrown into the most curious folds owing to the drying and shrinking of the subcutaneous tissues.

These observations on the obesity of ancient Egyptians I have been often able to confirm by the examination of mummies and dried bodies of all times. I have in my possession, for instance, the arm of a mummy of the XXIst Dynasty, which had been carefully packed with earth. It is a stout arm even now, though it is evident that the embalmer had not really restored the limb to its original shape, as deep folds of the skin, some more than one inch in depth, show that the arm was not fully distended by the embalmer's packing, and that it was much fatter than it looks now. The skin of the abdomen of a mummy of Persian times (500 B.C.), which looked terribly emaciated, was thrown into deep folds; the skin had evidently shrunk considerably during the mummifying process, and during life that person must have had an imposing abdomen.

[1] For the dates, I follow Breasted (*A History of Egypt*) whenever possible.

Similarly, in a Coptic body from Akhmin (400 A.D.) which looked like a skeleton, in spite of its sixteen hundred years' desiccation in hot sand, the skin of the buttocks showed the redundant folds of a stout person. Pieces of skin, soaked in proper softening fluid, swelled up to their original size and a large amount of subcutaneous fat was demonstrated.

The abdominal wall of another Coptic mummy, which had been simply dried, was more than two inches thick. Considering that the abdominal wall of dried bodies is not more than half an inch in thickness as a rule, the subcutaneous tissue of this man must have been very abundant. In some mummies of the XXIst Dynasty (about 900 B.C.), the embalmer filled out the cheeks of the person with a paste consisting of some fatty material and sawdust, or of sand, evidently with the idea of preparing a mummy bearing some likeness to the deceased. Some of these heads show greatly distended cheeks and a good deal of obesity.

The point is interesting as showing that many of these people did not die of wasting diseases such as phthisis, but of some acute disease. I have heard it stated that many of the statues now in the Cairo Museum have the typical phthisical look, and in a discussion which took place some years ago at the Institut Égyptien it was said that their appearance showed that the originals died of phthisis. The examination of mummies, however, points exactly to the contrary, as the majority were well-nourished persons.

In this connection I must allude to the mummy of Amenhotep III and to the bones of his son Ikhnaton, which are described in this memoir, as perhaps the most typical instance of pathological obesity is shown in the portraits of the heretic, King Ikhnaton (1375–1358 B.C.). According to Weigall, one reason why this monarch's almost ridiculous appearance is faithfully represented is that he introduced a very realistic form of art, destined, alas, to have but too short a life. Weigall says:

> In the drawing of the human figure, and especially that of the Pharaoh, there are three very distinct characteristics in this new form of art. Firstly, as to the head: the skull is elongated; the chin, as seen in profile, is drawn as if it were sharply pointed; the flesh under the jaw is skimped, thus giving an upward turn to the line; and the neck is represented as being long and thin.

Secondly, the stomach is made to obtrude itself upon the attention by being drawn as though from a fat and ungainly model. And thirdly, the hips and thighs are abnormally large, though from the knees downwards the legs are of more natural size. This distortion of human anatomy is marked in a lesser degree in all the lines of the body; and the whole figure becomes a startling type of an art which seems at first to have sprung fully developed from the brain of the boy-Pharaoh or from one of the eccentrics of the Court.

It may be that he had objected to be represented in the conventional manner and had told his artists to draw him as he was. The elongated skull, the pointed chin, and, even, perhaps, the ungainly thighs could only be accounted for by some radical deformity on the royal model, and that he was a well-made man in this respect the recently discovered bones most clearly show.[1]

Weigall also suggests that this way of depicting the king was due to a kind of renaissance, and to a return to the archaic form of art, in which many of the characteristics just described were prominent.

This last hypothesis appears to me unnecessary, and I am convinced that we are in presence of real portraits of the monarch. True, the abdomen is rather prominent in other people represented at Tell el Amarna, but this is due chiefly to the peculiar type of dress which, apparently consisting of a mantle firmly tied below the umbilicus, emphasised the lower part of the abdomen. In persons not wearing this dress the abdomen is flat, and even in men attired in the garment just described it is never as protuberant as in King Ikhnaton.

In one picture, the king is represented distributing collars of gold from a balcony, and his abdomen actually hangs over the edge of the balcony: a most realistic piece of portraiture.

The thighs of the queen and daughters are perhaps accentuated, but the abdomen is flat. One of the princesses, however, appears to have inherited some of her father's characteristics, as she is occasionally represented with very full, round thighs, contrasting with those of the sisters standing in front and behind her.

The very thin calves of Ikhnaton show that the artist faithfully copied nature, for great corpulency accompanied by very thin calves is not infrequent in the East nor even rare in Europe. Witness, for instance, the famous portrait by Valesquez in the Munich Gallery,

[1] Weigall, *Ikhnaton, Pharaoh of Egypt*, 1910.

in which the contrast between the truly enormous abdomen and the thinner lower extremities is striking.

The extreme corpulency of the king may have been responsible for his politics. On account of his obesity he probably disliked physical exertion, and this may have been the reason why he persistently refused to lead his army to war when the outlying provinces of his kingdom were threatened. Time after time he was appealed to for help, but he remained at home and thus became responsible for the loss of some of the foreign possessions of Egypt.

Another picture from Tell el Amarna may be referred to here (*El Amarna*, I, II, XVIII). It is divided into two halves, that on the left showing the household of Ikhnaton, that on the right the household of his predecessor Amenhotep III. It shows that Ikhnaton's obesity was inherited, for father and son show the same abdominal deformity. Indeed, the whole royal family is distinctly stout, in contrast with the three lean female servants on the extreme right. The mummy of Amenhotep III (1411–1375 B.C.) is among those examined by Elliot Smith, and, naturally, I looked with great interest to see whether the mummy would confirm the diagnosis made from the pictures. Unfortunately, the body was in such a wretched state that nothing could be deduced with certainty from its examination.

It may be noted that, according to Elliot Smith, the skull of Ikhnaton presents a number of interesting and significant features. The cranium is broad and relatively flattened, its measurements being 18.9 cm. in length; and 15.4 cm. in breadth; 13.6 cm. in height; 9.9 cm. minimal frontal breadth, with a circumference of 54.5 cm.

Elliot Smith adds:

> Although 15.4 cm. is quite an exceptional breadth for an Egyptian skull, all the other numbers are smaller than those obtained in the case of Amenhotep III. Nevertheless, the form of the cranium and the fact that it is exceptionally thin in some places, and relatively thick in others, indicate that a condition of *hydrocephalus* was present during life.

Professor A. R. Ferguson, professor of pathology in the Cairo School of Medicine, is of opinion that the signs of this disease are unquestionable. Whether the skull is Ikhnaton's or not, it is interesting to find that hydrocephalus existed about thirty-five hundred years ago.

The bones supposed to be Ikhnaton's are also in the Museum, and Elliot Smith fully discusses their authenticity. In my opinion, however, the evidence that they are Ikhnaton's is by no means conclusive, but not having had an opportunity of examining them, I leave this question for another occasion.

Death from violence.—The king Saknounrâ Tionâken (about 1870 B.C.), of the XVIIth Dynasty, died from injuries, and it is clear from the examination of his mummy that he met his death in an attack by at least two, and possibly more, persons armed with at least two (perhaps three or more) implements, one of which was probably an axe and another a spear. The absence of any injury to the arms, or to any other part of the body, shows that no resistance could have been offered to the attack. It is quite possible that the wounds may have been inflicted while Saknounrâ was lying down on the right side.

The mode of death of this king had been unknown before his mummy was examined. His wars against the Hyksos had not been forgotten, but it had never been ascertained that he had died in battle.

A wound probably caused by a fall backwards was found in the occipital scalp of Princess Meritamon. This had apparently been produced ante-mortem.

Mutilations.—Mutilations are rare. We note that there is no evidence that women were circumcised, but the bodies are in such a state that it would often be difficult to state with certainty whether such an operation had been done. The men, on the other hand, always appear to have been circumcised, and from the fact that a boy eleven years old, found in the tomb of Amenhotep II (1420 B.C.), was still uncircumcised, it may be argued that this operation was performed at a later age, as in present times.

The question of the treatment of the genital organs after death, whether, for instance, they were buried separately or not, is a difficult one. It is not always very easy to say whether the genital organs are present or not in mummies, and it has happened that two observers have come to different conclusions with regard to this apparently easily ascertainable fact.

The pudenda were present in Ahmose I (1557 B.C.), Thutmose IV (1411 B.C.), Amenhotep II (1420 B.C.), and Yuaa, and the state of affairs in Thutmose II, Thutmose III (1447 B.C.), and an unknown man in Nibsoni's coffin was uncertain. In the case of Seti I (1292 B.C.) the wrappings were not removed, and therefore no definite statement of the mode of treatment of the pudenda can be made.

A very curious feature of Merneptah's (1215 B.C.) mummy is the complete absence of the scrotum, but not of the penis. Midway between the root of the penis and the anus a transverse scar is visible. It represents the place from which the scrotal sac was cut away, but as it is now thickly smeared with balsam, it is not possible to say whether it was removed during life or after death. It was certainly done before the process of embalming was complete, because the wound is covered with balsam. The fact that there is a wound suggests that Merneptah was castrated either after, or shortly before death.

As Elliot Smith remarks:

It seems unlikely that in so important a matter as the treatment of the genital organs, the embalmers should suddenly have broken away from the convention of their time in the case of Thutmose II and III, but not in their immediate predecessors and successors, and again in the succeeding dynasty in the case of Ramses II. The absence of the genital organs in the latter Pharaoh seems to me due to accidental circumstances.

The scrotum of Ramses V (1157 B.C.) was large and baggy and had been pushed back and pressed against the perineum, the whole of which was covered by it. The great size of the scrotum suggested that Ramses V suffered from hernia and possibly hydrocele. Immediately below Poupart's ligament, in the right groin, there is a large, irregularly triangular, deep ulcer with thickened edges. It measures 0.2 by 1.8 cm., and is covered by a black, resinous paste, which prevents a minute examination of the character of the ulcer; but its situation suggests that it may represent an open bubo.

I may add that in no mummy that I have examined have I found any evidence that the genital organs had been interfered with after death.

The only other mutilation that is found frequently is the piercing of the ears for the introduction of earrings. The fashion appears to have changed with different kings, for whereas the perforations in some are very large, in others they are quite small. In one mummy of the XXIst Dynasty (about 1000 B.C.) that I examined, I found the lobule dragged down by the weight of the earring and the size of the hole was wide enough to allow the introduction of the whole thumb.

Baldness, etc.—Among pathological conditions affecting the cutaneous system is baldness, which was found in many of the men and not a few of the women.

Queen Nofritari's head, for instance, was bald on the vertex, and Queen Notmit also was bald. In most cases the baldness is central; occasionally scattered patches are found in the skull, showing that it may have been caused perhaps by some local parasitic disease. No examination appears to have been made for scalp parasites. Personally, I have not been able to find any in the mummies I have examined, except, in a few cases, the eggs of lice still adhering to the hair.

It is not clear to what the baldness was due. It may possibly have been caused by the wearing of the wig, just as the baldness of the modern Egyptian is generally attributed to the wearing of the tarboush and the turban. Indeed, upon the lateral aspects of one cranium there are large triangular depressions due to atrophy of the outer surfaces of the parietal bone, which may have been due to some heavy wig or headgear.

I would point out, however, in that connection that the Greek priests, who never cut their hair, and who never remove their heavy headdress except at the altar, have luxuriant tresses as a rule. I am therefore quite unable to account for the baldness of old and modern Egyptians.

Blackheads (comedones) are not rare in Egyptain mummies and well marked in the forehead of Ramses II (1225 B.C.). His finger nails exhibit very distinct longitudinal ridging, and, therefore, the king was probably ill for some considerable time before death. His Majesty's superficial temporal arteries are even now prominent and tortuous, and their walls undoubtedly calcareous. It will be remembered, in this connection, that the aorta of King Merneptah was calcified, and I have elsewhere drawn attention to the frequency of arterial diseases in ancient Egypt.

Ulcers are not infrequent. In a woman buried in the tomb of Amenhotep II, there is an elliptical ulcer (2.2 × 1.2 cm.) with indurated edges, and, on the inner surface of the same heel, a much larger ulcer (4.4 cm. in diameter). These wounds have all the appearance of ante-mortem injuries with inflammatory reactions around the edges. Elliot Smith thinks it possible, however, that if they were done immediately after death the action of the salt bath on these cut edges may have given rise to these appearances. He found in some other mummies of women the skin cut away from the heel. If these ulcers were not ante-mortem, they were certainly done before the embalming process was complete, because the linen was packed into them and is adherent to the bone.

An ulcer the nature of which is doubtful is to be seen in the body of Ramses IV (1161 B.C.). An elliptical piece of skin (1.8 × 0.7 cm.) was cut off the right side of the penis, at the junction of the glans with the body of the organ; this was done probably just after death and before the process of embalming, but it may possibly be an ulcer with clean-cut edges. An ulcer 2 × 1 cm. is visible on the back of the right scapula, extending from the posterior lip of the glenoid fossa to its lower half; its edges are raised, and the nature of the lesion is doubtful.

Skin eruptions.—Maspero had already noted that one of the thighs of Queen Anhapon (XVIIIth–XIXth Dynasties) showed "stigmata" arranged in groups similar to those left by lichen.

A curious appearance of the skin is seen also in the mummy of Thutmose II. The skin of the thorax, shoulders and arms, hands, the whole of the back, the buttocks and legs (including the feet) is studded with raised macules, varying in size from minute points to patches a centimetre in diameter. The skin of the head is not affected. A condition precisely similar to this is also found in the mummy of Amenhotep II, and in a less marked form in Thutmose III, and the question is whether these macules are due to some cutaneous eruption, or are the result of the action of the preservative bath post-mortem. On the whole, I am inclined to look upon them as the manifestation of some disease, the nature of which is not altogether clear, but the fact that this irregularity of the skin occurs in three successive Pharaohs suggests that it may be due to some irritant amongst the ingredients of the preservative materials employed by the embalmers at that particular time.

Very different is the eruption on Ramses V, in whom on the lower surface of the pudenda, lower part of the abdominal wall, and on the face there is a well-marked pustular eruption, which Professor A. R. Ferguson stated to be highly suggestive of smallpox. This rash is exactly similar to the one which Professor Ferguson and I described in our paper.[1] It may be remembered that Professor Unna of Hamburg criticised our view, and gave it as his opinion that: (1) the lesions were not characteristic of smallpox; (2) the appearance of the skin was due, not to disease, but to soaking in water (*durchnässt*); and (3) the bacilli found were of modern, origin.

I may be allowed to answer shortly Professor Unna's criticisms. In the first place, we did not say that the case was one of variola, but as the title of our paper stated we described "an eruption *resembling* that of variola." In our conclusions also, we wrote of the "probable existence of smallpox," and throughout we spoke of lesions "resembling" those of smallpox. We gave in full the description of the appearances which led us to this conclusion, and although we concluded that the bacteria were present at the time of death, yet we allowed that "they probably multiplied enormously after death."

We would remark that whereas our conclusions are based on a large number of sections, Professor Unna's are based on the examination of two sections only.

The mummy in question was one of the XVIIIth Dynasty, which had been removed from its rock-hewn cell at Deir el Bahri, and taken straight down to Cairo, together with a large number of other mummies. Deir el Bahri is one of the dryest spots on earth, where rain falls only about once in every two years, and where the average temperature in the tombs is 22° C. The tombs are about three miles in a straight line from the Nile, and certainly not less than a mile distant from the ground yearly inundated by the river; the floors of the graves are at least 25 m. higher than the highest level of the water. In such a tomb the mummy could not possibly have been "durchnässt," at any time, and other mummies from the same

[1] *Supra*, this volume, p. 32.

tombs, now at Kasr el Aini Museum in Cairo, are as dry as a bone, and none show a rash similar to the one described by us.[1] From Deir el Bahri the mummies were taken to the Museum in Cairo, and afterwards to the top floor of the Medical School, and there again it is absolutely impossible that they should have been "durchnässt." Lastly, during the softening of the object and the preparation of the sections, water was used twice only, namely, to remove the alcohol from the sections before staining, and to wash out the superfluous stain; in both cases for two minutes only. One can exclude, therefore the theory that these bacteria belonged to the twentieth century A.D., as Professor Unna suggests.

The discovery of these bacilli is not a solitary find, for I have stained bacteria in material dating from previous ages, e.g., in the intestinal contents of a body of the XIth Dynasty (2000 B.C.), in the sand of brick of Karnak Temple (which sand, let it be said by the way, was quite sterile when inoculated into gelatine or bouillon), in the mud with which the internal cavities of mummies were packed, in the lungs of mummies of the XVIIIth, XXIst, XXIId Dynasties, and of Greek, Roman, and Coptic times, in the kidneys of mummies of the XXIst Dynasty, in the livers of mummies of the XXIst Dynasty and of Coptic times, etc.

All the mummies were unrolled by me, and were perfectly dry. Several of them had been treated with hot gum, of which they contained considerable quantities.

After all, it is not very remarkable that bacteria like other vegetable tissues should be recognisable after several thousand years. I examined during the last two years sixteen bodies of Coptic times, in which the garlands of flowers round the neck, although dried up, were in a perfect state of preservation. I found that the garments covering these bodies were simply beautiful, with well-preserved coloured patterns; they even stood washing with soap and water. There are now about one hundred specimens of these embroidered garments, representing most diverse objects, in the Alexandria Museum.

[1] Since writing the above, I have found another dried body, also from Upper Egypt, which shows very much the same appearance as that described by Dr. Ferguson and myself. I hope to publish something more about it later on.

Linen bandages also, dating from the XXVIIth Dynasty, look almost as if they had just come from the maker, and I have in my private collection a beautiful specimen of Coptic embroidery which might have been made only a few years ago. The fringe is perfect, and the fine thread used for stitching the hem is very resistant and might easily be threaded and used again. Similarly, in some microscopical sections the nuclei of the cells, e.g., in the skin and liver, can be recognized still. There is no reason, therefore, why very resistant bacteria should not be seen now.

Lesions of the teeth.—Very various also are the lesions of the teeth.

In an unknown woman, perhaps the princess Meritamon(XIIth–XIIIth Dynasties, about 1900 B.C.), all the teeth of the upper jaw were carious, with the exception of the canine and third molar; and the first and second molars were reduced to mere carious stumps. An old woman called Houttimihou (XVIIIth Dynasty, about 1400 B.C.) had a carious first molar and an alveolar abscess at the root of the first molar tooth near it. Amenhotep III had teeth moderately worn. On the right side, though not on the left, the teeth of both upper and lower jaws were thickly encrusted with tartar, and there had been an extensive abscess below the right incisors, and a smaller one above the right upper canine. The upper incisor teeth had been lost before the death of Amenhotep, and the alveolar process absorbed in part; the right upper lateral incisor had been recently lost, for its alveolus and the perforation (facial) of a small alveolar abscess were still present. There is also evidence of suppuration around the anterior lateral root of the left lower first molar.

It appears to me that as caries of teeth is not mentioned, this loss of teeth and the multiple alveolar abscesses were probably due to pyorrhoea alveolaris. It is very strange that the lesions of periodontal disease, which are certainly very common from predynastic to present times, should hardly have drawn any attention as yet.

The above quotations show conclusively how much the ancient Egyptains, even of the best circles, suffered from their teeth. I have already in other papers drawn attention to the fact that many dental lesions could have been remedied by very simple operations, which, however, do not appear ever to have been undertaken. It shows conclusively that the stories copied from textbook to textbook about the wonderful knowledge of dentistry possessed by old Egyptians are not borne out by facts. It is impossible to believe that Amenhotep III would have endured the agony which he must have gone through if the court dentist had known how to pull out a tooth.

Talipes equino-varus.—A well-marked deformity was that of Siptah (1209 B.C.) whose left foot shows the characteristic deformities of talipes equino-varus. This malformation is one which was known to have existed in ancient Egypt, for Miss Murray[1] in her valuable monograph has described and figured it. On the walls of Egyptian monuments also representations of club-footed males and females have been found, and I have figured some of them in a previous paper.[2] These malformed people shared with dwarfs, if not the affection, at any rate the interest of kings and rich people, as they often formed part of some large household.

The facts enumerated above form an important addition to our knowledge of the diseases of ancient Egyptians, and seeing how much has been learned from the examination of a few mummies, one cannot help regretting that, in the past, much material should have been wantonly destroyed. Let us hope that this waste may be diminished in the future.

[1] Margaret Murray, *The Tomb of Two Brothers.*
[2] "On Dwarfs and Other Deformed Persons in Ancient Egypt," *Bulletin de la Société Archéologique d'Alexandrie*, No. 13 (1911), p. 1.

A TUMOUR OF THE PELVIS DATING FROM ROMAN TIMES (250 A.D.) AND FOUND IN EGYPT[1]

(Journal of Pathology and Bacteriology, Vol. XVIII [1914])

The bone which forms the subject of this note was found by us in the catacombs of Kom el Shougafa, in Alexandria.

The skeletons in the catacombs undoubtedly date from Egyptian-Roman times, and, most probably, from the middle of the third century after Christ, or from some time before that date. The specimen in question was discovered among a number of human bones, in a grave which had been thoroughly rifled some time ago. The other bones were heaped up in utter confusion at one end of the grave, and they were in such a bad state that it was impossible to gather together the rest of the skeleton to which this specimen belonged.

The grave had been opened for some time and was very damp, and all the bones had a tendency to break to pieces, even when treated with the greatest care. Often they were so fragile that the only method of preserving them was to plunge them into melted paraffin at 55° C.; when all the air bubbles had escaped (ten to thirty minutes), the paraffin was allowed to run off. Care was taken to dry them thoroughly before they were placed in the paraffin, all adherent sand and other foreign bodies being removed with a soft brush. The specimens so treated could then be handled with perfect safety.

DESCRIPTION OF SPECIMEN FOUND

We shall compare the bone to be now described with a control one, approximately of the same size and dating from the same period.

The tumour occupies the right os innominatum (Plate XLV, Fig. 1) and affects particularly the ischium and lower portion of the ilium. The os pubis is apparently normal.

```
                                                                   cm.
     Maximum vertical length, from iliac crest to tuber ischii ... 21.6
     Maximum vertical length of control...................... 21.4
     Maximum width from angle of pelvis to spine of ischium..... 12.5
```

[1] This paper was written with J. Graham Willmore as junior author.

Posterior portion of ilium, including articular surface, has been broken away along an irregular line drawn on antero-internal surface, from the angle of great sacro-sciatic notch to a point on iliac crest corresponding to middle of insertion of quadratus lumborum. On postero-external surface a large spike of bone, owing to fracture being obliquely directed from before and outwards to behind and inwards, projects nearly as far as postero-inferior spine. Spine of ischium is also broken away. Thus, the great sacro-sciatic notch, viewed from behind, appears far more nearly complete than it does when seen from interior of pelvis. Broken surface of bone is cancellous and apparently healthy, though perhaps rather more spongy than normal.

Ilium greatly thickened throughout. Crest smooth and rounded, measures at its thickest 1.9 cm., and at its thinnest 1.5 cm. across. Control pelvis shows evidence of osteo-arthritis, with thickening and roughening of crest, yet its corresponding measurements are 1.7 and 0.75 cm.

	cm.
Maximum vertical length of ilium, from crest to upper border of acetabulum	10.0
Corresponding measurement in control	14.4
Maximum horizontal measurement, from broken area near superior-posterior to superior-anterior spine	12.5
Control	13.0
From anterior-superior to anterior-inferior spine	4.0
Control	2.3
Depth of notch between the two	0.7
Control	0.8
Thickness of bone, from a point just above acetabulum externally to a little above bony insertion of the psoas parvus internally	2.3
Control	2.1

ACETABULUM

The cavity of the acetabulum is healthy:

	cm.
Maximum vertical diameter	5.7
Control	5.5
Maximum horizontal diameter	5.2
Control	5.5
Maximum depth	2.4
Control	3.7

In the control pelvis there is a good deal of osteo-arthritis, with lipping of the acetabular brim and thinning of the floor of the cavity.

	cm.
From anterior-superior spine to angle of os pubis	15.7
Control	13.5

TUMOUR OF THE PELVIS

The specimen was sawn across horizontally through middle of acetabulum, from just above the origin of the ischial spine behind to point of junction of horizontal ramus of os pubis with ilium in front.

The obturator foramen is left intact.

The line of section passes through the main mass of the tumour (see Plate XLVI, Figs. 2 and 3). The body of the ischium in particular is seen to be enormously distended.

	cm.
a)* The maximum antero-posterior diameter of tumour, as seen on the upper surface of the lower segment, measures..	7.0
b) The maximum traverse diameter......................	5.1
Control...	1.2
c) Maximum vertical length approximately...............	11.0
Control identical.	
From centre of the acetabulum transversely across to the inner surface of the pelvis...........................	2.5
Control...	0.1
From the acetabulum across to the obturator groove, the thinnest part of the tumour, is.......................	1.3
Control...	0.3

* Line (a) (7 cm.) is taken from posterior border of body of the ischium to its junction with horizonta ramus of the os pubis. Ramus of pubis is spongy, but while there is no very definite wall between the two, the process seems to have stopped short at this point, i.e., the obturator groove.

Line (b) (5.1 cm) is taken from posterior brim of the acetabulum to the inner surface of the bone just above the origin of the ischial spine.

Line (c) is taken from 1.0 cm. above lower border of ischial tuberosity, which does not appear to be involved, to a point 1.0 cm. above upper border of acetabular brim.

It will thus be seen that the tumour has encroached upon the cavity of the acetabulum, while in the control, in connection with the osteo-arthritis, there seems to have been some rarefying process at work which has unduly thinned the acetabular floor and rendered its cavity deeper than normal.

	cm.
From a point on the outside just below acetabular margin to a corresponding point on inner surface of body of ischium..	4.9
Control...	2.8
From the posterior border of the ischium to most prominent part of anterior margin (i.e., about the middle of the posterior border of the obturator foramen)..............	6.0
Control...	3.6

The tumour does not appear to involve either the tuberosity or the ramus of ischium. A line drawn from the posterior border of the acetabular notch to the lower border of, and at right angles to, the ramus of the ischium, measures only 5.4 cm. as compared with 5.8 cm. in the control; whereas a line drawn from the same point—i.e., the acetabular notch—to the nearest part of obturator foramen measures 3 cm., as compared with 1.2 cm. in control.

The obturator foramen is greatly encroached upon; it is crescentic in outline, the two horns pointing backwards and upwards, and backwards and downwards, the enlargement forward of body of ischium being most marked between these horns. The transverse breadth of the foramen at its middle part is only 2 cm. as compared with 4.5 cm. in the control; longitudinally, it measures 5.5 cm. as compared with 5.3 cm. in the control. Thus, it is evident that the tumour, starting probably in the body of the ischium, has spread forwards so as to encroach on the obturator foramen, and also sideways, expanding particularly within the true pelvis. The expansion upwards, therefore, has not been so great, and forwards and downwards it has been still less.

Examined from inside the true pelvis, the bone presents a rounded, polished surface, bulging into the pelvic cavity, with seven grooves on it which converge into one large groove passing backwards and outwards under ischial spine. On the inner side these radiate forwards and spread out fanwise, the uppermost vertically upwards for about 3 cm. in front of the ischial spine; the second towards the ileo-pectineal line; the third, indistinct, is lost on the bulging surface of the tumour; the fourth, very well defined, deep and narrow (0.5 cm.) passes forwards and slightly upwards and outwards over the body of the tumour and apparently leads directly into the acetabulum. The fifth (1.5 cm. broad in its widest part) is separated from the preceding by a well-marked ridge of bone 0.6 cm. broad, curves upwards and outwards almost parallel to the preceding, and is lost near the posterior margin of the obturator foramen. The sixth, indistinct, runs to the lower angle (or horn) of the obturator foramen. The seventh, well defined, pursues the usual course of the groove for the pubic vessels and nerve. It is probable that all these grooves were formed by enlarged blood vessels.

On section (Plate XLVI, Figs. 2 and 3) the tumour is seen to consist of compact bony tissue with numerous cavities interspersed. One of them, situated near the inner surface, extends from in front of the centre of the acetabulum to near the origin of the ischial spine, and is of considerable size. It measures 2.1 cm. in length, 1 cm. in breadth, and 2 cm. (approximately) in depth. The cavities are in some places smooth and shining, in others they show numerous fine trabeculae which branch and project into the interior and form a delicate honeycomb. These trabeculae are very soft and friable, even after treatment with paraffin.

The cavities above mentioned have no obvious communication with the exterior, and in no way resemble those produced by osteophagous insects, samples of whose work are sometimes to be seen on the surface of certain bones; moreover, they are situated in the midst of hard and massive compact tissue, not in the cancellous tissue.

Microscopically, nothing new was ascertained, chiefly because the sections proved exceedingly unsatisfactory.

PLATE XLV

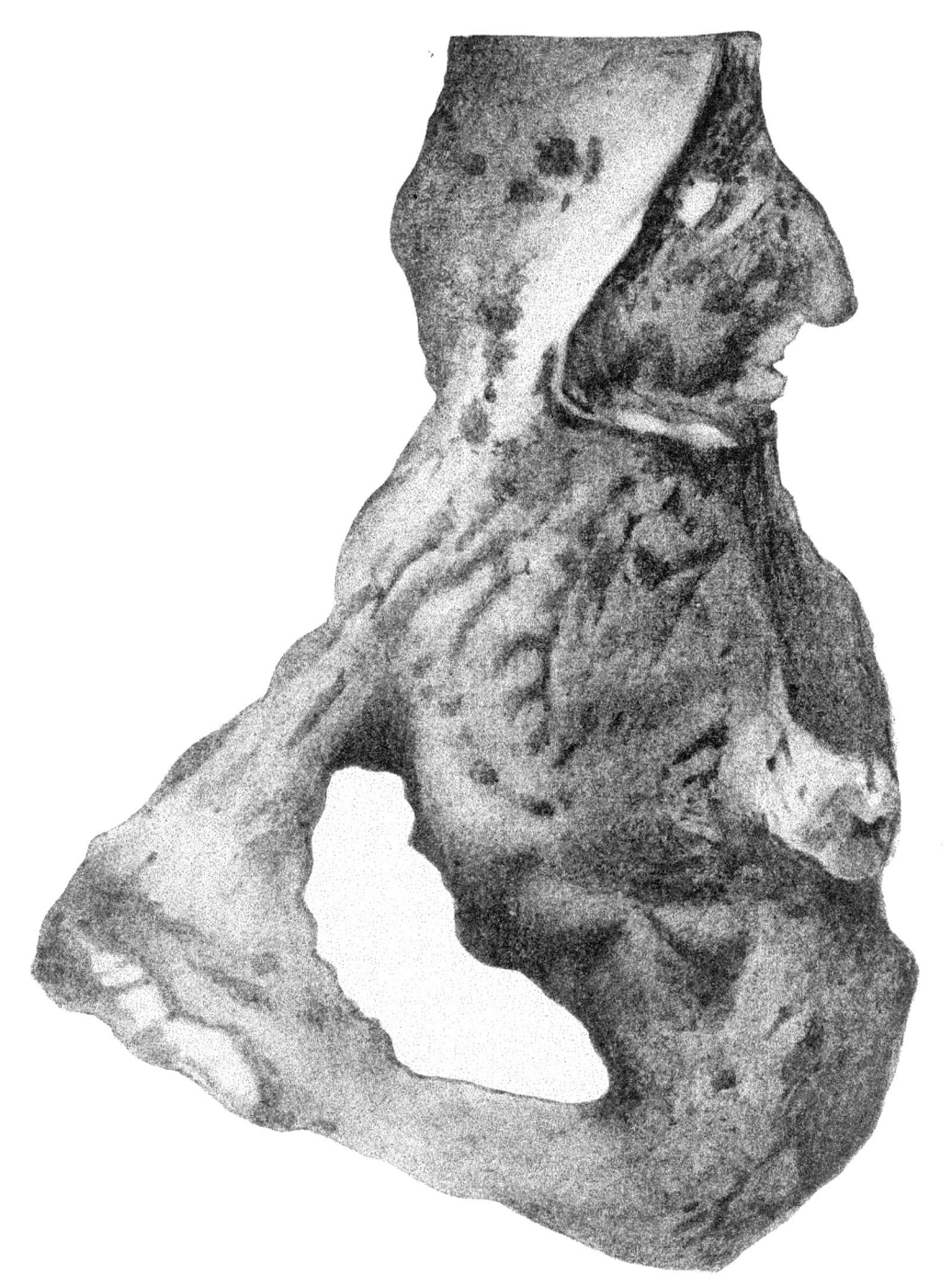

FIG. 1

PLATE XLVI

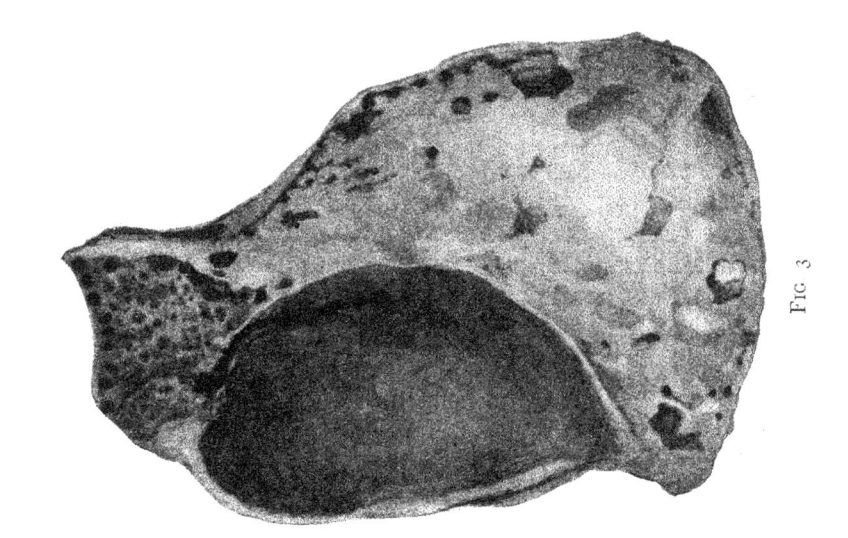

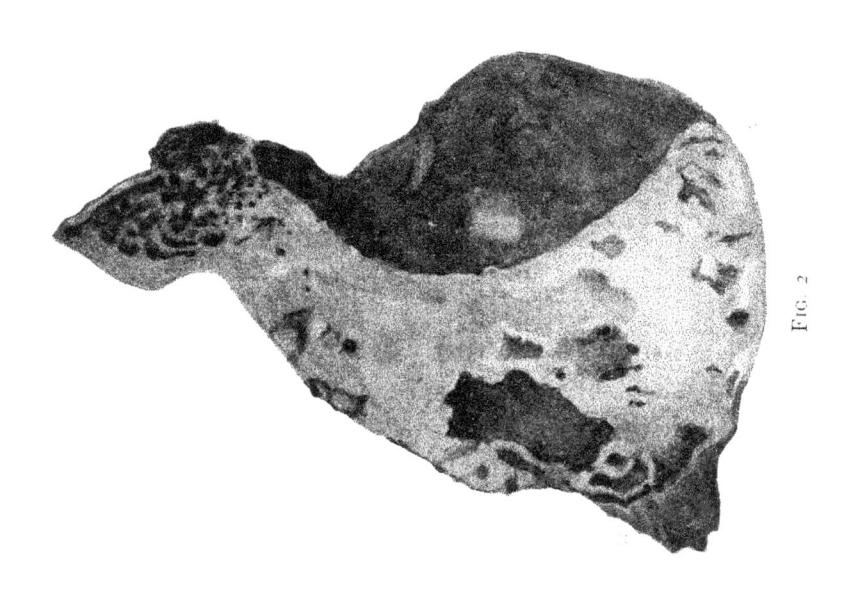

Fig. 2

Fig. 3

SUMMARY

We are here in presence of a tumour which has started in the cancellous tissue of the pelvis. Its growth has caused (1) a very marked expansion of the bone, noticeable chiefly in the body of the ischium and ilium; (2) great deformation of the obturator foramen; and (3) it has encroached to some extent on the acetabulum. Judging from the numerous grooves on the surface, it is very probable that this tumour was highly vascular, and that very soon it would have involved the more superficial parts of the bone, which had remained intact so far.

The exact nature of the tumour must remain uncertain. It is clear, however, that the swelling was not due to any of the infective agents, such as tubercle, syphilis, actonomycosis, etc. From the fact that the larger part of the tumour is solid, secondary carcinoma can also be excluded.

Taking into consideration the fact that the swelling is deeply seated, partly solid and partly cystic, and had evidently been growing fast, we are of opinion that the tumour was most probably an osteosarcoma, of which the bony substance has resisted the effects of time, whereas its soft parts have disappeared.

It is not possible, however, to say whether the tumour was primary or secondary.

DESCRIPTION OF PLATES XLV-XLVI[1]

PLATE XLV

Fig. 1.—Tumour in situ.

PLATE XLVI

Figs. 2 and 3.—Section through the tumour.

[1] The blocks have been prepared from paintings by M. A. Cooper. The drawings are exactly natural size.

A PATHOLOGICAL SPECIMEN DATING FROM THE LOWER MIOCENE PERIOD[1]

The typical lesions of chronic joint disease have been discovered in European skeletons dating from remote antiquity, as, for instance, in the skeleton of a man from the Quaternary station of Raymonden, a village situated in the commune of Chancelade, seven kilometres to the northeast of Périgueux. This skeleton now occupies a place of honour in the museum of that town, and its anatomical and pathological peculiarities have been fully described by a competent observer.[2]

The bones are those of a man who was about fifty years old at the time of death, and who, long before his end, had suffered from an extensive fracture of the right temporal region, which had completely healed. All the maxillary teeth had been lost during life. The arthritic lesions consist of:

1. Very wide enlargement of the costo-transverse articulation of one rib, with articular exostosis typical of chronic osteo-arthritis.

2. Enlargement of the transverse diameter of the glenoid cavity of the right scapula, of which only fragments remain. This enlargement was probably due to osteo-arthritis of the humero-scapular articulation; few traces of periarticular pathological osseous formations are noticeable round this articulation, and the head of the right humerus presents the characteristic lesions of dry arthritis. The articular surface of the bone is encircled by an osteophyte cushion, 0.009 m. wide and 0.008 m. thick, and the many vascular orifices opening on it show clearly that the movements of the joint had been affected by pathological changes in the cartilage, which probably had been completely absorbed during life.

[1] This paper first appeared as an appendix to a work by R. Fourtau, *Contribution à l'étude des vertébrés miocènes de l'Égypte*, which was issued by the Geological Survey Department of Egypt, 1920.

[2] L. Testut, "Recherches anthropologiques sur le squelette quaternaire de Chancelade, Dordogne," Extrait du *Bulletin de la Société d'Anthropologie de Lyon.*

The occurrence of osteo-arthritis in prehistoric people has been known for a long time, and in 1881 J. le Baron[1] wrote an interesting memoir on this subject. Since then evidence proving that this disease was very common during the Stone Age has been gradually accumulating. In the Neolithic burials of Vendrest in the Vendée, for instance, Baudouin[2] found specimens of osteo-arthritis of the cervical vertebrae, atlas, atloaxoid articulations, knee-joint, ribs, lower end of the fibula, third right metatarsal, first phalanx of the toes, first phalanx of the right hallux, and second phalanx of the toes and probably of the vertebrae also.

The Neolithic ossarium of Bazoges en Pareds (Vendée) yielded to the same observer human bones with typical osteo-arthritic lesions of the fibula (four cases), patella, ulna, clavicle, axis, hallux (three cases), phalanges of foot, etc.[3]

The museums of the Anthropological School and of the Jardin des Plantes, Paris, and many of the interesting anthropological collections in provincial French towns contain numerous anatomical specimens showing that for thousands of years many inhabitants of Gaul were crippled by osteo-arthritis.

In England also the disease appeared very early. The prehistorical remains of Caithness[4] show pathological lesions probably due to osteo-arthritis. In one case exostoses were discovered on the front spaces of the pubic bones near the symphysis, and on the ilium and sacrum in the region of the synchondroses. It was certainly prevalent during the Bronze Age.[5] An old man found near Broadstairs, for instance, suffered from "osteitis of the vertebral column, pelvis, and shoulder girdle,' and some of the vertebrae of a middle-aged male Jute from a neighbouring grave were ankylosed by spondylitis.

[1] J. le Baron, *Lésions osseuses de l'homme préhistorique en France et en Algérie*, thèse de Paris, 1881 (8vo). See also J. le Baron, "Sur les lésions osseuses préhistoriques," *Bulletin de la Société d'Anthropologie de Paris*, IV (1881), 596.

[2] Marcel Baudouin, *Diseases of Bones*.

[3] Baudouin, "Les affections osseuses découvertes dans l'ossuaire néolithique de Bazoges en Pareds (Vendée)," *Arch. Prov. de Chirurgie*, Vol. XXIII (1914), No. 1, p. 22.

[4] Samuel Laing, *Prehistoric Remains of Caithness*, with notes by Th. H. Huxley.

[5] F. G. Parsons, "On Some Bronze Age and Jutish Bones from Broadstairs," *Journal of the Anthropological Institute of Great Britain and Ireland*, XLIII (1913), 550.

The Germans of pre-Roman days did not escape. The long bones of a skeleton from a tumulus[1] at Klein Asbergle-Ludwigsburg, were disfigured by excrescences typical of arthritis chronica deformans. Rough, warty, comblike outgrowths were obvious in the posterior side of the femur and humerus, especially in the neighbourhood of the joints and along the muscular insertions.

Arthritis deformans has been described in a series of Swedish skeletons dating from Neolithic times.[2] It was prevalent in Scandinavia at the time of the Vikings and a well-marked case was discovered[3] in a Viking ship dating from the tenth century A.D. The subject of the disease was an old man about fifty years old.

It is very interesting to note that also by the excavation of the tumulus where our last viking ship, the Osberg-ship, was found in the year 1904, there were also removed from the ship fragments of a female skeleton (also probably fifty years old) which was showing traces of *arthritis deformans*. I have also by examination of many hundreds of skeletons from the anatomical collections in Lund and Upsala (Sweden) seen several specimens with the same disease.[4]

Arthritis of prehistoric Danish bodies also has been described,[5] and was very common, as the majority of adult skeletons are attacked.

Elliot Smith and Wood Jones[6] showed the great frequency of osteo-arthritis among ancient Egyptians in Nubia and Upper Egypt. Later on, Rietti and I[7] described many specimens dating from the

[1] H. von Holder, "Untersuchungen über die Skelettfunde in den vorrömischen Hügelgräbern Württembergs und Hohenzollerns," *Fundberichte aus Schwaben*, II (1895).

[2] C. M. Furst, *Skelettfunde aus Steinzeitgräbern in Nerike, nebst einigen über Steinaltersvolkes Krankheiten und Verletzungen*, Fernwannen, 1914. See also *Mitteilungen zur Geschichte der Medizin und der Naturwissenschaften*, Vol. XIII, No. 4, p. 515.

[3] N. Nicoloysen, *The Viking Ship Discovered at Gothstadt in Norway*, Christiania, 1882.

[4] Private letter from Dr. Fredrik Gron of Christiania.

[5] H. A. Nielsen, Ref. in *Mitteilungen zur Geschichte der Medizin und Naturwissenschaften*, IV, 377.

[6] G. Elliot Smith and F. Wood Jones, *Archaeological Survey of Nubia, Report for 1907-8*, Vol. II, "Report on the Human Remains."

[7] M. Armand Ruffer and Arnoldo Rietti, "On Osseous Lesions in Ancient Egyptians," *Journal of Pathology and Bacteriology*, XVI (1912), 439. M. A. Ruffer, "Studies in Palaeopathology in Egypt," *ibid.*, XVIII (1913), 149. "Notes on Two Egyptian Mummies," *Bulletin de la Société Archéologique d'Alexandrie*, No. 14 (1912), p. 1. "Note on the Diseases of the Sudan and Nubia in Ancient Times," *Mitteilungen zur Geschichte der Medizin und Naturwissenschaften*, Vol. XIII (1914), No. 4.

Meroitic kingdom of the Sudan, and Greek and Roman Alexandria and early Christian Upper Egypt.

The cave bear, *Ursus spelaeus*, lived in the caves before man. It is found in the Lower Palaeolithic epoch and is occasionally though rarely met with during the Reindeer period, especially at Bassompuy and in many Solutrean and pre-Solutrean strata. The Herm grotto in the Ariège contained very many skeletons of this animal. Drawings of the cave bear adorn a slate plate discovered in an Upper Palaeolithic stratum, and the wall of a grotto at Combarelles (Dordogne).

This enormous beast, when erect, sometimes measured as much as 2.5,[1] m. and though herbivorous chiefly, probably fed on carrion also, and on game now and then.

The naturalist Saak,[2] in 1824, collected from the Sundvich caves, near Iserlohn, many bones of *Ursus spelaeus* exhibiting pathological changes which were studied afterwards by Nöggerath,[3] and especially by von Walther.[4] The latter correctly described the lesion of osteo-arthritis and spondylitis, and the investigations of Virchow on *Höhlengicht*, which are always quoted, were not published till more than fifty years afterwards.

The last student of this disease in cave bears has described the following pathological lesions:[5]

1. *Bear A.*—Seventh cervical vertebra. Large osteophyte of the body. Osteitis of transverse processes.

2. *Bear B.*—Dorsal osteophyte of posterior part of body *en bourrelet*.

3. *Bear C.*—Dorsal vertebra. Posterior region of thorax. Right and left osteophytes of the inferior face of the body.

4. *Bear D.*—Dorsal vertebra. Osteophyte of body localized on the left side.

5. *Bear E.*—Ankylosis of two lumbar vertebrae. Median osteophyte of body. Vertebral superior and inferior osteo-arthritis. Superior ankylosis.

[1] Hugo Obermaier, *Der Mensch aller Zeiten*, p. 91.

[2] Iwan Bloch, *Der Ursprung der Syphilis*, p. 320.

[3] Nöggerath, *Archiv für die gesamte Naturlehre*, Vol. II (1824), No. 3, p. 323.

[4] Fr. von Walther, "Ueber das Altertum der Knochenkrankheiten," *Journal der Chirurgie und Augenheilkunde*, VIII (1825), 1.

[5] Marcel Baudouin, "La spondylite déformante à l'époque néolithique et chez les animaux préhistoriques," *Arch. Prov. de Chirurgie*, 1912, p. 274.

6. *Bear F.*—Inferior ankylosis of two successive lumbar vertebrae. Central region. Median osteophyte of the body encroaching on neighbouring bodies. Inferior and posterior vertebral osteo-arthritis. Inferior ankylosis.

The osteo-arthritic lesions of the vertebrae of cave bears which, thanks to the kindness of Professor Cartailhac, I had an opportunity of examining in the museum of Toulouse, are identical with those of spondylitis deformans in early or modern man. The lipping of the vertebrae, the osteophytes on the borders of the vertebral bodies, the pathological changes in the articulating surfaces, and the ankylosis resulting from these various lesions, all are typical of spondylitis deformans. Pathological changes in the teeth attributable to pyorrhoea were present in one skull only, in which the fangs of the molars and premolars on one side were partly bare.

A tibio-tarsal articulation of a *Bos primigenius* in the same museum showed well-marked signs of periarthritis. The tibia of a cave hyena in the museum at Foix, in the Pyrenees, shows severe osteo-arthritic lesions, and I have seen similar specimens in several other provincial museums of France.

Spondylitis was not uncommon in the sacred monkeys of the ancient temples near Thebes. The large articulations of a young Cynocephalus, for instance,[1] were surrounded by huge osseous "vegetations," and several dorsal and lumbar vertebrae of this animal were ankylosed. Six vertebrae of the lumbar region of another monkey were similarly affected, the three lower lumbar vertebrae forming a solid block, owing to the ossification of the anterior vertebral ligament and neighbouring fibrous tissue. The layer of new bone, hard as ivory, was from 0.003 to 0.004 m. thick, and extended as far as the transverse processes. A large number of the lumbar and caudal vertebrae of another monkey also were ankylosed.[2] Without hesitation this pathological condition has been attributed to life in cold and humidity, regardless of the fact that the rainfall at Thebes is practically nil, and the average temperature of the cold and sunless temples is 20° C.

Sheep and oxen were not immune in ancient Egypt.[3] The last dorsal and four first lumbar vertebrae of a sacred sheep, for instance,

---

[1] Lortet, *La faune momifiée de l'ancienne Égypte*, Série II, p. 2.
[2] *Ibid.*, Série III, p. 2.   [3] *Ibid.*, p. 9.

were so firmly ankylosed that all movements must have been extremely difficult. The vertebral ligament, ossified on the internal (?) side, was from 0.003 to 0.005 m. thick. No trace of ulceration existed. The pelvic bones of a *Bos africanus* also were deformed by numerous vegetations and exostoses.

The facts just related show clearly that, from the earliest times, osteo-arthritis attacked men and animals living under the most different climates and conditions and eating most dissimilar food.

It will be noticed that all the examples given so far date from comparatively modern times, or from the Quaternary period, and that little or nothing is on record concerning osteo-arthritis in animals which lived before the Quaternary period. M. Fourtau, however, has drawn my attention to a paper by L. Mayet[1] in which this author mentions and gives a photograph of the right foot of a rhinoceros, showing ankylosis of the metatarsal bones with the tarsus, with surrounding exostoses. No details of this find are given.

The specimen to be described now was discovered by M. Fourtau, of the Geological Museum, Cairo, near Hateyet el Mogharah, a lake of the Mariut desert. He informed me that the specimen was lying in a Burdigalian stratum of the Lower Miocene period, and that it is not less than 900,000 years old and very probably much older. I may be allowed to express to M. Fourtau my best thanks for handing this unique specimen over to me.

The two bones are completely petrified and in an excellent state of preservation, the cancellous structure of the bone being perfect, and though the specimen had been broken into two pieces when lifted out of its bed, its fractured surfaces are perfect and were afterwards glued together with excellent results. Unfortunately, it is not possible to make sure to which of the two kinds of petrified crocodiles occurring in this stratum these bones belonged.[2]

The specimen comprises two vertebrae which may be either the last lumbar or the first caudal vertebrae. Judging from their size, it may be assumed that the length of the animal was not less than

[1] L. Mayet, "Étude des mammifères miocènes des sables de l'Orléanais et des faluns de la Touraine," *Ann. de l'Université de Lyon*, nouvelle série, No. 24 (1908).

[2] It is most probable that these vertebrae belonged to the species of "gavial" now described by Mr. Fourtau under the name of *Tomistoma Dowsoni*.

5 m., including a tail about 2.5 m. long. The body of the anterior vertebrae measures 0.5 m., and that of the second 0.54 m. from above downwards, and the antero-posterior diameter of the anterior vertebrae o 054 m. from before back, and 0.058 m. from side to side at the superior border. Owing to the presence of new bone, the corresponding measurements of the posterior vertebra remain doubtful. The greater part of the two spinous processes and of the transverse processes, with the exception of the left anterior process, is broken off. The bases are smooth, without noticeable lesions.

A thick band of osseous tissue, obviously pathological, firmly binds together the vertebrae. It extends to the left side at A (Plate XLVIII, 4) for about 0.05 m., the point B (Plate XLVIII, 4) being 0.05 m. over the median line. From the point A (Plate XLVIII, 4) the osseous band running upwards forms a sinuous, raised border gradually melting into normal bone at the base of the transverse processes. The convex superior border extends to within 0.005 m. (Plate XLVII, 1 B and Plate XLVIII, 4 C) of the anterior border of the vertebral body. From the point B (Plate XLVIII, 4) the new bone runs almost perpendicularly downwards to C (Plate XLVII, 1) for almost the whole length of the body of the posterior vertebra.

On the right side (see Plate XLVII, 2), the pathological osseous band extends to the base of the transverse process of the posterior vertebra, crosses over the intervertebral space at B, spreading then over the right side of the bodies of both vertebrae. At B (Plate XLVIII, 4) the new bone is more than half a centimetre thick.

At E (Plate XLVII, 1) there is a loss of substance evidently due to a post-mortem traumatism, whereas the hole F (Plate XLVII, 1, 2) has all the characteristics of a large blood vessel.

A distinct pathological osseous arch with its concavity towards the intervertebral space bridges over the latter. The concave space thus formed between the pathological band and the vertebrae was full of fine sand, and, when this had been washed away, the vertebrae underneath the band were found normal.

Plate XLVIII, 5, represents the anterior surface of the anterior vertebra and it shows the enormous mass of new bone which had developed along the lines *ab* and *ad*. This figure may be usefully compared with No. 6 (Plate XLVIII), the photograph of the inferior surface of the body of a dorsal vertebra of an ancient Egyptian, with the lesions of spondylitis deformans.

In both, the new bone is sharply separated from the bodies of the vertebrae, superadded to them, so to speak, and is thickest on one side. The surface covered by the cartilage is normal and other pathological alterations are absent. No. 5 (Plate XLVIII) shows that part of the bone has broken after death, leaving a surface which is apparently free from disease.

REMARKS

The first idea to suggest itself was that the lesion might have been caused by a traumatism, a blow, for instance, and that the new bone was simply callus. This diagnosis is shown to be fallacious by the fact that pathological lesions which could be attributed to a traumatism, severe enough to produce the development of thick layers of bone, e.g., sinus, spiculae of new bone, loss of substance, etc., are totally absent. On the other hand, the changes characteristic of spondylitis deformans, as observed in ancient and modern human skeletons, are conspicuous.

In man, the first and most characteristic lesion of spondylitis deformans is the growth of an osteophyte from the antero-lateral border of the body of one or more vertebrae. As a rule, three, four, or five, or more vertebrae are thus attacked, and, very occasionally, the disease is limited to one or two vertebrae (see Plate XLVII, 3). Fig. 3, for instance, represents two Egyptian human vertebrae with spondylitis deformans, dating from the Roman period. The osteophytes from the neighbouring vertebrae have grown until their gradually narrowing extremities have met at *a*, whereas their bases are broader. The bridge thus formed forms an arch, the concavity of which is turned towards the intervertebral space. The rather soft new bone is not eburnated, and this is the case even when it has attained a considerable size. The upper and lower borders of the osteophyte, not more than two or three millimetres thick, are usually prolonged in this case for a few millimetres on the body of the vertebra, and, as a rule, the osteophytes are situated uni- or bilaterally, hardly ever centrally, and the posterior border of the vertebrae is attacked only when the disease has made some progress already.

In a later stage the base of the osteophytes spread out on the anterior surface of the bodies until those from the superior and inferior borders coalesce. In bilateral disease, the osteophytes ultimately extend laterally, cross the middle line, and the anterior and lateral surfaces of the body may thus be covered by a thick ring of bone.

In man, osteophytes springing from the posterior border of the body are never more than 0.001 m. or 0.002 m. thick, and therefore do not press on the spinal cord, although they may ultimately coalesce with the anterior and lateral osteophytes, and then a complete ring of osseous tissue surrounds the vertebrae and the intervertebral spaces. The spinal foramen of the crocodile also is not narrowed, and its walls show no pathological changes.

Intervertebral discs have been found in position in mummified bodies, and in cases of spondylitis the discs, though shrunk, appear normal. The intervertebral spaces of skeletons with spondylitis are neither diminished in size nor altered in shape.

This description applies exactly to the specimen which forms the subject of this paper, and the two photographs (Nos. 3 and 6) demonstrating the changes due to spondylitis in human dorsal vertebrae show the great resemblance between the lesions of this disease in man and those seen in our crocodile. The disease in the crocodile evidently began on one side, spread to the middle line, and was extending on the other side at the time of death. The bone had developed in the antero-lateral ligament, or, at any rate, in its close proximity, and had spread along the anterior surface of the body of the vertebra and formed a typical arch over the space for the intervertebral disc. The articulating surfaces showed no pathological alterations, and the borders of the spinal foramen were intact.

In the crocodile as in man, therefore, the disease is more marked on one side, the bone forms an arch over the space for the intervertebral disc, and the upper and lower surfaces of the body and the spinal foramen are untouched.

PLATE XLVII

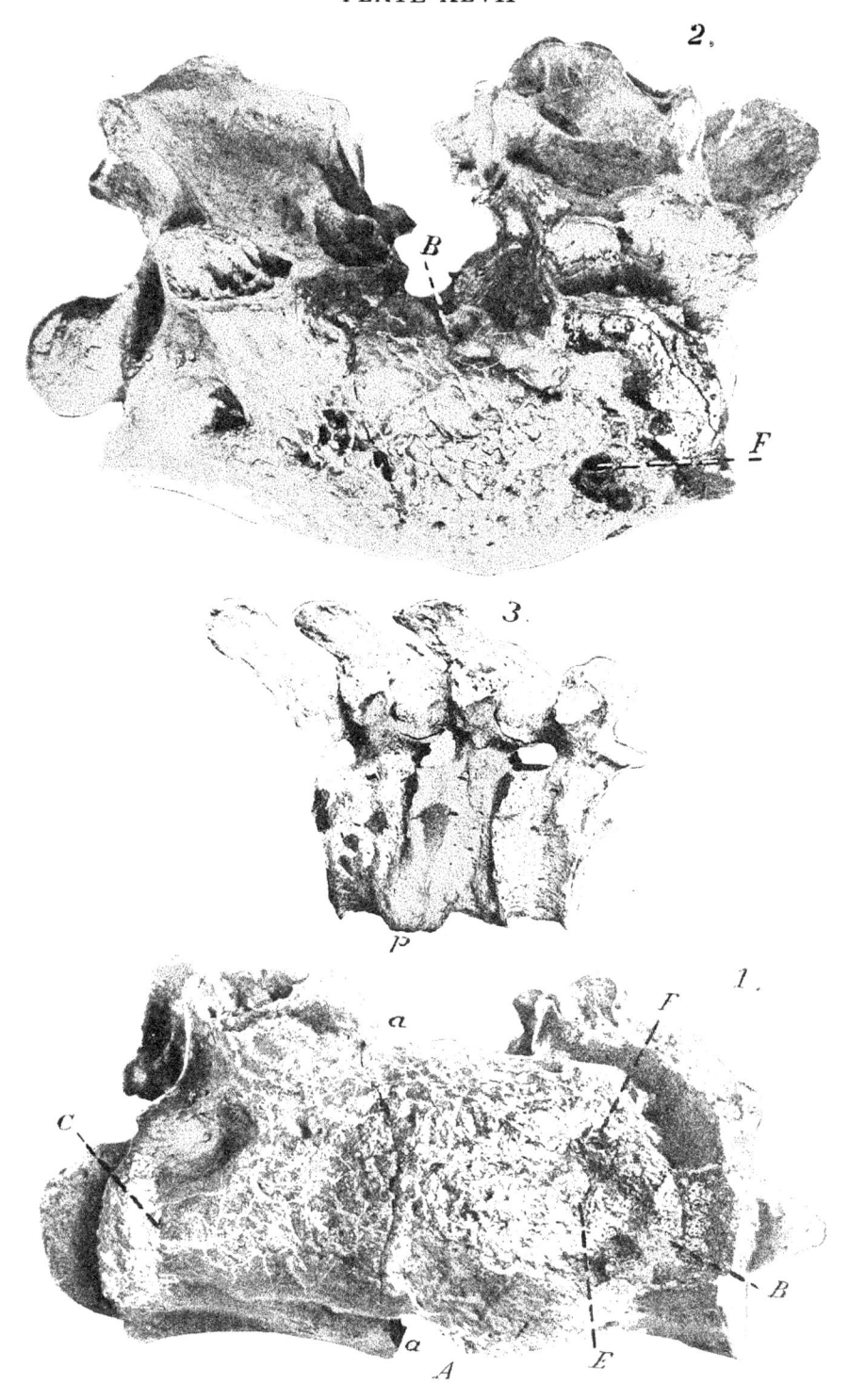

PLATE XLVIII

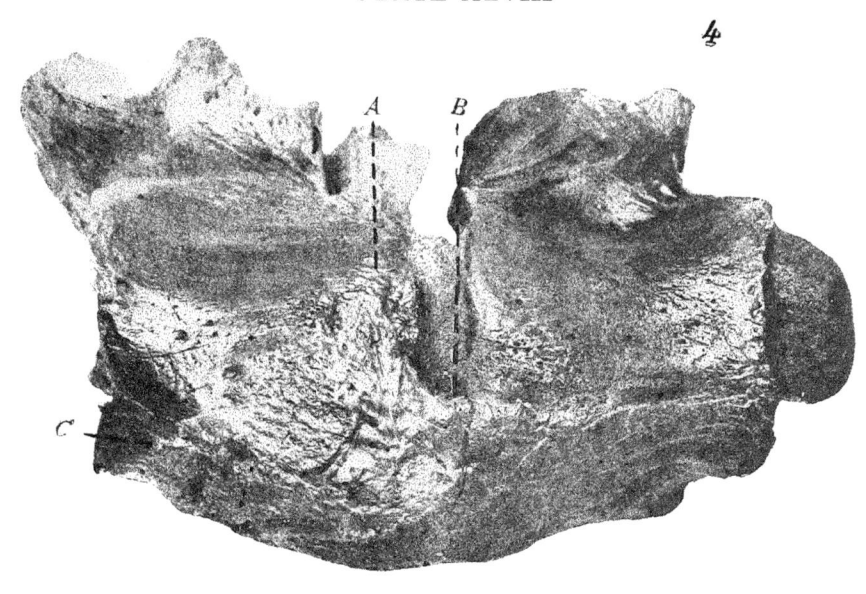

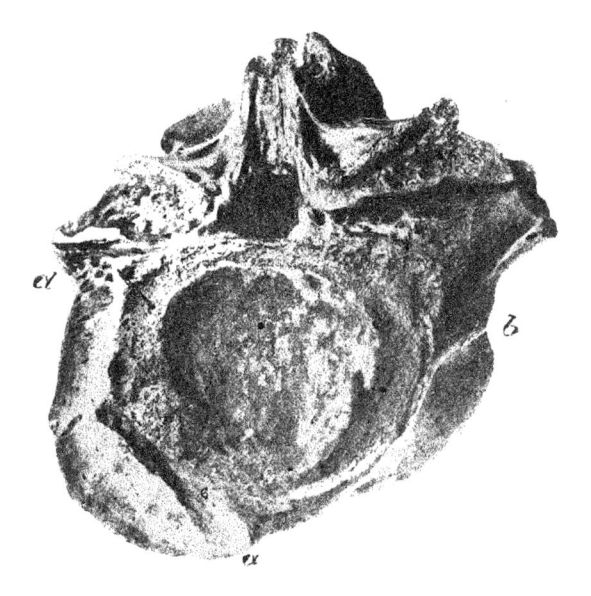

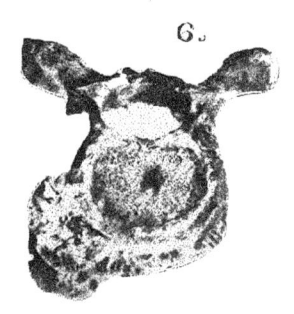

I conclude that the pathological lesions which crippled the vertebral column of a crocodile living not less than 900,000 years ago are exactly similar to those seen in modern human beings.

DESCRIPTION OF PLATES XLVII–XLVIII

PLATE XLVII

Fig. 1.—Ventral view of posterior lumbar or anterior caudal vertebrae of a fossil crocodile (possibly a gavial of the species *Tomistoma dowsoni*), from the Lower Miocene Period of Egypt, showing at the letters A, B, C the limits of the growth of new bone due to spondylitis deformans. a marks the inferior and superior points where the lines of new growth converge. E marks a point at which there has been some loss of substance, possibly due to post-mortem traumatism. F indicates a rounded opening, possibly occupied by a bloodvessel.

Fig. 2.—Right lateral view of same vertebrae, showing at B the new bony growth, and at F the vascular opening.

Fig. 3.—Lesions of spondylitis deformans, at p, in the thoracic vertebrae of a man of the Roman period in Egypt. Note the similarity in lateral development of the lesion in man and crocodile.

Figures about ⅔ natural size.

PLATE XLVIII

Fig. 4.—Left lateral view of vertebrae of fossil crocodile showing extent of osseous lesions at A, B, C.

Fig. 5.—View of anterior end of anterior vertebra of fossil crocodile showing development and overlipping of the osseous lesions of spondylitis deformans along the lines a-b and a-d.

Fig. 6.—Posterior aspect of dorsal human (Egyptian, XXIId Dynasty) vertebra showing lesion of spondylitis deformans at the lower, left angle.

Figures about ⅔ natural size.

SOME RECENT RESEARCHES ON PREHISTORIC TREPHINING

(*Journal of Pathology and Bacteriology*, Vol. XXII [1918])

PREFATORY NOTE

When my husband left last winter on the mission to Salonika which ended in his death at the hands of the enemy, he left with me several unfinished works, most of which he intended to issue under the title of "Studies in Palaeopathology." Some of the series had been published prior to his death in the *Journal of Pathology and Bacteriology* (XV [1911], 1; XVI [1911–12], 439; XVIII [1913–14], 480), and elsewhere.

According to my husband's instructions, I have filled up certain lacunae in the present paper, and made various necessary alterations. He did not profess that it contained anything new, but it is a compilation of several authors' investigations into this subject, to be used as a reference.

It is perhaps, owing to the untimely death of the author, not exhaustively complete, but matter of interest may still be found in this paper of Sir Armand Ruffer's on "Prehistoric Trephining."

ALICE RUFFER

The facts relating to this science are scattered through anthropological, ethnological, and historical memoirs, and especially through papers describing excavations of ancient sites. The pathologist, therefore, unless in touch with anthropology and allied sciences, does not become acquainted with the latest pathological finds, and yet it is only by the patient accumulation of such observations that the science of the history of disease can be established on a firm basis. The object of this paper is to put on record, for the benefit of pathologists, observations bearing on their science made during the last few years, but which are scattered through various publications. I have added a few facts observed by myself.

RECENT OBSERVATIONS ON TREPANNING

Trepanning the skull was an operation frequently performed in Neolithic times, especially in western Europe, and quite lately Baudouin[1] has again found in western France a number of trepanned skulls dating from prehistoric times, which are interesting from the

[1] Marcel Baudouin, "Étude d'un crâne néolithique à double trépanation," *L'homme préhistorique*, V (1908), 207.

fact that some had been trepanned twice, thrice, and even four times. Evidence has now been forthcoming that the operation was not limited to western Europe, but was performed also in Bohemia at a very early period.

The results of prehistoric surgery were sometimes very good. The cicatrisation is often so complete that no doubt can exist regarding the patient's survival for many years. In some skulls, however, evidences of repair are completely, or almost completely, absent, either because the patient died shortly after the operation, or, as some authors maintain, because the bone was removed after death.

My impression is that the majority of the openings which have been supposed to have been made post mortem were really made during life, and that in these cases death supervened very shortly after the trepanning. This hypothesis is certainly correct in cases when, in a skull with two or more trephining holes, one or more are cicatrised, whereas one opening alone shows no signs of repair. The probability then is that the subject was trephined several times for chronic, acutely painful disease, e.g., tumor cerebri, and that the last operation was fatal. On the other hand, when the greater part of the temporo-parietal region or nearly the whole of one side of the cranium had been removed, the possibility of this having been done on the living is very slight.[1]

It has been suggested that post-mortem operations on the skull were made with the object of obtaining pieces of cranial bones to be used as amulets. Indeed, pieces of bone detached by trephining ("rondelles") were carefully preserved, for not only are some of them pierced for suspension, but their smooth borders indicate long friction against the skin. Powdered cranial bones were supposed to possess curative properties in the remote past and up to the Middle Ages, and rondelles were certainly worn as ornaments or as amulets as late as Gallic times.

Discovery of trephined prehistoric skulls.—The discovery of the first trephined prehistoric human skull dates from 1685; it was found at Cocheral.[2] It had been twice "perforated," and these

---

[1] I have seen in some anthropological museums skulls labelled as "trephined post mortem" in which I could not find any real evidence of ante- or post-mortem operation.

[2] Cartailhac, *La France préhistorique*, Paris, 1889, p. 281.

perforations are now considered to have been caused by a surgical operation, which the patient survived long enough for his wounds to heal. In 1816 another trephined prehistoric skull was discovered at Nogent-les-Vinages, in an ossarium containing no less than nine hundred skeletons. The opening in this cranium measures about 3 by 2 inches, and at the time the skull was found the loss of substance was considered as due to a wound or fracture, which had completely healed. Indeed, Cuvier, who examined this skull, estimated that the patient survived the injury for a dozen years. It is now recognised that the aperture was due to a trephining operation, and not to an accident. In 1872 Prunière drew attention to the many trephined Neolithic crania discovered in ossaria, grottos, or dolmens of the Lozère region, and since that time many trephined skulls have been brought to light in divers places.

French discoveries of trephined skulls.—The largest number of trephined prehistoric heads have been found in France, e.g., at Enteroches (Charente), Moret (Seine et Marne), Tour-sur-Marne, Bougon (Deux Sèvres), Petit Morin (Marne), Vienne, Marennes (Puy de Dôme), Sorde and Fondonneau (Basses-Pyrénées).

A short account may be given of a few particularly interesting trephined skulls lately found in that country. The skull of a man who died when about fifty years old, found at Crécy-sur-Serre (Aisne), was pierced by two trephining holes.[1] The first was situated on the antero-superior angle of the left parietal bone near the anterior fontanelle, and the second was above the right temporal fossa, almost in the middle of the inferior border of the right temporal bone. Absence of any signs of repair suggested to the discoverer of these skulls that both operations had been performed after death. In my opinion the possibility of the operation having been done during life, and having been followed very soon by death, cannot be denied.

At Montereau-sur-Seine,[2] almost sixty miles from Paris, two trephined heads were discovered in a prehistoric burial. No details concerning them are available so far.

[1] Marcel Baudouin, "Étude d'un crâne néolithique à double trépanation," *L'homme préhistorique*, V (1908), 207.

[2] Berthiaux, "Le préhistorique à Montereau," *L'homme préhistorique*, VI (1908), 85.

A cranium[1] of an adult female with three trepanations is probably Neolithic, but, unluckily, its origin is somewhat obscure. The patient survived the three operations long enough for a small exostosis to form on the border of one opening. The holes are small and close to one another, the first being situated in the antero-superior parietal region; a second in the same region on the right side; and the third not far behind the second. The diametres of the openings (13 and 15 mm.) somewhat exceed that of the crown of the usual modern trephining instrument, and the sloping borders of these orifices indicate that the operations were performed by scraping horizontally with a sharp flint, and not by cutting with a saw. The only striae present are on the posterior margin of the third hole, and indicate that an instrument had been used vertically in that situation.

Six trephined heads,[2] unearthed in one locality, are good examples of the skill of Neolithic surgeons. A piece of bone 90 by 57 mm. had been removed from the right parietal bone of the first cranium, and the absence of any signs of cicatrisation proves that death supervened soon after the operation. In the interior of the second cranium, which presented a similar lesion, a very perfect rondelle was found, which measured 60 by 10 mm. and from 10 to 7.5 mm. in thickness. Some striae on the superior surface of the rondelle are so sharp that they might have been made with a graver's tool. The context and illustrations, however, leave one in doubt as to whether the rondelle belonged to this cranium or not. The third cranium had been trephined twice. A festooned opening measuring 90 by 50 mm. is situated over the right temporal and parietal bones, and another, almost round, measuring 36 by 30 mm., occupies the vertex just behind the left parietal bone. Both these apertures show no signs of repair. A typical trepanation, measuring 20 mm. in diametre, with borders showing evidences of almost complete repair, occupies the upper part of the occipital bone of the fourth cranium. The fifth cranium shows a deep depression,

---

[1] Marcel Baudouin, "Études d'un crâne préhistorique à triple trépanation executée sur le vivant," *Bulletin de la Société d'Anthropologie*, 1908, p. 436.

[2] Émile Schmit, "Présentation de quelques crânes néolithiques trépanés," *ibid.*, 1909, p. 206.

measuring 90 by 55 mm. on the occipital protuberance, in the centre of which there is an artificial aperture probably made by a process of scraping. A sixth cranium was discovered in a grotto close to that in which the five others had been buried. On the left parietal bone of this skull there is a D-shaped opening, 50 by 57 mm., due to a trepanation. The patient survived the operation for a long time, as the borders are completely healed.

Trephined crania lately discovered in other parts of Europe.— During the last forty years, trephined crania have also been unearthed in Switzerland, Bohemia, Poland, Denmark, Thuringia, Sweden, and from the pile dwellings on the lake of Brienne, at Chavannes, Sutz, and Locres, and quite lately a few more have been discovered in countries other than France. A skull trepanned for injury has been found in a Neolithic grave at Höckergrab in Bohemia.[1] It was that of a powerful man aged between fifty and sixty years, and a hole, measuring 40 by 60 mm., caused by a blow or a fall, was situated on its superior part. The anterior border of this hole showed the action of pus, and the discoverer of this skull believes that an operation with the object of coping with suppuration had been performed on the posterior border, and that cicatrisation had progressed far, when death supervened.

The very numerous trephined skulls of the ossarium of Sedec (Bohemia), though probably very ancient, are not accurately dated.[2] A skull,[3] found at Mahren, of a girl approximately ten years old at the time of death, had a frontal scar, possibly the result of a surgical trepanation. This cranium dates from the Bronze period, and, if the diagnosis be correct, the case is of some importance, as trephined skulls of children from that period are very rare. Unfortunately, details regarding this and the preceding cases are wanting.

Naked-eye appearances of apertures due to trephining.—The holes due to the operation are usually described as being fairly regular, more or less ellipsoid, and measure, on an average, about 4 cm.

[1] F. V. Grüngel, "Einige prähistorische Funde aus dem Saager-Land," *Prähistorische Zeitschrift*, CXI (1911), 304.

[2] D. Dudik, *Ethnologische Zeitschrift*, 1878, p. 227.

[3] This skull was discovered by Wankel, and described by Dudik, *loc. cit.*

across. The borders are sharp, oblique, bevelled from without inwards, and very often the singularly compact surfaces produced by the growth of fresh bone prove that cicatrisation took place, and that the patient survived the operation for a long time.

Reasons for trephining in prehistoric times.—Common and widespread as trephining was in Neolithic times, yet very little is known concerning its purpose or concerning the modus operandi of the prehistoric surgeon.

According to the theory usually accepted, the operation was first performed from time immemorial on sheep for relief of "staggers," and, later, man extended the application of this veterinary method to his species—firstly, for relief of severe and persistent headache due to causes unknown to him; and, secondly, for the removal of the splinters of a fractured bone. The theory of the veterinary origin of trephining is based on pure hypothesis, and I know no facts in support of it.

Broca suggested that the operation was performed on young epileptic or mad subjects, to rid them of the "genius," the "demon" causing the dreaded symptoms. Assuming that the ideas of Neolithic men resembled those of some modern, partly civilised peoples who honour an epileptic or lunatic as a holy man, he maintained that the convulsive accidents, on account of which trephining was performed, endowed the patient with a religious character. The patient benefited by this superstition, for both he and his cranium were regarded as objects of reverence. The fact that, as we have seen, rondelles were perforated in order to be worn lends some support to this theory. The full discussion of Broca's views, however, would entail entering into questions outside the scope of this present paper, and must therefore be left for the present.

LUCAS-CHAMPIONNIÈRE'S MEMOIR

A paper by the late Lucas-Championnière[1] contains some valuable facts regarding the methods of the Neolithic surgeon, and of his contemporary rival in Kabylia. The author emphasised the fact that, until quite lately, trephining had fallen completely into

---

[1] Lucas-Championnière, *La trépanation préhistorique*, Paris, 1878; *Les origines de la trépanation compressive*, Paris, 1912.

disrepute in modern Europe, so much so that, in 1874, Stromayer taught that, in cases of comminuted fracture of the skull, the best treatment was to wait for the elimination of bony splinters by suppuration. Lucas-Championnière maintains that in Neolithic times this operation was based partly on empiric knowledge and partly on a regular and extended series of observations; that it was probably performed for many reasons, and that the modern operation for fracture of the skull is but a survival of an old custom.

Geographical distribution.—The author lays stress on the fact that the geographical distribution of the operation is peculiar, for

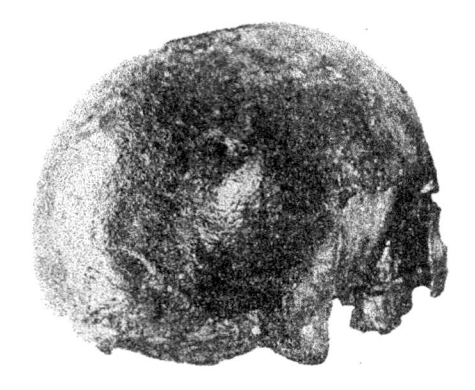

there is no evidence that the Hindoos or Chinese ever practised it, and no specimens of trepanning have been met with in Egypt,[1] nor among the Greeks or Romans. Some trepanned crania, however, have been discovered in Gaul, belonging to an epoch corresponding to that of Roman civilisation.

In America, previously to the arrival of Europeans, the operation was not known among the Redskins of the North, but existed in the empires of Mexico, Central America, and was especially prevalent in Peru. The contemporary hill tribes of Daghestan, the

[1] No case of trepanning in ancient Egypt has been published, but lately Dr. Arnoldo Rietti and I found at Alexandria a skull dating from 200 A.D. which appears to have been trepanned. We hope to publish the case in full before long. (NOTE.—Dr. Rietti tells me that owing to pressure of work consequent on the war, he has hitherto been unable to attend to this matter, but hopes to write the paper shortly. The photograph printed herewith is of the skull in question.—Alice Ruffer.)

natives of Tahiti, the Polynesians and Loyalty Islanders, the Kabyl tribes (but not the Arabs or Negroes in contact with them), and Montenegrins practise this operation, and thus show their belief in its efficacy.

Lucas-Championnière's experimental investigations.—The author then discusses the results obtained by several modern observers, who, using Neolithic flint instruments, have experimented on the dead body, in order to discover, if possible, the modus operandi of the prehistoric surgeons.

Three methods based on these studies have been described:

1. *Müller's method.*—The bone is slowly scraped away. The sloping border so produced is enormous as compared with the aperture, and therefore unlike that of the majority of Neolithic skulls.

2. *Capitan's method.*—A series of straight or curved lines having been drawn on the skull, a sharp flat instrument is first passed and repassed along these lines until the bone between them becomes loose and can be removed. The objection to this method is its tediousness and the time it takes—more than one hour for a small opening. Moreover, the borders of the hole thus made are sloping, bevelled, smaller than in prehistoric European trephined skulls, but not necessarily smaller than the openings found in trephined Peruvian crania.

3. *Lucas-Championnière's method.*—The operation is performed in several stages. (1) The bone is perforated by rotating the point of sharp flint. (2) A circle of perforations extending to the inner table is made, so close to one another that the perforations run into each other. (3) These openings are further connected by cuts with a sharp instrument, the cutting edge of a flint for instance, so as to obliterate the dentated border more or less completely.

The edges of the opening in trephined prehistoric, or modern, savage skulls are always bevelled, and the loss of substance in the external table therefore exceeds that in the internal table. The orifice is triangular, or square, or irregular, but rarely quite round, and this irregularity of the openings may have been the reason why many trephined prehistoric skulls passed unnoticed in the early days of anthropology. In some Neolithic skulls a smaller opening is present near the larger one, and the object of this is unknown.

In Peruvian skulls, on the other hand, the borders of the opening are often festooned; and it did not escape Lucas-Championnière's notice that this operation, in prehistoric times, was not necessarily fatal, for the obliterated osseous canals of the bevelled edge and the smooth, compact bone prove that the patient long survived the trepanation. Repair, however, was not always uniform. Multiple trepanations, though not rare in Neolithic times, are seen more frequently in Peruvian skulls, and still more often in contemporary Kabyls.

Lucas-Championnière's investigations in Kabylia.—Lucas Championnière was led to study trephining among the contemporary Kabyls, and he describes two methods used in Kabylia. The first consists in cutting through the cranial bones by making straight strokes with a short rectilinear saw. In the second method the surgeon, using an instrument like a gimlet, makes a complete circle of small perforations, then connects them all by short cuts with a saw, and finally removes the piece of bone thus circumscribed. Sometimes both methods are combined. It must be noted, however, that Lucas-Championnière never saw the operation actually performed by Kabyls (see also below).

Lucas-Championnière's views regarding incomplete operations.—The author insists that the evidence as to the superstitious use of cranial rondelles as amulets is not altogether satisfactory. He explains incomplete trephinings in Neolithic times by supposing that the operation was perhaps divided into two stages (see below), and that, in some cases, after the removal of the external table, the second part of the operation was not carried out. It is by no means clear, however, how the external table alone could be removed by Lucas-Championnière's method. Incomplete trepanations also are not rare in contemporary Kabylia.

Lucas-Championnière's views regarding the operation on children.—The theory that trepanation was performed on children (Broca) is not supported by evidence, as only one trephined infantile skull dating from Neolithic times has been found in France, and none have been discovered in Kabylia, America (before the conquest), or Montenegro. On the other hand, several trephined skulls were those of extremely old people.

Lucas-Championnière's views regarding site, etc., of operation.— The favourite situations for trephining in prehistoric times were the posterior part of the frontal, and especially the parietal bones as far as the occipital bone, on which the operator never trespassed much. The sagittal suture was avoided so carefully that it has been suggested that at a time when man was unacquainted with the use of iron, he knew enough anatomy to avoid the longitudinal sinus, and some authors have gone so far as to believe that Neolithic man had some knowledge of the motor centres. The Kabyls choose the same regions for the operation, and they also have learnt how to keep clear of the dangerous region, the longitudinal sinus.

As a rule, no traces of an accident are noticeable in trephined Neolithic skulls, and the operation therefore either was not done for traumatism, or, if performed for that reason, the splinters were carefully removed with the neighbouring bone.

No information exists regarding the dressing, if any, used by prehistoric peoples. Kabyls apply to the wounds: (1) tar; (2) honey which has been cooked; (3) butter melted and cooked (Lucas-Championnière).

Discussion of modus operandi of prehistoric people.—Discussing the various methods supposed to have been used by prehistoric peoples, Lucas-Championnière rejects the theory that the aperture was made by simple scraping, for the following reasons: (1) such an operation would take a very long time; (2) it would be attended by much haemorrhage; (3) a rondelle could not be removed in that way (this last argument appears to me conclusive as far as a large number of cases is concerned); (4) this technique would be useless when the bone to be trephined was really hard; (5) the cranial openings would be unlike those actually found; (6) the bevelled border would be much wider than is usually the case.

Lucas-Championnière admits that some operation resembling Capitan's process may have been used where the cranial openings are square, but maintains that his own method was the one generally used. The fact that the opening is not festooned (as it should be if Lucas-Championnière's method had been used), this author endeavours to explain by the supposition that, after the operation, the surgeon had taken the trouble to "correct" these irregularities, though in my opinion such "corrections" would have served no useful purpose, and would have caused a good deal of unnecessary pain.

Lucas-Championnière's views regarding the reasons for the operation.—The author points out that the evidence of the superstitious use of cranial rondelles as amulets is not altogether satisfactory. He believes that the only object in view was the cure of disease supposed to have its seat in the head, and especially of the diseases usually attended by severe headache. The relief afforded by the removal of splinters from a fractured skull may possibly have suggested an operation in cases where the pain was due to hidden disease, and on this theory surgeons may be said to have practised "cerebral decompression" as early as Neolithic times.

The Kabyls trephine sometimes for accidents, and more often for persistent headache. Such is their confidence in the beneficent results of this operation that, should it be unsuccessful once, they willingly undergo another. Sometimes the external table alone is removed. We may point out, however, at once that later investigations do not confirm this author's accounts of Kabyl methods. The art of trephining is a family craft, and the operators believe in it most thoroughly; for the *hakeem* (medical practitioner), Lucas-Championnière's informant, had been trephined three times, and his father twelve times. Three of his brothers were operators also. The author mentions that the Cornish miners, at the beginning of last century, thought so little of the operation that they insisted on being trephined after accidents to the skull, and proceeded home immediately after the operation. One Cornish surgeon had operated sixty times, and another had assisted during his apprenticeship at forty trephinings. He supposes that in Cornwall the custom dated from prehistoric times.

Objections to Lucas-Championnière's suggested method of trephining.—There are several objections to Lucas-Championnière's conclusion that a similar method was used by prehistoric surgeons. In the first place, the rondelles which I have seen in French and other collections are never notched, as they would be had this method been used. Secondly, I have not seen dentated borders of a trephine wound except in one Peruvian skull. Lucas-Championnière gives a photograph of this skull in his memoir and admits that this patient must have died very soon after the operation, as all signs of repair are wanting. For my part, I consider it far more probable that this opening was made after death by the embalmer in order to remove the brain. The Egyptian embalmers, it is well known, extracted or washed out this organ through the nose. It is true that Lucas-Championnière succeeded in trephining a skull by this method so skilfully that the borders of the opening were not festooned. This fact does not meet the objection just raised, for what may be comparatively easy to a skilful surgeon of the nineteenth century may have been impossible to a Neolithic surgeon. The borders of an opening thus made must have been festooned unless our prehistoric colleague took great pains to round off the aperture after the operation, and, personally, I can think of no reason for his doing so. Thirdly, in Lucas-Championnière's diagram of the operation, no less than thirteen perforations are indicated. Granting that no such large number would be required, yet an operation requiring several perforations of both tables of the skull with a sharp instrument must have been a most dangerous one, each drilling increasing the chances of wounding the dura mater. Even the Kabyls carefully avoid wounding this membrane. Fourthly, it is extremely difficult, if not impossible, to perform by this method an operation limited to removal of the external table of the skull, and we have seen that such incomplete operations were by no means rare.

Proof that Lucas-Championnière's method was not always used.— There are two facts which show that two methods entirely different from Lucas-Championnière's were occasionally used.

Firstly, before the European invasion, this operation was sometimes performed in Peru by marking off a small area of the skull with straight lines, and then incising with a powerful instrument along these lines. This method is clearly shown in a skull in the Trocadère Museum (Paris) which exhibits four deep cuts, and from between them a piece of bone, almost round, has been removed. The incisions were made with a very sharp and powerful cutting instrument, and not with a scraping instrument, and the operation had evidently been bungled by the surgeon, whose incisions were too long and too close together. I have seen no incision resembling it in European skulls, and the scars suggest a technique and instruments very different from those used in Europe.

Secondly, a prehistoric skull in the Lisbon Museum shows clearly that the area of bone to be removed was first circumscribed with a powerful instrument, e.g., a strong flint knife. On the top of this skull, a deep, ellipse-shaped furrow encloses a piece of the bone measuring about 50 by 40 mm., but the furrow does not penetrate the whole thickness of the bone, and lines and scratches round this groove demonstrate that the instrument often slipped during this operation. For some unknown reason, the trephining was never completed, although the patient apparently survived for some time. In this case Lucas-Championnière's method was certainly not used.

HILTON SIMPSON'S INVESTIGATIONS IN KABYLIA

Recent observations on the modern modus operandi in Kabylia and New Caledonia throw some light on the question of the technique used in ancient times. The facts relating to Kabylia were observed by Mr. Hilton Simpson[1] during a stay of more than two months at El Kantara, "the mouth of the Sahara," and during a journey of one month's duration, in the spring of 1913, among the Shewia Berbers of the Wady Abdi, and the Valley of Bouzina, in the western parts of the Atlas Mountains.

The author gives a description and illustrations of a complete set of Kabyl trephining instruments, nine in number, and all bearing unmistakable signs of having been used. Marks of burning upon their wooden handles which from their appearance could scarcely have been made when the blades were hafted, showed that apparently these instruments had been passed through the fire.

These instruments are: (1) Scalper (Arabic name, *matabaa*): A cylinder of iron about 1⅛ inch in depth and 1¾ inch in diameter, made of a strip of iron with one sharp edge, bent round until the ends touch without being joined. Where the ends meet, one is joined by fusion on its blunt edge to a round bar of iron about 13 inches long, so that the cylinder is at right angles to the bar. The

---
[1] Hilton Simpson, *Journal of Anthropology*, 1914.

other end of the bar passes through a round wooden handle 4 inches in length, and is bent round at right angles to prevent this handle from slipping off. (2) Retractor (Arabic name, *shefira*): An iron blade $2\frac{1}{2}$ inches in length was fitted into a round wooden handle $3\frac{1}{8}$ inches in length. The blade where it joins the handle is rectangular in section and about $\frac{1}{8}$ inch wide, but it gradually becomes flatter and wider until at the distal end it is about $\frac{3}{8}$ inch wide, the end being slightly rounded at the corners and presenting a fairly sharp edge. This end is bent over at right angles to the rest of the blade to form a hook. The whole blade slopes slightly backwards for the handle. (3) Retractor (Arabic name, *shefira*): An iron blade projecting about $1\frac{3}{4}$ inch of its length, the blade is rectangular in section and about $\frac{1}{8}$ inch wide, but the distal end is flat, widening to a width of $\frac{3}{8}$ inch, is bent round at right angles, forming a hook, the fairly sharp edges of which are slightly rounded at the corners. (4) Hook or Retractor (Arabic name, *mongash*): An iron blade about $1\frac{5}{16}$ inch long, inserted in a lathe-turned wooden handle, presumably of European origin. Where it joins the handle the blade is rectangular in section and about $\frac{1}{4}$ inch wide, but it narrows to the distal end, which is little more than $\frac{1}{16}$ inch in width. The distal end is bent sharply round to form a small hook. (5) Drill, also used as an elevator (Arabic name, *herwerl*): An iron blade about $2\frac{3}{4}$ inches long projecting from a round wooden handle $3\frac{1}{4}$ inches in length. Where it joins the handle, the blade is $\frac{1}{4}$ inch wide, and it gradually increases to a width of $\frac{3}{8}$ inch near the distal end; it narrows abruptly, leaving a "shoulder" on each side, at the distal end, so that the last $\frac{3}{16}$ inch of the blade is only $\frac{1}{8}$ inch wide. This end is rounded and has a cutting edge. The "shoulders" on the blade would serve to prevent too large a hole being made through the skull when the instrument is used as a drill. (6) Saw (Arabic name, *monshar*, or *manshar*): Consists of an iron blade projecting $3\frac{7}{8}$ inches in length, fixed into a round wooden handle $2\frac{7}{8}$ inches long. The blade is rectangular in section where it joins the handle, and is about $\frac{1}{8}$ inch wide. It curves downwards almost at right angles, 2 inches from the handle, and then curves outwards again at the distal end, where the blade is flat with a serrated lower edge containing eleven teeth. The serrated edge forms a segment of a circle, the teeth being upon the convex. (7) A second saw (very similar to No. 6): An iron blade $4\frac{5}{8}$ inches long and in a wooden handle about $2\frac{3}{4}$ inches long. The curves in this saw are not so sharp as in No. 6, there are thirteen teeth on its convex edge. Neither of these two saws is sharp. (8) A third saw: An iron blade $2\frac{1}{4}$ inches in length with a round wooden handle $3\frac{7}{8}$ inches long. The blade for $1\frac{1}{3}$ inch from the handle is rectangular in section, and about $\frac{1}{8}$ inch wide; the last $\frac{7}{8}$ of the blade is a flat rectangular surface with three serrated edges. The teeth are fine and sharp. (9) Elevator (Arabic name, *mhez*): A flat iron blade about $3\frac{3}{16}$ inches wide, protruding about $1\frac{3}{4}$ inch from a round wooden handle $2\frac{1}{2}$ inches long. The distal end curves very slightly indeed, and is fairly sharp. The corners are not rounded, but one of them has been broken off.

The method of trephining used by the Kabyls is as follows:

The first stage of the operation consists in removing a portion of the scalp in order to expose the place to be trephined. This is effected by making the "funnel-like" instrument (*matabaa*) white hot and placing it firmly, like a branding iron, on the head; a flicking movement of the instrument then removes the piece of scalp thus burnt round. The great heat, as well as sterilising the *matabaa*, also prevents excessive bleeding from the scalp. The retractors (*shefira*) are then used to draw away the scalp around the place to be trepanned, in order to give room for the use of the saw. Presumably the hook (*mongush*) is also used for the same purpose. A hole is then drilled in the skull by spinning the drill (*herwerl*) between the palms of the hands. This is to let out any pus and blood that may be under the skull, but the hole thus made would also be useful as a starting-place for the saw. The saw is then applied to the "good" bone just clear of the injured part. Only a very small amount is sawn through, after which the elevator on the hook is inserted in the incision, and, if possible, the "bad" bone slightly raised to let out pus and blood. Great care is taken that the dura mater is not pierced, for the operator thinks that the patient must die if this is done.

Only the small incision, with the saw described above, is made on the first day, but on the next and each succeeding day the process is repeated until the whole of the "bad" bone has been removed. So little is sawn through each day that it takes from fifteen to twenty days to remove a portion of skull as large as a penny piece. The part sawn away is lifted from the head by the elevator or the hook.

When the "bad" bone has at last been removed, no artificial bone or plate is placed over the cavity, and the skin is induced to grow again over the wound by the daily application of fresh dressings of a mixture of honey and butter, and the stem and leaves of an herb, powdered as fine as snuff. This herb grows locally upon the hills, and belongs to a species of labiatae. The daily dressing is continued sometimes for as long as one month, at the end of which time the patient is cured. No form of anaesthetic is used. There is no evidence of any attempt to sterilise the saw, the retractors, or the elevator (unless we accept the burns on the handles of the instruments as an indication that they have been purposely sterilised by heat), and the rags used as bandages are of the dirtiest description. The surgeon does not wash his hands, as a rule, before or after dressing a wound.

A native surgeon stated that he trephined as many as five or more heads annually, the reason for the operation being usually heads "broken" by blows from sticks or stones. Operations for the removal of damaged bone from the arms and legs were performed in the same manner and with the same instruments.

The Kabyl operation, therefore, according to this author, is performed to remove splinters of bones after accidents. It is difficult to reconcile this statement with Lucas-Championnière's assertions, firstly, that some patients have been trephined twice; and secondly, that the Kabyls trephine chiefly for headaches. Neither of these authors mentions whether Kabyls attach any religious importance to the operation, nor whether they regard the removed bone as a charm or an amulet.

TREPHINING IN NEW CALEDONIA

G. Nicolas gives an account of a totally different method in use among the contemporary New Caledonians. The operator makes a crucial incision on the scalp with the sharp edge of a large broken bottle or a razor, and, having turned the flaps aside with his fingers, files away the bone with a cutting and sharpened shell. The operation is often badly carried out, for it may be incomplete, or, contrariwise, the membranes of the brain may be injured. The wound is then closed by placing a shell over it, and Nicolas himself has felt such a shell in situ. The cutaneous flaps being turned back a dressing of certain chewed herbs is applied. The chief indication for the trephining is persistent headache, and a man who had suffered excruciating pains after a fall on the head reported that he had been completely cured by the operation.

Trephining is carried out fairly often. One skull completely and another incompletely trephined were found in a cave containing some hundreds of skeletons.

CONCLUSIONS

The conclusions to be drawn from the new facts related in this review are as follows:

1. The operative methods of Neolithic people are very imperfectly known.

2. Further investigations with regard to Kabyl methods are necessary, as the Kabyl methods described by the French author are not identical with those mentioned by the British traveller. This may be due to the fact that the observations of the two authors were made in different parts of Kabylia. Both may therefore be right.

Contemporary Kabyl methods differ greatly from those used in contemporary New Caledonia. Neolithic people therefore may have employed not one but several methods, either at the same time or consecutively, or in different regions.

3. Contemporary Kabyls trephine for accidents, and, according to Lucas-Championnière, for persistent headache also. Contemporary New Caledonians trephine chiefly for the relief of headache. Similarly, Neolithic people may have trephined for injuries, but as most of the trephined skulls show no signs of accidents, headache was very probably the chief indication for this operation. No fresh evidence has been obtained to show that a religious signification was attached to trephining.

4. Lastly, I would suggest that the trephining hole is situated in the upper and posterior part of the parietal bone, probably because this region was most easily accessible to the operator in a period when beds and chairs were not used. The contemporary barber-surgeon in the East when operating invariably squats in front or behind the patient, and in thus doing copies his colleagues of ancient times. A picture on a tomb at Beni-Hassan, dating from over three thousand years, shows the barber-surgeon squatting before a man on whose head he is performing some kind of operation. The walls of a tomb of Sakkarah are decorated with bas-reliefs representing operations, and among them some operation on the penis of a youth.[1] In this bas-relief also the surgeon squats down before the sufferer, whose hands are held before his face by a man standing behind, who thus not only prevents untoward movements, but also hides the operation from his prisoner. In another bas-relief, the patient, still standing up, rests his right hand on the squatting operator's head. Other bas-reliefs of the same tombs are not sufficiently well preserved to allow a diagnosis of the operation to be made, but in all the surgeon either squats on the ground or sits on a low (stone?) stool either before or behind his patient. The Neolithic surgeon probably took up the same position, and the patient's head was either held by an assistant or by the operator himself, and, like his contemporary Egyptian

---

[1] The picture is supposed to represent a circumcision, but I can see no evidence of that.

colleagues operating on the scalp, he encircled and held the head firmly with his left arm, and operated with his right hand.

Excellent hold is obtained on a person's head either in this manner or by fixing the head between the knees. It is best for the operator to sit a little higher than the patient, e.g., on a stone, and for the patient to squat between the operator's legs. Whether the surgeon sits before or behind the patient makes no difference, for, in either case, the upper parietal region is the region most easily reached.

In order to study the question experimentally, I have asked several people, ignorant of surgery and not acquainted with my object, to sit in the position thus described. I then asked one of them (the operator) to catch hold of the other person's (the patient's) head and pretend to drill a hole in it. The point invariably chosen for this drilling was the parietal region, and, strangely enough, not the vertex but the side of the parietal bone, and usually the left side. These points correspond almost exactly with those which were most often trephined in prehistoric skulls, and I suggest therefore that the reason why prehistoric surgeons trephined most often the parietal region of the skull was because that region was by far the easiest to operate on, when both patient and operator squat on the ground.

ARTHRITIS DEFORMANS AND SPONDYLITIS IN ANCIENT EGYPT

(*Journal of Pathology and Bacteriology*, Vol. XXII [1918])

PREFATORY NOTE

When starting in December, 1916, on a mission which was evidently attended by dangers and which finally proved fatal to my husband, he left with me instructions as to various unfinished papers at which he and I had worked together.

It was his written wish that the present part of his "Studies in Palaeopathology" should be submitted to his friend and former assistant, Captain J. G. Willmore, R.A.M.C., who has kindly devoted his short leave during the summer of 1917 to assisting me to prepare this paper on "Arthritis Deformans." We have decided to eliminate certain short passages wherever we had doubts as to Sir Armand's intention rather than give a possibly erroneous impression. We have not, however, attempted to write a summary or conclusions, such as my husband would certainly have given, since the paper speaks for itself, and we preferred not to add any matter which he had not time to prepare.

Captain Willmore undertook the arduous task of supplying references, which my husband left to be filled in, searching for suitable illustrations, etc.

My very sincere thanks are due to Captain Willmore for this labour of love, undertaken for his former chief in the Quarantine Service of Egypt. Without his valuable help, I might never have been able to give to the world this part of Sir Armand Ruffer's "Studies in Palaeopathology."

ALICE RUFFER

December, 1917

INTRODUCTION TO THE STUDY OF ARTHRITIS IN ANCIENT EGYPT

Arthritis deformans is a chronic, painful, debilitating disease, which in many cases goes steadily from bad to worse. The lesions in the neighbourhood of the articular surfaces cause pain in the joints and tendons, together with muscular spasms whenever the articulations are moved.

The vertebral lesions of spondylitis deformans gradually disqualify a patient from earning his living by agricultural pursuits, hunting, netting fish, or indeed by any manual labour, or any pursuit requiring even moderate physical exertion.

The pain in many of the ancient Egyptians whose lesions have been described must have been very severe. As the lumbar spine was the part most frequently involved, it follows that these people suffered severely from lumbago, sciatica, pains and cramps in the lower limbs. The skeletons do not show any lesions proving that the spinal nerves were pressed upon, but the osseous lesions are only a fraction of the pathological alterations present during life, and the vertebral lesions were undoubtedly surrounded by a wide area of inflammatory exudate which pressed heavily on the spinal nerves (Plate XLIX, Fig. 1) and possibly caused intense pain during life. The sleepless nights due to the pain coming on suddenly during sleep, the alterations in the general nutrition due to the intense suffering, must have sufficed to alter profoundly the physical and mental well-being of the ancient Egyptians.

The limitation of movement caused by the pressure of spondylitis deformans was very great in some cases, and the aspect and carriage of the patient must have varied according to whether the intervertebral cartilages had been absorbed or not.

When the absorption had taken place in the lumbar or cervical regions, the favourite places for such alterations, the collapse of several intervertebral spaces undoubtedly caused marked deformity. When, on the other hand, there was no absorption of the vertebral cartilages, considerable stiffness unaccompanied by deformity was the result. A large number of ancient Egyptians, therefore, were considerably crippled, the majority of these by changes in the vertebral column, and a minority by lesions of the peripheral articulations.

The pathological lesions in the dorsal region, though not conducive to much deformity, were very important on account of their interference with respiration. When the costo-vertebral articulations were attacked, as was often the case (Plate XLIX, Fig. 2), the pain on respiration must have been extremely severe, and the thoracic movements rendered almost impossible. Moreover, the periarticular lesions of the costo-sternal articulations undoubtedly added to the difficulties in respiration. Abdominal respiration also was occasionally rendered difficult and perhaps painful by the lesions on the anterior surface of the vertebrae having involved the tendons of the diaphragm.

Respiration, then, was difficult and painful, but must have been almost impossible whenever any bronchial or lung attack called into play the muscles which are only used in forced respiration, the attachment of which, as has been shown often, were extensively ossified. Cough was extremely painful, and any disease causing even moderate dyspnoea must have proved fatal in people whose respiratory muscles were unable to respond to the extra strain put upon them.

The lesions of arthritis deformans in peripheral joints gave rise to pain, limitations of movement, etc., and were in themselves sufficient to prevent any active exertion on the part of the patient. When the temporo-maxillary joint was attacked, difficulty in taking nourishment became an important and distressing symptom.

In a paper[1] on the lesions of teeth in ancient Egyptians, I drew attention to the very common occurrence of pyorrhoea alveolaris in people with spondylitis and other manifestations of arthritis deformans, and dental disease added to the joint lesions must have rendered the patient's life well-nigh unbearable.

In spite of these serious and unsatisfactory conditions of health, some of the patients lived for a long time. Even in the predynastic period many lived long enough to have the vertebral column ankylosed from end to end. For instance, the old woman from Thebes,[2] whose case has been put on record, was certainly confined to her bed for months or years before septic poisoning from a huge bedsore proved fatal to her.

Every Nubian or Egyptian village contained within its walls a fairly large number of people, chronic invalids, who could do little work, and a few completely crippled who were unable to earn their living by agricultural pursuits. Some may have engaged in light pursuits, such as cooking, tailoring, etc., which required little exertion, but in an agricultural community only a very small proportion could have earned their living in that way. The rest, when not wealthy, were dependent on the charity of their friends, and as they lived a long time in this crippled state, it follows that to assist one's friends and neighbours was already a duty in predynastic times.

[1] Sir Armand Ruffer, "Studies in Palaeopathology: Lesions of Ancient Egyptian Teeth," *Journal of Pathology and Bacteriology*, XVIII (Cambridge, 1913-14), 149.

[2] Elliot Smith, "A Contribution to the Study of Mummification in Egypt," *Mémoires présentés à l'Institut Égyptien*, Tome V (1906), fasc. 1.

ARTHRITIS DEFORMANS AND SPONDYLITIS

Lesions such as we have described could not have occurred in uncivilised people, for the patients would have died of inanition before the changes could have proceeded so far, and their existence is the best possible proof of the high degree of civilisation to which ancient Egyptians had attained.

Chronic articular and periarticular disease, therefore, has existed in man and animals for many thousands of years.

In this paper I intend to give an account of chronic, non-suppurating, articular, and periarticular disease as it occurred in Egypt and Nubia during the last eight thousand years or more.

The material is the same as that on which my paper on the pathological lesions of the teeth of ancient Egyptians was based, namely:

1. Skeletons and mummies, dating from various periods of Egyptian history, given me by the late Sir Gaston Maspero, Professor Flinders Petrie, Mr. Wainwright, Professor Breccia, and others.

2. The large collection of predynastic and later skeletons in the Museum of the Medical School of Cairo.

3. Fragments of skeletons from Merawi (Sudan) and Faras (Nubia), kindly handed over to me by Professor Griffith (Oxford).

4. Skeletons of the Macedonian soldiers buried at Chatby, in Alexandria.

5. Skeletons of Alexandrians (Greeks, Egyptians, etc.) from the catacombs of Kom el Shougafa and Ras el Tin.

6. Coptic mummies.

7. Last, but not least, the field notes of Dr. Wood Jones, published in the *Archaeological Survey of Nubia*, Vol. II, "Report on Human Remains," and Professor Elliot Smith's papers.

The existence of arthritis deformans and spondylitis in ancient Egyptian skeletons has been noted by Elliot Smith, who described[1] a male body of the Ancient Empire from the Giza pyramids with complete bony union of every vertebra in the entire column.

Wood Jones[2] has given a complete and excellent account of this disease as it existed among ancient Nubians. It was found that the

---

[1] Elliot Smith, *Archaeological Survey of Nubia*, Bull. No. 2 (Cairo, 1908), p. 59, n.

[2] Wood Jones, *Archaeological Survey of Nubia, 1907–8*, Vol. II, "Report on Human Remains" (Cairo, 1910), 273 f.

disease might exist in every joint, including the temporo-maxillary articulation.

Disease of the knee-joint was perhaps less common than might have been expected. He states that in by far the greater number of affected joints (knee-joints) eburnation is not a conspicuous feature, whereas the irregularity of the articular surface is marked. Wood Jones says:

> It would seem that the disease may take one of two forms: one in which the bony outgrowth and a great roughening of the articular surfaces are the most notable features; and one in which the eburnation of the opposed ends of the bones is most pronounced. The first form tends in a very great number of cases to bony ankylosis of the affected joints.

I would rather, instead of speaking of two forms of the disease, look upon these two forms as two "stages" of the disease.

He describes the changes found in the elbow, head of the humerus, hands, hips (including coxa vara), etc., and points out that the periarticular changes and lesions of parts of the bone away from the joint are as important as, if not more important than, those in the articulations themselves. Further, he gives a very accurate description of the changes found in spondylitis deformans.

In several cases spondylitis deformans coexisted with arthritic disease in other parts of the body.

Wood Jones's memoir is, further, very interesting on account of the field notes which are a perfect mine of information.

The type of the disease in ancient Egypt was distinctly peripheral; that is, the chief changes were in the ligaments, the capsules of the joints, but not in the joints themselves. Whether the articulating surfaces of the vertebral column, the hip-joints, knee-joints, or the smaller joints be examined, the larger number of cases show no alterations whatever in the articulating surfaces. When the latter are eburnated, or simply show signs of wearing, as in the acetabular cavity of the hip-joint, then, in every case, the lesions of the disease at the periphery of the joint were intense, and the lesions of the articular surfaces appeared to be late lesions coming after the periarticular changes had prepared the ground, so to speak.

Very possibly the articular lesions during life were very marked and left but little trace after death. Profound changes in the synovial membrane, in the ligaments, in the cartilages even, may have been conspicuous in the living and yet have left no trace in the skeleton.

All that can be said for certain, therefore, is that although, very possibly, the articulations and articular surfaces during life may have been the seat of extensive lesions, these left no trace after death in the bony structure. The peripheral changes, on the other hand, were extremely marked and in themselves must have produced extremely severe symptoms.

The question now arises as to what variety of arthritis deformans, as varieties exist now, the Egyptian form belongs.

Thomas M'Crae[1] divides arthritis deformans into three groups:

1. A form in which the changes predominate in the structures, apart from the bony parts of the joint, although the cartilages are frequently involved to some extent. The degree of change varies greatly. This group is termed "periarticular" and is the commonest of all.

2. A form in which the chief change consists in marked atrophy of both bones and cartilages. With this there are usually marked atrophic changes in the muscles. This is termed the "atrophic" form, and appears to be comparatively rare.

3. A form in which hypertrophic changes are the most prominent. There may be marked bony overgrowth, which may occur at the edges of the articulating surfaces especially, or in the spine, involving the cartilages and ligaments.

but not as common as the first.

These forms, however, are not so fixed that one can always say with certainty that a given case belongs to one group rather than to another; these forms may pass into one another. Moreover, it is by no means clear what is meant by bony overgrowths at the edges of the articulating surfaces, or in the spine, involving the cartilages and ligaments. As we have seen, such bony overgrowths (leaving out the cartilages) are common in our cases, but they appeared to us to be more of the nature of a deposit of bone in inflamed tissue than an osseous overgrowth from pre-existing bone.

Very difficult, also, is the diagnosis of this disease in the spine. The term spondylitis deformans, which I have used throughout this paper, denotes[2] an arthritis of the spinal joints, changes in them

[1] Osler and M'Crae, *System of Medicine*, VI, 505.   [2] M'Crae, *op. cit.*, p. 535.

which are frequently associated with proliferation of bone, atrophy of cartilages with its replacement by bone, and osseous changes in the ligaments. These last are apparently involved very frequently, perhaps the anterior lateral ligament most often of all. The extent of involvement varies greatly, and the process may extend along several vertebrae, making practically a solid column for some distance, or a process of one vertebra may be joined to that of the next one. The transverse processes are not infrequently involved. The lesions may be symmetrical or asymmetrical; in the lower spine the process is frequently most marked on one side, in the cervical region much more often on both sides.

This condition of the spine may be the only manifestation of spondylitis deformans, or may be associated with arthritis of the peripheral joints. M'Crae states that in thirty-nine out of eighty-one cases of spondylitis the spine alone was involved, and in forty-two this was associated with arthritis elsewhere.

He also maintains[1] that the joints of the vertebrae may be involved in a general polyarthritis, and apparently need not be described now, as, for obvious reasons, the pathological changes of this polyarthritis would not be noticeable in skeletons.

One point, which is not usually mentioned in the papers on spondylitis, has obtruded itself, and that is the very important lesions at the points of muscular attachments on the skeleton. These lesions in some parts of the body, as, for instance, in the lumbar and pelvic regions, were so severe that they must have crippled the patient almost completely. A man whose vertebral groove was filled with ossified muscles would have had a "poker spine" even in the absence of any other lesions (Plate XLIX, Figs. 3 and 4). Similarly, the man whose muscular attachments to the pelvic or to the upper part or lower ends of the femur or upper end of tibia were more or less ossified must have had his movements considerably impaired. The lesions, moreover, which are seen in the skeletons are probably slight, as compared with those which existed during life but left no trace in the skeletons after death. It is practically certain that the inflammatory process which gave rise to roughness and osseous deposits at the point of attachment of the

[1] *Op. cit.*, p. 529.

muscles spread for some distance along the tendon and even into the muscular fibre. When both ends of a muscle were attacked, as was sometimes the case, the action of such muscle must have been considerably interfered with. It may be that the atrophy of muscles—an atrophy which does not appear to be caused by mere disuse—may be due in some cases to these lesions, but there is no proof of it; moreover, the fact that this atrophy is sometimes marked in cases in which the chief change is advanced atrophy of bones as well as cartilages—a change which did not exist in our cases—is distinctly against this theory.

On the other hand, the involvement of the muscles may perhaps account for the severe pains of obscure origin which many of these patients suffer from. It seems to me probable that many cases of so-called muscular rheumatism, associated or not with arthritis deformans, may be due to such changes.

The lesions of the vertebral column leave no doubt regarding the nature of the disease. The cases were typical cases of spondylitis deformans, or "poker spine."

The only difference between the disease in modern and ancient people lies in the fact that in modern people the cartilages are often ossified, whereas in the few mummies examined by me and in skeletons no evidence of ossification of the cartilages could be obtained.

This objection is probably of little value, for several reasons. In the first place, the cases in which the cartilages were still present were so few that no conclusions could be drawn. In the second place, marked ossification may have been present, but unless the cartilage was so completely ossified as to form a solid block, nothing of it would be found in the sand more or less filling the grave.

It has been shown in the course of this paper that in some skeletons there were distinct signs of ossification of the fibrous part of the intervertebral disc, and that in others, especially in the cervical region, the cartilages had evidently been absorbed during life—the vertebrae falling together. It is evident, therefore, that some very serious changes had taken place in the cartilages, the lesions being of such a nature, however, as to leave no trace in the skeletons. In the cervical and lumbar regions the vertebrae occasionally fell together, the deformity implying a disappearance of the cartilages through some profound pathological change.

The disease in ancient Egyptians was perivertebral rather than vertebral, that is, as in modern people, the ligaments, and more especially the anterior common ligament, were most affected.

The material at our disposal was not such as would easily settle the question as to whether the spondylitis deformans was or was not accompanied by arthritic or periarthritic changes in other parts of the body. It was but seldom that the whole skeleton was obtained, and in most cases only a few bones were present, so it was not possible to say whether other joints besides those actually discovered suffered or not.

Certain it is, however, that whenever a complete skeleton was discovered with lesions of spondylitis deformans, so often were one or more of the distant joints affected. In many cases, therefore, spondylitis was complicated by peripheral articular disease, as it is at the present day.

I. MATERIAL EXAMINED AND ITS CHRONOLOGY

The first skeleton to be described is that of Nefermaat, discovered by Wainwright[1] in a IIIrd Dynasty mastaba at Meydum. The tomb had been rifled at the time of burial by the workmen, who had desecrated the body and considerably damaged the skull and many of the bones.

The body had been enclosed in a coffin, which had disappeared, and some time after burial the tomb had been filled with mud which had penetrated into all the foramina of the bones, and it was supposed that the body had been first dismembered and the bones then wrapped up in bandages. The bones, extremely fragile, were covered with thick incrustations of salt, and the mud still filled all the spinal foramina and the interstices between the bones. There was nothing to show that the salt had been added as a preservative, and most probably it had crystallised out of the surrounding mud and been deposited on the bones during the four thousand years or more which had elapsed since burial.

[1] Wainwright, "Meydum and Memphis, III," *Report of the British School of Archaeology in Egypt*, 1910.

The spinal column from the fourth cervical vertebra to the coccyx had been converted by disease into a rigid block, which at some time or other after death had been accidentally broken into several pieces.

The atlas, axis, and third cervical vertebrae were absent. The first piece consisted of the cervical vertebrae, from the fourth down to the first dorsal inclusively. The vertebrae of this first piece were firmly tied together by solid new bone which had developed in the anterior common ligament, and this osseous bridge formed a distinct arch over each empty intervertebral space. The intervertebral discs were never ossified, the surfaces of the bodies of the vertebrae were smooth, and the empty intervertebral spaces were not narrowed. So much could be seen through the gaps left here and there. The posterior common ligament, completely ossified, did not bulge into the canal, and, therefore, did not press on the spinal cord. Numerous osteophytes developed from the inferior-anterior border of the first dorsal to form a bony bridge with similar prolongations from the superior border of the second dorsal vertebra.

The whole dorsal region displayed similar lesions, the anterior and posterior borders of the vertebral bodies being firmly bound together by the ossified anterior and posterior common ligaments, and the articulating surfaces with few exceptions solidly united by periarticular osseous overgrowths. Most of the spinous processes were broken off; the few still present were normal, with the exception of the eleventh and twelfth, which were connected by a strong, bony bridge.

Similar alterations were present in the lumbar region. The right vertebral groove opposite the twelfth dorsal and first and second lumbar vertebrae was filled with a mass of somewhat spongy bone, about 3 cm. broad, extending laterally over the articulating surfaces, which are covered everywhere with thick new bone. A similar mass, somewhat smaller, occupied the left vertebral groove. The posterior spinous processes were not ossified. The fifth lumbar vertebra was firmly fixed by new bone to the sacrum, which was otherwise normal.

The pathological changes in the acetabula were limited to the formation of a few small osteophytes at the junction of the articular and non-articular portions (Plate XLIX, Fig. 5).

The head of the right femur was broken off post mortem. A slight deposit of new bone at the junction of the head and neck showed that this bone also had suffered. The lesions of the right femur also were limited to slight thickening of the anterior border of the articulating surface of the knee.

The scapulae, which were the only bones of the upper extremity that were discovered, were healthy except for some very slight roughness due to chronic inflammation round the scapulo-humeral articulations.

The manubrium sterni showed curious lesions. On the right side the first rib was firmly ankylosed with it, and about $1\frac{1}{2}$ inch from the sternum it had evidently been badly broken, and, owing to want of surgical knowledge, perhaps, a false joint had been the result of the accident.

Enough of the costal cartilages was left to prove that they had been completely ossified.

The few bones of the skull which were left showed no alterations, except that the internal surfaces of both condyles had been rendered uneven by old periarticular inflammation.

The skeleton of this man therefore exhibited the signs characteristic of severe spondylitis of the vertebral column throughout its whole length.

The lesions were especially marked in the anterior and posterior vertebral ligaments, but whereas in the former the inflammatory process had led to the formation of large bulging osteophytes, the surface of the latter was even and smooth. and very probably therefore the spinal cord had not been pressed upon. The intervertebral discs had certainly not been ossified, and the upper and lower surfaces of the bodies were apparently free from disease.

The articular surfaces, on the other hand, were practically immobilised by the complete ossification of the fibrous tissues round them, and all these changes had made the whole vertebral column incapable of flexion, extension, or lateral movements. This condition, sufficiently serious in itself, had been aggravated by the extension of the disease to neighbouring tendons and muscles. The vertebral groove in the lumbar region being filled by a mass of spongy bone. and the dorsal and cervical regions being affected by lesions similar, though less severe, the muscles originating from the lumbar region—the latissimus dorsi, serratus posticus inferior, spinalis dorsi, erector spinae, interspinal muscles, etc.—have been considerably interfered with. Similarly, the attachments of the dorsal and cervical muscles were not normal, and their efficiency being lessened thereby, the movements of the arms, neck, and thorax were certainly rendered more difficult. The movements of the head also had been affected by the extension of the disease to the internal borders of the condyles.

Respiration, already impeded by the rigidity of the vertebral column and the pathological changes in the spinal muscles, was impeded still further by the ossification of the costo-vertebral articulations and costal cartilages and by the old fracture of the first right rib. The patient's misery had been increased by the pain accompanying the movements of the pelvis, hip-joints, knee-joints, shoulder-joints, and of several other articulations. The head, neck, back, and limbs were motionless, and the man, unable to turn round on his couch, to sit up, to attend to any necessities of life without assistance, was a typical chronic and helpless invalid for years before death.

Perhaps in this case the disease did not extend to the smaller articulations, in contrast to the following case, in which the smaller articulations had been undoubtedly attacked. The fragments of this second skeleton, found by Professor Flinders Petrie in a tomb of the IIIrd Dynasty near the Fayoum pyramid, were those of a short adult, whose age and sex are not ascertainable, and were remarkable on account of the gravity of the pathological lesions.

Some osseous overgrowth existed at the point of attachment of the cervical transverse ligament, and was most marked on the left side, where the new bone formed a kind of cushion about 4 mm. long, 3 mm. broad, and 3 mm. thick, projecting upwards from the anterior arch on the same side. The tubercle on this arch was greatly thickened, whereas the superior articulating surfaces were normal. The odontoid process of the axis was very irregular in shape and was capped by an osteophyte quite 5 mm. long. The inferior-anterior border of the body was prolonged into a spear-shaped point. The articulating surfaces were normal.

The fourth (?) cervical vertebra was much thickened round the body, especially anteriorly. The inferior-anterior border sent off a thick prolongation downwards, and the worm-eaten and rough appearance of the body suggested that there were some pathological changes in the intervertebral discs also. The cervical vertebrae (fifth and sixth) were firmly joined by the anterior and posterior common ligaments. The disease had not extended to the articulations.

Only two of the dorsal vertebrae were found, and both showed great thickening on the anterior and lateral borders of the body, where the new bone measured as much as 4 mm. in thickness. The only lumbar vertebra present, namely, the first, had a mass of new bone, 8 mm. thick, occupying the superior left lateral border.

Only one metatarsal bone and two phalanges were discovered. The metatarsal bone was greatly thickened at both ends, and the second and terminal phalanges of one finger were firmly ankylosed in a fixed position.

The pathological changes in this skeleton resemble those of the first. The anterior and posterior common and periarticular ligaments were ossified throughout the whole length of the vertebral column, and the articulations of the smaller bones of the hand and foot of the second skeleton were attacked also. The disease had probably attacked many of the small joints, as the only two bones that were found showed severe pathological alterations.

Although both these bodies dated only from the IIIrd Dynasty (2980-2900 B.C.), osteoarthritis existed long before that period in Egypt and in Nubia.

The specimens next to be described were discovered in the necropolis of Kawamil,[1] and were examined by my friend, the late Dr. Fouquet, who described under the name of *mal de Pott* the typical pathological alterations of spondylitis deformans.

Kawamil is situated 515 km. south of Cairo, and the district contains many necropoles and *kjoekken-moeddings* dating from the Neolithic and the first Pharaonic periods. Two cemeteries near the village of Aoulad-Haroun are of special interest: the first on the north side, with some thousands of native tombs and pottery characteristic of the Neolithic epoch; the other more to the south, with graves less ancient, containing bodies skeletonised before inhumation in cysts made of clay or crude bricks, or in large pots.

Kjoekken-moeddings with worked stone implements, fragments of bones, vases, and small bronze objects, are found in the desert between the two cemeteries, and one little hillock is made up of an enormous quantity of droppings of antelopes and gazelles.

The age of the bones discovered at Kawamil is therefore somewhat uncertain, and the difficulty is increased by the fact that in his papers Dr. Fouquet did not say in which cemetery the bones described by him were found. In conversation, however, my late friend told me that the bones came from the predynastic cemetery on the north. An estimate of six thousand years for the age of these bones is therefore not exaggerated.

The bones to be first described belonged to a man supposed to have been approximately forty years old at the time of his death. The specimen consisted of two lumbar vertebrae, the bodies of which were strongly united by massive bilateral bridges of bone and by an anterior median band, "séparant 2 ouvertures d'abcès par congestion, dans le canal desquels on aperçoit des bourgeons osseux en voie de formation." These layers of new bone were fairly thick with powerful exostoses, whereas the transverse and spinous processes were normal.

[1] De Morgan, *Recherches sur les origines de l'Égypte*, Paris, 1897.

The drawing illustrating Fouquet's paper shows no sign whatever of an "abcès par congestion." There is no appearance of ulceration nor of any lesion of the bodies of the vertebrae, and the new bony growth is confined entirely to the ligamentous structures binding together the vertebrae. The intervertebral space was not narrowed, and appeared to be normal.

The second specimen also consisted of two lumbar vertebrae, enclosing a patent and not narrowed intervertebral space. The bodies of the two vertebrae were immobilised on the right side by an irregular bony bridge and by a similar narrow, smooth, and very prominent bridge on each side in front, whereas the articular surfaces were fixed by irregular, thin, narrow, osseous bands. The vertebral bodies were solid and resistant and the spongy tissue was not rarefied. In several places, and especially anteriorly, there were depressions hollowed out by small vessels, around which there were doubtful traces of suppuration. The specimen apparently came from a man (?) who died young. The third specimen also presented lesions similar to those of the first, that is, lesions typical of spondylitis deformans.

On the whole, therefore, the lesions of the Kawamil vertebrae, dating from the epoch of chipped flints, greatly resemble those of the vertebrae from the IIIrd Dynasty.

The remains of many of the Nubian skeletons of the late predynastic and early predynastic periods had lesions typical of spondylitis deformans, and so common was this disease in early Nubian epochs that "in the prehistoric cemetery in the main street of Shellal near Assuan, no adult body failed to show some traces of its presence." The lesions naturally differed greatly in severity, varying from a mere lipping of the adjacent edges of individual to the involvement of several vertebrae, and even to the ankylosis of a series (Plate XLIX, Fig. 6). Very commonly two or more lumbar vertebrae of prehistoric skeletons were held together by connecting, irregular, osseous bridges, which, however, were sometimes limited to one side of the anterior surface (Plate XLIX, Fig. 7).

Proof has already been adduced that, in Egypt, the disease appeared very early, but the extent of its spread cannot be estimated. For example, the fifteen predynastic bodies unearthed in

Tourah, near Cairo,[1] were normal; and of the IIIrd Dynasty skeletons from the same place only one showed "lipping" and "absorption" of the vertebrae from the second cervical vertebrae downwards. The old pyramid builders paid their tribute to spondylitis, and in one case the whole spinal column was found converted into a solid block.

The evidence regarding the existence in the Delta of this disease in very ancient times is not forthcoming, because, for obvious reasons, ancient skeletons have not been found in the Delta; but, considering it was not rare in that part of the country during the Greek, Roman, and early Christian periods and is fairly common now, it is more than probable that it was not rare during the dynastic era. The frequent occurrence of spondylitis deformans in Nubia during the early periods has been alluded to already, but it must not be assumed, as has been done more than once, that every Nubian was thus afflicted.

The new cemetery (17) at Shellal, for instance,[2] situated on the east bank of the river at Khor Baha, contained the remains of people of the early and middle predynastic times, which were in a poor state of preservation, and skeletons of early dynastic times (A group) and late Ancient Empire periods (B group). Of the one hundred and four graves, six contained fragments, six contained children, and three were occupied by dogs, and not by human skeletons. Four cases of spondylitis were found in the eighty-nine graves remaining, and of these one had arthritis of the knee and other articulations as well.

The cemetery of Dabod contained a series of archaic remains, ranging from the late predynastic period on to the Middle Empire, and a group of bodies dating from the New Empire.

The archaic series included bodies belonging to the late predynastic and early dynastic times (A group), and to the archaic Nubian Middle Empire periods (or C group), and the characteristics of these bodies closely agreed with those of the remains of similar dates found near Shellal. The late predynastic and A-group

---

[1] Derry, *Denkschrift d. k. Akad. d. Wissensch. in Wien*, 1912.

[2] Elliot Smith and Wood Jones, *Archaeological Survey of Nubia, 1907-8*, II, 116.

skeletons conformed to the predynastic Egyptian type, whereas the archaic and middle Nubian people had been evidently tinged with Negro blood.

An analysis of the notes showed that in thirty-four undated graves three skeletons showed lesions of spondylitis. The lesions of the vertebrae were complicated by osteitis of the pelvis and arthritis of the knees in one case, and by arthritis of the metatarsals in another.

After a large number of burials had been eliminated, because they contained either children or animals, there were left: twenty-five archaic bodies with ten cases of spondylitis; seven middle Nubian bodies with two cases of spondylitis; twenty-seven New Empire bodies with three cases of spondylitis.

Forty per cent of the archaic inhabitants, therefore, had been attacked by spondylitis, sometimes complicated by other severe arthritic lesions, such as arthritis of the knee (Plate L, Fig. 8) and osteitis of the pelvis, arthritis of the left shoulder-joint (Plate L, Fig. 9), accompanied by great eburnation, and ankylosis of the pelvis (Plate L, Fig. 10).

Cemetery 30, on the eastern side of the river, included skeletons from the middle predynastic and early dynastic periods, and from the Middle Empire C group and the New Empire group. The predynastic bodies were in a fair state of preservation, in contrast with those of C group and New Empire date, which were not so useful for our purpose.

The New Empire graves need not be considered, as there are no notes concerning them; four cases are also useless for other reasons; and there remain notes of five archaic skeletons, of which three had spondylitis, and of twelve middle Nubian bodies with four cases of spondylitis.

Cemetery 40 included burials from the early dynastic, New Empire, and Christian periods, but the notes of the early dynastic series alone are available for our purpose. Of the twenty-nine bodies mentioned, two must be eliminated, and there are then left twenty-seven skeletons with nine cases of spondylitis.

The incidence of this disease during predynastic and dynastic times in Upper Egypt is not known, but for reasons to be explained afterwards it can be assumed that the incidence was probably very great.

It will be convenient here to study this disease as it appeared in Nubia and in Alexandria during the period beginning at the time of the Greek occupation 332 B.C. to about 300 A.D., that is, roughly six hundred years. The huge gap this left in our historical study will be filled up later on, as far as possible.

The examination of the mummies found in Cemetery 3, on the island of Hesa, in Nubia, gives an idea of the conditions prevailing in Nubia during the Ptolemaic period. The mummies had been put into coffins of stone or pottery, which had been buried in chambers carved out of a granite hill. The bodies were those of the priests of Philae and of their women and children, who lived during the second or third century B.C. The information concerning the pathological lesions in these people is not very satisfactory, as, owing to the bad preservation of the bodies, complete examination of them was impossible. Still, the fact remains that five skeletons with spondylitis, sometimes very severe, were found among sixty-four skeletons examined.

Farther south, in a Roman cemetery (14), which contained but few bodies, several skeletons with spondylitis were discovered. A young man, whose lumbar vertebrae showed much lipping, had also characteristic arthritis of the knee and elbow. Two lumbar vertebrae of another man with extreme spondylitis were firmly ankylosed, and he had suffered also from some inflammatory process in both tibiae and fibulae.

In the Romano-Nubian group (X group) of Cemetery 13, situated higher up on the river and dating approximately from the second to sixth century A.D., several cases of spondylitis were found.

On the west bank of the Nile, opposite the island of Markos, the field notes referring to a group of twenty-four bodies (Cemetery 42), dating from the Byzantine period, mention one case of extreme spondylitis and one of arthritis of the knees.

A few personal observations made at Meroë in the Sudan and at Faras may be mentioned here, although they refer to a somewhat earlier period, namely, to that of the Meroitic kingdom.

During the winter of 1913, the writer had an opportunity of witnessing for a few days the excavations then in progress at Merawi (Sudan). Professor Griffith, of Oxford, who was directing the work, gave every facility for studying the skeletons still in the graves, and the skulls and bones which he had collected at Merawi, and also the specimens which he had dug up at Faras in 1912.

Merawi is situated on the Nile (18° N.) close to the ancient Napata, and must not be mistaken for another village of the same name which is situated farther south; Faras lies a few miles north of Wady Halfa, not far from the Second Cataract of the Nile.

At Merawi, owing to the very bad state of the bones, no case of arthritis was met with, until at length three lumbar veretebrae with marked lipping of the anterior borders of the bodies were found in one grave. Two lumbar vertebrae in another grave showed some lipping of their borders, and were held together on one side by a strong bridge of new bone, measuring about 15 mm. in width and about 5 mm. in thickness.

At Faras, the vertebrae were very few and badly preserved. Three sacra, however, showed signs of spondylitis deformans. The disease, therefore, existed at Merawi and Faras, two of the hottest and driest places in the world.

The skeletons from Alexandria, with the coldest and wettest climate of Egypt, came from many graves and belonged to various nationalities.

The first part of this material was found at Chatby, near Alexandria, about two minutes' walk from the sea, in the tombs of the Macedonian soldiers of Alexander the Great and Ptolemy I. In view of the constant growth of the modern town, which will soon extend over the whole of this region, the Municipal Commission ordered an archaeological survey of this site. The work was entrusted to Professor E. Breccia, who gave Dr. Rietti and myself permission to examine most of the bones found in the necropolis and to be present during the excavations. Professor Breccia has since given a full account of his work in two magnificent volumes.[1]

Owing to a lawsuit, the work has been suspended for a time; this delay is specially unfortunate, because the names of the tombs to be

[1] E. Breccia, *Le necropoli di Sciatbi.*

yet opened indicate that these contain the skeletons of the ladies of pleasure who accompanied the Greek army. Here, if anywhere, evidence of gonorrhoea and syphilis should be found, if venereal disease really existed at that period.

The bodies were in rock-hewn graves, the first grave being an ossarium, measuring about 2 c.m., filled with sand and bones, and closed with a stone slab, the edges hermetically sealed with mortar. The bones, after the bodies had undergone decomposition elsewhere, had been thrown pell-mell into the ossarium, and evidently little care had been taken, for the femur of a horse was found among the human bones.

The other sepulchres were horizontal shafts, 3.5 feet high, 6 feet deep, and about 3.5 feet wide, cut into the sandstone rock in the same manner as the ossarium. Very rarely, such a tomb contained but one body lying on a layer of sand about 6 inches deep; as a rule, several skeletons, five, six, or even more, were present. The small size of the shafts was proof positive that the bodies had not been put in together, and that putrefaction had destroyed the soft parts of the first body before the second had been introduced.

Funereal urns filled with ashes or half-carbonised bones were also discovered. The Greeks of that period, therefore, were eclectic in their customs, some families burying, others burning their dead.

Unfortunately, the level of the land had sunk several feet since the last inhumation. Hence some tombs were partially filled, others merely infiltrated with sea water, and the bones were often found lying in thick, wet mud. Such skeletons were in very bad condition, and most of the smaller and some of the larger bones could not be found, even when the slush was removed carefully by hand; but although, as might be expected, the bones in dry graves were naturally rather better preserved than those in a wet bed, yet this was by no means the rule. The skeleton of a female, for instance, lying on a bed of dry sand, was so fragile that some of the bones were broken when their careful removal was attempted; on the other hand, bones lying in liquid mud were sometimes very hard, while others from the same grave broke as soon as touched.

Sometimes the soldiers had been buried with their wives and children. It is much to be regretted that infantile skeletons were useless for pathological research, as hardly a single one of their bones was preserved sufficiently well for examination.

A superficial examination sufficed to show that various races were represented. Some of the thirty-two skulls examined had high-bridged noses, others remarkably flat ones; some were brachycephalic, others markedly dolichocephalic, and two were evidently negroid. The variations in stature were also considerable, some men being very tall, others small. These differences are not to be wondered at considering that from the start Alexander's army was distinctly a "mixed" crew. Of the 30,000 foot soldiers who left Greece with Alexander, only 12,000 were Greeks (Smith's *Classical Dictionary*); the others were foreigners, chiefly Thracians.

It is highly probable that the Greek and foreign soldiers settled in Egypt had intercourse with and often married native women, just as their successors have done in modern times. The present Berberine, especially when coming from Korosko, often boasts that he is a descendant of a Turkish soldier and a native woman; and the term Turk, as used by the Berberine, includes Greek, Herzegovinian, Bosnian, Bulgarian, and Serbian—in fact, any one who has served in the Turkish army. Similarly, the population of Alexandria under the Ptolemies included Macedonians, Greeks, Syrians, Jews, Persians, etc., and the nucleus for the future population of Alexandria already existed in Alexander the Great's time.

Mahaffy draws special attention to the false impression given by most authors that Alexandria was a city in which the Jews and Greeks counted for everything, the natives for nothing. On the contrary, the majority of the poorer classes was from the beginning Egyptian, and to the last the city remained very different from other Hellenistic foundations. The native element, though at first thrust out from power and influence, gradually reasserted itself, and the city that opposed Caesar was probably far more Egyptian than that which opposed Antiochus Epiphanes.

Old Alexandria, therefore, may be compared to the modern town, where, although the greater part of the wealth and power is in the hands of the Europeans, any law repugnant to native ideas or customs speedily becomes a dead letter.

The extent of intermarriage between the various people inhabiting Alexandria cannot be estimated, but that they did live in very close association is shown by the fact that, during the Roman period, many inhabitants had two names, one Egyptian and the other foreign.

The possible influence of race and environment on the pathology of ancient Egypt may perhaps be discussed on another occasion, but these few lines suffice to prove that an attempt to unravel this question by the study of material collected in Alexandria can lead to no practical conclusion.

The catacombs of Kom el Shougafa, situated close to Pompey's pillar at Alexandria, date from the second century A.D., and most of the skeletons were those of the members of a mixed Graeco-Egyptian population. The tombs contained hundreds of skeletons, most of which, owing to the gradual infiltration of water, were practically useless for our purpose. The supposition that these catacombs contained the skeletons of the Alexandrian youths massacred by Caracalla is disproved by the fact that many skeletons were those of women and children.

The mode of burial was almost identical with that at Chatby. The first body had been placed on a layer of sand about 4 inches thick, and later on it had been pushed aside to make room for a second occupant. The loculi contained fragments of eight and ten bodies, and as the size of the tombs precludes all possibilities of more than two or at most three bodies having been buried at any one time, it follows that this process had been repeated more than once. So far the writer has seen no trace of cremation or mummification at Kom el Shougafa.

In 1912 very few of the skeletons had been examined for pathological lesions. Since then, fragments from over 150 adults have been studied, but the state of the skeletons was such that not a single skull could be reconstructed. Some of the loculi had been rifled by tomb robbers in ancient times and by modern archaeologists, and in both cases the result had been the same: the bones had been thrust aside into a heap in one corner of the tomb and most of them had been broken. No statistics, therefore, were available, concerning the incidence of any disease.

At Ras el Tin, in a garden of His Highness the Sultan's palace, a workman engaged in sinking a well suddenly slipped into a catacomb in which many hundreds of bodies had been placed. This catacomb is made up of a number of passages, lined on each side with loculi containing skeletons. A full archaeological account will be given later on by the curator of the Alexandria Museum, who allowed me to remove some of the bones in the short time during which the underground passages remained open.

Archaeological observations make it certain that the people buried there were Egyptians, and that the tombs date from the days of Cleopatra. The Egyptian origin of the skeletons is confirmed by the fact that most of the bodies had been embalmed, for the majority of the skulls had been perforated for the removal of the brain, according to the classical Egyptian method. Remnants of embalming material were entirely absent, except for a few very small fragments of plaster masks and mummy cases, and some small amount of gummy material in a few skulls. The bandages wrapped round the body had not been proof against the dissolving action of the wet sand, which in the course of twenty centuries had filled the catacombs. This state of things is to be regretted, the more, since practically nothing is known of the methods of the embalmer's craft in the Delta; but as the embalming material disappeared quickly it probably consisted of some easily putrescible substance such as linen, and not of earth, sand, resin, pitch, bitumen, nor any resistant vegetable matter. Whatever the method may have been, it proved a complete failure.

The loculi were roughly 6 feet long and 3 feet high, and five or six perforated skulls and the remains of a like number of skeletons were discovered in some. By no amount of force could such a number of bodies have been squeezed into that space; clearly, therefore, the first and second mummified bodies had fallen to pieces before the third and any of the others were introduced. Another unavoidable conclusion is that the loculi were in use for a fairly long time, some centuries possibly.

Spondylitis deformans was obviously very common among the people buried at Chatby, though, for reasons just explained, this conclusion cannot be based on accurate statistics. The thirty-two skulls found do not represent the truth, and a larger number were undoubtedly buried, as the number of skulls does not agree with that of the mandibles or right femurs. Judging from the number of the latter, it is certain that at least forty adults or fragments of forty adult bodies were put to rest in the graves examined at Chatby.

One complete skeleton was obtained. It was that of a young woman whose third molars had not quite emerged, and was in a very bad state of preservation, the skull and smaller bones falling to pieces when a careful attempt was made to remove them. The whole spinal column from end to end showed early signs of spondylitis deformans, namely, overlapping of the anterior borders of the vertebrae, and enlargement, eburnation, and ankylosis of the articulating surfaces.

In other graves many vertebrae were found ankylosed, or, when separate, in such a position that there could be no doubt that they belonged to the same body. A few typical examples of these lesions are now given.

Ankylosis of the articulating surfaces between the axis and the third cervical vertebra was the characteristic lesion of one skeleton. Moreover, the posterior borders of the bodies were firmly bound together by new bone which had developed in the posterior common ligament. The odontoid process was very rough, especially at the lower borders of the groove for the transverse ligament, and its rough and asymmetrical tip was capped with newly formed bone (Plate L, Fig. 11). The inferior articulating surface of the third vertebra was greatly enlarged and surrounded by osseous outgrowth, and a long spur of bone projected from the inferior-anterior border of the body.

The third, fourth, and fifth cervical vertebrae of another skeleton were firmly joined together. The upper and lower borders of the bodies, especially those of the sixth, though somewhat thickened, were otherwise practically normal. The disease was chiefly confined to the articular surfaces, which with two exceptions were almost double their normal width, flattened and fixed to one another by thick new bone.

Similar changes disfigured the dorsal region of many spinal columns. One osseous block consisted of three dorsal vertebrae.

The upper border of the body of the highest vertebra was thickened, especially in front, where the new bone was at least 5 mm. thick. The right lower border had thrown out a flat osteophyte, 10 mm. long and 20 mm. broad, which met another osteophyte projecting upwards from the vertebra below, and the upper and lower articulating surfaces were very rough, irregular, and enlarged. Similar lesions were present in the next vertebra, and, further, the border of the surface articulating with the tubercle of the rib was deformed. The roughened superior-anterior border of the last vertebra had thrown out a strong osteophyte which met a similar projection from the preceding vertebra. The superior and inferior articulating surfaces showed all the changes characteristic of spondylitis deformans. The costo-vertebral articulating surfaces were enlarged, rough, and almost worn away.

Such ankylosed masses were of common occurrence, and the large majority of the dorsal and lumbar vertebrae showed more or less profound inflammatory changes. Two lumbar vertebrae, for instance, were firmly bound together by a strong mass of new bone extending right round the bodies of both, and strong prolongations at each extremity proved that the disease extended to the vertebrae both above and below.

The disease also attacked the sacrum and pelvis. Firm ankylosis between the sacrum and the right iliac bone existed in two cases, and in two others the fifth lumbar vertebra and the sacrum were firmly joined by strong osteophytes. In another skeleton a strong osteophyte extended upwards from the left anterior-superior border of the sacrum to the fifth lumbar vertebra.

Typical spondylitis deformans, therefore, existed among the Greeks and other settlers in Egypt at the time of the Ptolemies.

The manifestations of the disease in the mixed population buried at Kom el Shougafa were not less interesting. Two tombs containing eight adult bodies were examined in the first investigations of this catacomb, and no less than four skeletons exhibited typical lesions of spondylitis deformans.

One skeleton resembled that of the IIIrd Dynasty described above, the whole vertebral column having been converted into a rigid block. The anterior, posterior, and lateral common ligaments in the cervical and lumbar regions were so completely ossified that a glimpse into the intervertebral spaces was obtainable here and there only. Similarly, all movements of these regions were arrested owing to the articulating surfaces being tightly held by dense new bone. The spinous processes of the cervical vertebrae were normal, whereas those of the lumbar vertebrae were connected by a strong bridge of bone which had developed in the supraspinous ligament. The lesions of the dorsal region, though severe, were on the whole less serious than those of other parts of the vertebral column. The limitation of movements due to the strong osseous bridges connecting the bodies of the vertebrae anteriorly was undoubtedly very great, but there was not that complete ossification of all the ligaments which was conspicuous both above and below that region. In fact, the borders of the bodies of the dorsal vertebrae were free from disease for more than two-thirds of their lengths. The articulating surfaces also were not so tightly bound together, though bony excrescences due to severe inflammation were conspicuous. The costo-central and the costo-transverse articulating surfaces were normal, whereas the periarticular ligaments were ossified more or less completely.

Other tombs of Kom el Shougafa, cleared in 1913, yielded the fragmentary remains of over two hundred adults, and ten axis vertebrae, out of forty which were collected, showed distinct pathological changes. The articulating surface of the odontoid process with the atlas was sometimes enlarged and sometimes eburnated, the tip was often capped by new bone, very irregular in shape, and sometimes curved like a Phrygian cap.

The sacrum was affected by osteo-arthritis in the same proportion, namely, 25 per cent, and the proportion of diseased cervical, dorsal, and lumbar vertebrae was nearly 40 per cent.

The contemporaries of Cleopatra buried at Ras el Tin, two centuries previously, were similarly affected. The whole lumbar and dorsal vertebrae of one case were firmly bound together by osseous bridges, and in consequence the curvature of the vertebral column was such that the patient must have been doubled up when he stood (Plate XLIX, Fig. 3). More probably, however, he could not stand up at all. Numerous osseous blocks were found consisting of two, three, or more vertebrae from various parts of the vertebral column (Plates L and LI, Figs. 12 and 13), and from an examination of a considerable number of fragments the conclusion was reached that the incidence of this disease was not less than 30 per cent and was probably somewhat higher.

About eighty miles west of Alexandria, the traveler finds the ruins of the ancient sanctuary of Abou Menas, which, during the early Christian period, was a pilgrimage place visited by sufferers. The crowds of sick pilgrims brought back to their friends holy water contained in special bottles, which have been discovered as far as Mainz in Germany, and in England, France, etc., and this fact clearly proves the high esteem in which the Abou Menas water was held. The exact date of the foundation of this ancient Lourdes is not known, but it was certainly not later than the fourth century A.D., and the popularity of the shrine lasted until its destruction by the Arabs.

The archaeologist who brought these ruins to light, laboriously noted every bit of glazed pottery or fragment of stone, etc., which littered the site, and recorded his observations in a very elaborate illustrated work. His soul, however, was clearly above such trifling things as human remains, for, one year after he had left, a number of skulls, vertebrae, and limb bones were found thrown about the passages and elsewhere, but most of the contents of the graves are lost forever. A similar state of things exists at Abou Sir, where the graves near the sea, dating from a perhaps slightly earlier period, have also been rifled almost completely. A few bones alone had been left in situ by the tomb robbers.

This neglect is all the more regrettable in that many skeletons must have been those of patients who suffered from some chronic disease for which they had sought relief at this miraculous spring, and an examination of their skeletons would have revealed curious facts concerning the pathology of early Christian times.

Among the very few vertebrae discovered at Abou Menas were: (1) an axis, with a typical cap of new bone of the odontoid process, and signs of inflammation on the outer border of the inferior articulating surface; (2) a cervical vertebra, probably the fifth, with its left upper articulating surface greatly enlarged and eburnated, and much osseous overgrowth round its inferior border; the right lower articulating surfaces showed similar changes (Plate LI, Figs. 14 and 15); (3) three dorsal vertebrae from one grave with marked thickening of the anterior borders, and inflammation round the costo-vertebral articulation; (4) four lumbar vertebrae with great thickening and formation of osteophytes of the anterior borders; the interspinous ligaments had also been affected, for the spinous processes were very rough.

It has been shown that spondylitis deformans existed in Nubia from the earliest periods down to the Christian era, that is, for a period of eighty centuries at least. In Lower Egypt, that is, round Alexandria, it has been traced from the time of Alexander down to the time of Abou Menas, that is, for another period of eight hundred years. The data regarding the incidence of this disease in Upper Egypt may now be examined.

Facts previously enumerated prove that the disease existed in the predynastic period, at the time of the pyramid builders and in the IIIrd Dynasty, and, indeed, the case of Nefermaat, a rich man of that dynasty, is one of the most typical on record.

The lesions now to be described were observed in the skeleton of a mummy of the XIIth Dynasty (2000–1788 B.C.), given to me by the late Sir Gaston Maspero.

This woman had died at an advanced age, for the sutures of the skull, with the exception of the squamous suture, were ossified. The teeth were deeply worn, and the alveoli of the left maxillary, first premolar, and all three left molars, and the right second and third molars were obliterated. The left maxillary canine was carious.

The first four cervical vertebrae were normal; on the fifth there was a strong osteophyte growing from the anterior-inferior part of the body. The sixth cervical was normal, whereas a strong osteophyte occupied the left anterior-inferior border of the seventh.

The dorsal vertebrae were healthy, with the exception of the ninth and tenth, the adjoining borders of which were united in the middle line by a thick osteophyte about 15 mm. long and 3 mm. broad at its base. The second and third lumbar vertebrae showed some lipping. The spinous processes from the tenth dorsal to the second lumbar vertebra were joined together by a bridge of new bone.

The lesions, therefore, though not severe, were typical.

Skipping a period of a thousand years, let us now examine a skeleton from the XXnd Dynasty (945–743 B.C.) given me by Professor Flinders Petrie. The vertebral column showed the following changes:

The atlas was normal except that a flat osteophyte, almost 10 mm. long, surrounded nearly half the outer border of the right upper articulating surface. Another small osteophyte protruded from the posterior border of the left upper articulating surface.

The extremity of the left transverse process of the atlas was much thickened, and was longer and broader than its fellow of the right side. The foramen for the left vertebral artery was not completely closed.

Distinct rough new bone extended along the inferior-posterior border of the body of the fifth cervical vertebra, and all round the superior and inferior borders of the body of the sixth. Each vertebral foramen was divided into two unequal parts by a thin spiculum of bone.

Seventh cervical.—New bone extended round the upper border of the body, and was more marked on the right side. The foramen for the right vertebral artery was narrowed by osseous growth to one-fourth the size of that on the left side.

First dorsal (Plate LI, Fig. 16).—Rough new bone along the superior-anterior border, extending for about 3 mm. down the body of the vertebra. The left costo-vertebral articulating surfaces of the first, tenth, and eleventh dorsal vertebrae showed marked signs of inflammation.

First lumbar.—Distinct thinning of the body.

Second lumbar.—Distinct roughening and formation of osteophytes on the borders of both superior and on the right inferior articulating surfaces.

Third lumbar.—New bone round the anterior part of superior border. A thin ridge of bone was prolonged on the left of the middle line along the anterior part of the body into a thick osseous excrescence which almost surrounded the lower border; this was especially marked on the left side. The right superior articulating surface was very rough, and its borders were surrounded by a ring of new bone (Plate LI, Fig. 17).

Fourth lumbar.—A very thick layer of new bone extended round the anterior border, especially on the left side, and in the middle for some distance on the body of the vertebra down to the left lower border. Much new bone had formed at the base and behind the left superior and inferior articulating processes.

Fifth lumbar.—New bone right round superior border extending downwards along body nearly for 10 mm.

We now again skip a period of approximately five hundred years, and examine a skeleton dating from the time of the Persian occupation of Egypt (about 500 B.C.).

All the vertebrae were present, except the axis and the seventh cervical, which could not be found.

Atlas.—The facet for the odontoid process was surrounded above and laterally by a strong layer of rough new bone. From the shape of the facet, it was evident that the odontoid process, instead of pointing directly upwards, was bent slightly backwards. The right tubercle for the attachment of the transverse ligament and the bone just below the right condylar process were slightly roughened. The foramen in the right transverse process was not completely closed.

Third cervical vertebra (Plate L, Fig. 11).—The upper and lower surfaces of the body were deeply hollowed, especially the former, the hollow of which was nearly 10 mm. in depth. Its upper surface was very rough. Some formation of new bone along the anterior lower border, where the new bone was approximately 2 mm. thick. The whole body was very thin, measuring about 5 mm. in thickness, and there had been a good deal of absorption of bone on the inferior surface laterally.

Fourth cervical.—This showed the same lesion, but the osteophyte along the anterior-inferior border was stronger and irregular. The body was distinctly atrophied and less than 5 mm. thick.

Fifth cervical.—Marked hollowing of upper surface of the body. Formation of new bone along the upper anterior border, and, to a less extent, along the upper posterior borders. Lower surface practically normal. Thickness of vertebra = 6 mm.

Sixth cervical.—No new bone; the body about 12 mm. thick.

Seventh cervical.—Missing.

Sixth dorsal.—The left lower articulating surface very irregular in shape, rough, and nearly double the size of its fellow, on account of the formation of new bone around it.

Seventh dorsal.—The right upper and lower articulating surfaces very irregular in shape and double the size of their fellows. The bodies of both these vertebrae were somewhat thinner on the right side.

Eighth dorsal.—The left inferior articulating surface was greatly enlarged and very irregular, with some thick new bone growing round it. The anterior-superior border of the body was somewhat rough. The inferior border of the body was rough and there was an osteophyte 3 mm. thick and about 10 mm. long on the right side. Both upper articulating surfaces were very irregular and rough, owing to formation of new bone, especially on the left side. Right side of body distinctly atrophied.

Ninth dorsal.—Lower articulating surface was very rough and irregular, especially on the left side. Upper articulating surfaces fairly smooth but very irregular in shape. Upper border of the body had thrown out an osteophyte (25 mm. long and 10 mm. broad), which met a similar osteophyte projecting from the vertebra above. Distinct atrophy of the right side of the body of the vertebra. Lower border of body had thrown out an osteophyte similar to that from the upper border, the two being joined by a strong pillar of new bone. The upper costo-central facet was enlarged, rough, surrounded by new bone and so altered as to be almost unrecognisable.

Tenth dorsal (Plate LI, Fig. 18).—On the right superior border, a strong osteophyte met one descending from the vertebra above. Upper articulating surfaces irregular, but almost normal otherwise. Distinct atrophy of right side of body. Some slight formation of new bone along the right inferior border of body.

Eleventh and twelfth.—Practically normal.

First lumbar.—Normal, except for some slight thickening round the left superior articulating surface.

Fourth and fifth lumbar.—Some thickening around upper border of body.

The lesions in these three skeletons, though not so marked as in others already described, are quite typical and prove the existence of spondylitis in Egypt during the period of roughly fifteen hundred years, extending from 2000 to 500 B.C.

We will now pass over another thousand years and examine some Coptic bodies found at Antinoë, and dating from about 500 A.D.

In the first, the spondylitis was limited to the first five cervical vertebrae. The atlas showed slight thickening of bone on the anterior side round the facet for the odontoid process. The axis was normal, except that the tip of the odontoid process was covered by a cap of new bone measuring 3 by 3 mm. The upper articulating surfaces of the third cervical vertebra were enlarged as compared with the corresponding lower ones, the left upper surface being only slightly enlarged, whereas the right measured 15 by 13 mm. Bone had been deposited on the borders, and the articulating surface itself had a worm-eaten appearance. The right upper and left lower articulating surfaces of the fourth cervical and the left upper articulating surface of the fifth were greatly enlarged and honeycombed, whereas the lower articulating surface of the fifth and the vertebral column generally were normal.

In the next case, in which arthritic lesions in other parts of the body were severe, the alterations in the spinal column merely consisted of some lipping between the adjoining borders of the second and third, and between the sixth and seventh cervical vertebrae, and in the dorsal and lumbar regions from the seventh dorsal to the fourth lumbar. The lesions were most marked in the dorsal region where the new bone formed a thick irregular festoon round the anterior border. The last lumbar vertebra, the sacrum and coccyx were normal. Another case was that of a very muscular man, whose ensiform cartilage showed a curious defect in ossification (Plate LI, Fig. 19).

Cervical vertebrae, atlas.—Formations of new bone from superior border of anterior arch, so that the tip of the odontoid process was overlapped (Plate LI, Fig. 20) by bone growing from the atlas. Inferior articular facets of the third cervical vertebra greatly enlarged especially on the right side, where they were rough and irregular, with a thin line of new bone on the inner border. The superior articular facets of the fourth cervical vertebra were correspondingly enlarged, especially the right one, which measured 20 mm. from above downwards. The third dorsal vertebra had a strong anterior median ridge of new bone projecting for about 12 mm., which fitted in with a similar ridge on the fourth. Similar lesions existed from the sixth to the ninth dorsal vertebrae, both inclusive, and were especially marked on the two last, where these ridges formed a lateral prolongation 10 mm. broad at the base and projecting externally for 12 mm.

The lesions of osteo-arthritis in the vertebral column of Copts were sometimes slight, consisting merely of some lipping of the anterior borders of two, three, or more vertebrae. The lesions in one vertebral column were limited to periarticular inflammation of one (twelfth) costo-vertebral articulation, which was enlarged, white, and ivory-like. The head of the corresponding rib was enlarged and showed strong periarticular exostoses.

To sum up: spondylitis deformans has existed in Nubia and Upper Egypt during the predynastic periods, in the early, old, middle, and new dynastic and Ptolemaic kingdoms, during the Roman occupations, and later.

II. LESIONS IN THE VERTEBRAL COLUMN

Osteo-arthritis of the vertebral column having been proved to exist in Egypt from the earliest times, the more minute description of the lesions in the vertebral column may now be proceeded with. No attempt to deal with the subject in a chronological order will be made, as the facts just enumerated have shown that, in the main, the lesions of chronic articular or periarticular disease present the same characteristics in archaic Nubians as in predynastic, dynastic, and Ptolemaic Egyptians, the inhabitants of Alexandria during the Greek and Roman periods, and the Copts of early Christian times. The pathological anatomy of spondylitis did not vary during this period of eight thousand years. Further, it is clear that geographical distribution did not influence the course or incidence of the disease, since specimens from Lower Egypt, Upper Egypt, and Nubia showed that the frequency, nature, and severity of the lesions were unaffected by varying climatic conditions.

Probably the earliest and certainly the most characteristic lesion was the growth of an osteophyte from the antero-lateral borders of the body of one or more vertebrae. As a rule, three, four, five, or more were attacked, although very occasionally the disease was limited to one or two vertebrae. When the disease had started from the borders of two neighbouring vertebrae, the osteophytes thrown out from each ultimately met, forming an osseous bridge; whereas the bases of the osteophytes on the vertebral borders were from 2 to 3 mm. broad and were prolonged for a few millimetres only on the bodies of the vertebrae. This intervertebral bridge formed an arch, the concavity of which was turned towards the intervertebral spaces (Plate LI, Fig. 21). The new bone was rather soft and spongy and not eburnated, even when it attained a considerable size. The osteophytes were usually situated unilaterally or bilaterally, hardly ever centrally; and the posterior border of the vertebrae was never attacked until the disease had made considerable progress elsewhere.

This manner of onset was the rule for the dorsal and lumbar, but not for the cervical vertebrae, the periarticular borders and articular surfaces of which were often attacked when the bodies were still normal.

At a later stage the bases of the osteophytes spread on the vertebral bodies until those from the superior and inferior borders coalesced. In bilateral disease the osteophytes sometimes extended from each side until they met in or near the middle line, so that the anterior and lateral surfaces of the bodies were covered by a thick ring of bone (Plate XLIX, Fig. 4, and Plate LII, Fig. 22).

When the posterior border of the body was attacked, the layer of new bone along the vertebral canal was never more than 1 or 2 mm. thick, and therefore could not have pressed on the spinal cord during life. Sometimes the layer thrown out from the posterior borders coalesced with those coming from the anterior round the vertebrae and intervertebral spaces.[1]

Admitting, then, that the pathological process attacked the ligaments chiefly if not solely, it is logical to consider whether the immunity of the central parts of the bodies may not be explained by the anatomical connections of the vertebral ligaments. In this connection it may be remembered that the superficial fibres of the anterior common ligament extend from one vertebra to the fourth or fifth below, passing over the bodies of one or two vertebrae without touching them, whereas the deepest fibres are attached to adjacent vertebrae; and also, that the fibres adhere more closely to the intervertebral discs than to the bones, and are stretched across the transverse depression over the middle of the bodies without being attached to the latter. Some thin and scattered fibres on the sides of the bodies reach from one bone to the other. Lesions of the anterior common ligament starting in the superficial fibres would be most evident, firstly, near the upper and lower borders of the vertebrae; and, secondly, opposite the vertebral discs, where the anterior common ligament adheres most closely to the bodies of the vertebrae; that is, just where, as a matter of fact, the lesions are

[1] NOTE BY J. G. WILLMORE.—It has already been pointed out that in ancient Egyptians as in modern races the disease began and spread in the ligaments, i.e., that in its inception, at all events, it was perivertebral rather than vertebral. Analysis of the specimens already described affords, I think, sufficient ground for this contention, since it was invariably the ligaments, and more especially the anterior common ligament, which were the first to be attacked and showed the most advanced pathological changes.

most marked. During life, or before putrefaction has proceeded far, slight lesions of the anterior common ligaments would probably have been discovered opposite the bodies of the vertebrae; but in the graves, these small and delicate osteophytes, not being in close contact with the vertebrae, doubtless fell to pieces and were lost. In severe cases, on the other hand, the lesions still subsisted thousands of years after death.

The fact that the disease generally started from the anterior border laterally, and not centrally, may perhaps be explained by the very close adherence of the ligamentous fibres to the lateral vertebral borders; whereas the slightness of the lesions near the transverse process was perhaps due to the thinness and scarcity of the ligamentous fibres in that neighbourhood.

The intervertebral discs, which, though shrunken, were found in mummified or dried bodies with severe spondylitis, were apparently normal, and as a rule the intervertebral spaces were not altered in size or in shape. For example, a vertebral column from a "pan grave" at Ballalish, dating from the XIIth to XVIth Dynasties, showed very severe lesions of spondylitis (Plate LII, Fig. 23), and yet the intervertebral discs, though shrivelled from desiccation, were not otherwise altered. When moistened, the discs were easily split up into two thick laminae, enclosing a smooth-walled cavity, and there was no trace of new bone.

The laminae of a normal disc, which are arranged concentrically, consist mainly of parallel fibrous bundles, running obliquely between the vertebrae and attached firmly to both. The outermost layer is made up of ordinary fibrous tissue, the deeper and more numerous laminae of cartilage, and the central part of a pulpy and elastic, material. A thin cartilaginous layer on the lower and upper surfaces of each vertebra gives attachment to the discs, which are thickest in the lumbar region, thinnest in the intervals from the third to the seventh dorsal vertebrae, and form together about one-fourth of the length of the movable part of the column. The curvature of the cervical and lumbar portions of the vertebral column is due principally to the form of the discs, which are much thicker in front than behind.

In cases of spondylitis among ancient Egyptians no part of the discs was ossified, except the ring of fibrous tissue and cartilage in contact with the borders of the vertebrae. Nevertheless, some of the intervertebral discs were occasionally absorbed, with the result that the vertebrae fell together; and, owing to the anatomical peculiarities noted above, the removal by disease of the cervical and lumbar discs caused very severe deformities, such as the falling forward of the head on the chest (Plate XLIX, Fig. 3).

The articulations of the vertebrae were characteristically affected. Each articulation presents a synovial cavity surrounded by a fibrous capsule composed of ligaments, which are longer and looser in the cervical than in the dorsal and lumbar regions.

The periarticular borders of these articulations were often studded with large osteophytes which developed in the fibrous capsule. They doubtless caused great inconvenience, for the extent of the movements of the vertebral column, other than extension and flexion, are determined chiefly by the position of the articular surfaces. In the dorsal region these allow a certain degree of rotation; in the lumbar region lateral flexion but not rotation is possible, although by combining this lateral with antero-posterior flexion some degree of circumduction is produced. Severe lesions of the articular surfaces in several regions of the vertebral column, therefore, immobilised the whole of the spine, and, when limited to the cervical column, they prevented all movements of the head and neck, even when the other parts of the vertebrae remained healthy. New osseous tissue might surround the joint, and yet the articulating surfaces often remained untouched by disease, except in the instance which will be described further on.

The articulating surfaces of the atlas with the skull were generally normal, even in the rare cases when the borders of the condyles were distorted by periarticular inflammation, so that ankylosis of the head with the atlas was rare. In six thousand bodies examined in Nubia,[1] only one case of ankylosis of the occipito-atlantal articulation due to spondylitis was discovered.

In this case complete fusion existed between the right occipital condyle and the corresponding articular surface of the atlas, and the left atlantal facet was fused partly to the condyle, and partly to the lower surface of the jugular process of the occipital bone. The skull in this last case was firmly ossified with the upper cervical vertebra, and the resulting deformity was very great.

[1] Wood Jones, *Archaeological Survey of Nubia, 1907-8*, II, 244.

The spinal canal formed an obtuse angle with the foramen magnum, and the man's chin must have almost touched his chest. On the other hand, the articular surfaces between the atlas and axis were often enlarged, irregular, eburnated, and immobilised by a powerful ring of new bone. The surfaces for the insertion of the occipito-atloid ligaments often showed inflammatory changes.

Very peculiar were the alterations in the articulating surfaces of the odontoid process and of the atlas. The articulating surface of the process, and the facet for the latter on the arch of the atlas were eburnated and their borders rough, ragged, and irregular; the rounded tubercle for the attachment of the transverse ligament was similarly altered.

A very striking product of chronic inflammation was the little cap of osseous tissue frequently crowning the tip of the odontoid process. This little bony prominence, resembling a Phrygian cap (Plate LII, Fig. 24) nicely balanced on the tip of the process, was doubtless what remained of the attachments of the bands of the more or less ossified ligaments which united the process firmly with the neighbouring parts and certainly interfered considerably with movement. The atlanto-axial articulation allows the movements of rotation of the head and of the atlas on the axis, with the odontoid process as a pivot, the movements being checked by ligaments; while the occipito-atlantal articulation allows only very slight rotation but considerable flexion and extension of the head upon the vertebral column. As the axi-atlantal articulations were frequently attacked while the atlanto-occipital articulations usually escaped, rotation of the head was often abolished when nodding movements remained free.

A further impediment to the lateral movements and rotation of the head was the ossification of the transverse and cruciform ligaments at their points of attachment, and especially the very severe lesions of the articulation between the odontoid process and atlas. The movements of the head were hindered most by the pathological changes in the odontoid process; and the small cap of new bone, often crowning this process, at the point of attachment of the anterior and posterior occipito-axial, occipito-atlantal, and atlanto-axial ligaments, bears witness to the gravity of the pathological alterations in these important structures. The movements of flexion and extension of the head, therefore, were sometimes interfered with, but rotation was probably more often and more completely abolished when the atlanto-axial articulation was ankylosed.

The periarticular and articular changes also interfered with freedom of movement, for even in unilateral disease the neck was immobilised and the patients assumed the curious bird-like attitude of sufferers from cervical spondylitis deformans.

When the anterior part of the vertebral bodies and the transverse processes were involved, the action of the muscles, such as the longus colli, attached to the bodies and transverse processes of the cervical vertebrae, was certainly interfered with.

The bodies of the cervical vertebrae often appeared to be atrophied—an illusion caused by the growth of strong osteophytes on the anterior and posterior borders, which made the concavity and the upper surface appear deeper and the bodies thinner than they really were. One peculiarity of the disease in that region was that it was sometimes limited to one or two articulations on one side.

The shrinking of the intervertebral cartilages, accompanying or resulting from these lesions, inevitably produced several deformities. In the first place, the patient's height was diminished. In the second place, owing to the greater thickness of the anterior part of the normal cartilage, shortening was more marked anteriorly, and the head easily followed its natural tendency to fall forward on the chest, the patient then assuming the attitude usually supposed to be typical of old age.

The lesions of the cervical vertebrae, even when limited to the neighbourhood of the articulating surfaces, were almost always extremely severe. From being roughly oval, the articulating surfaces became irregular in shape, often enormously enlarged and, owing to the formation of new bone, almost convex, with a "worm-eaten" appearance due to enlargement of the blood vessels. Eburnation of these surfaces was more common than in any other region, and the fibrous capsule was often converted into a ring of dense new bone, which effectually put a stop to all movements. All these lesions finally converted all the structures composing this part of the cervical column into a rigid block, obliterated the normal curvature of the cervical spine, and thus led to great deformity of that region.

The spinous processes of the cervical and dorsal regions, rough in some cases, were usually normal. The supraspinous ligament between two or three lumbar vertebrae was often ossified, and occasionally this alteration extended to all the lumbar vertebrae;

on the other hand, the ligamenta subflava, composed of yellow elastic tissue, always remained free. The muscles lying in the vertebral groove suffered severely; an imposing mass of new bone sometimes filled up the whole groove, and firmly bound together the smaller muscles and the tendons of the muscular masses attached to the vertebrae.

The disease in the dorsal region was often limited to the bodies of the vertebrae, the osteophytes on the posterior and anterior borders being sometimes almost as thick as the antero-posterior diameter of the vertebral bodies themselves (Plate XLIX, Fig. 7).

The costo-central and costo-transverse articulating surfaces were often normal, even when, as often was the case, their borders were disfigured as the result of intense inflammation followed by deposit of new bone.

In other cases these articulations were the site of lesions which are of special interest in view of their severity.

In some specimens the morbid process, proceeding as far as marked eburnation, extended to the articulating surfaces; but these articular lesions were always accompanied by very marked periarticular changes and appeared to be secondary to them.

The costo-central articulation unites the heads of the majority of the ribs with two vertebral bodies in two distinct synovial joints, supported by ligaments which complete the capsule of the joint. An interarticular ligament divides the articulation into two parts, each lined by a separate synovial membrane. The costo-transverse articulation unites the tubercle and neck of the rib to the corresponding transverse process in an arthrodial joint; the neck of each rib is also united by a powerful ligament to the transverse process of the vertebra above. The articulation of the ribs to the spinal column behind and to the sternum in front allows a double movement of these bones,[1] but every such movement produces some friction in the costo-central and costo-transverse articulations. On the other hand, the muscles which elevate the ribs in respiration (external intercostals, scalenus anticus, serratus posticus superior, and the levatores costarum) were apparently not often involved. The lesions in the tendons of the diaphragm will be discussed with those of the lumbar region.

[1] Schäfer, *A Text-Book of Physiology*, p. 275.

The lesions of the articular surfaces and periarticular borders, though more common, were hardly ever as severe as in other parts of the spine. The movements of the dorsal vertebrae being limited in extent, profound changes in the anterior and posterior ligaments did not necessarily interfere with the movements or posture of the body, and the health of the patient suffered only from difficulties in respiration due to the involvement of the costo-vertebral articulations.

Pathological lesions of the intervertebral discs of the dorsal region were absent even in cases otherwise severe.

The lumbar region was most often and most characteristically attacked. Complete ossification of the anterior and posterior common ligaments was not rare, resulting in the lumbar vertebral column being converted into an immovable mass. Further, in severe cases, the upper and lower articulating surfaces were surrounded by mushroom-like, bony excrescences; the transverse processes were covered with flat stalactites of osseous tissue (Plate LII, Fig. 25), the vertebral grooves were filled with masses of spongy bone enclosing all the muscular attachments in that region, and the spinous processes were rough and firmly held together by the completely ossified supraspinous ligament. The intervertebral discs alone usually escaped.

As flexion and extension in the lumbar spine are comparatively important movements, and as ossification of the anterior and posterior ligaments was often extensive just in that part, the movements of the whole body were considerably interfered with; the ossification of the supraspinous ligament alone was sufficient to prevent any approximation or separation of the spines of the vertebrae, that is, all movements of extension or flexion. Lateral flexion also was rendered difficult, nay impossible, by periarticular inflammation and secondary changes in the articulating surfaces.

Very far-reaching in their effects were the pathological changes in the tendons of the muscles attached to the lumbar spine. The diaphragm, the most important of these muscles, on account of the part it plays in respiration, is attached to the spine by its crura or pillars, which lie on both sides of the aorta on the bodies of the lumbar vertebrae. These, at their origin, are tendinous in structure:

the right crus, larger and longer than the left, arising from the anterior surface of the bodies and intervertebral substances of the three and four upper lumbar vertebrae; the left from the two upper, both blending with the anterior common ligament of the spine.[1] As it was precisely the anterior ligament that was most often ossified, the crura of the diaphragm were necessarily involved in many cases, and difficulty in respiration, with all its attendant evils, was the result.

The pathological alterations in the many muscles attached to the lumbar vertebrae were of the greatest importance. The bending of the thigh on the body, and of the body on the thigh, all very important movements, were rendered difficult by the lesions in the attachments of the psoas to the transverse processes of the bodies and to the intervertebral discs of the lumbar vertebrae.

The erector spinae, a large muscular mass, was not infrequently involved, and in some cases all the attachments of this muscle were ossified, so that it was practically put out of action. Similarly, the disease involved the multifidus spinae, which occupies the vertebral groove by the side of the row of spinous processes from the sacrum to the axis, and which is attached also to the spinous processes of several vertebrae. The smaller rotatores dorsi, interspinalis and intertransversalis muscles often shared the same fate.

The muscles of the back come into play simultaneously in extension of the head and, on one side only, in lateral flexion of the column. The oblique muscles rotate the head and spinal column, and when the spine is fixed, some of the erector muscles may depress the angles of the ribs, and thus assist in forced expiration. Ossification of the attachments of these muscles interfered to some extent with all these movements. The capsular ligaments not infrequently showed lesions severe enough to immobilise the lumbar spine.

The lesions of the anterior parts of the bodies of the vertebrae often extended so far down the spine that a strong osseous bridge joined the anterior-inferior border of the fifth lumbar with the anterior-superior border of the first sacral vertebra. Complete ossification of the sacro-lumbar and ilio-lumbar ligaments was not rare,

[1] Gray, *Anatomy*.

and must often have interfered with movement, even when the sacro-iliac articulation was normal.

III. LESIONS OF THE PELVIS AND LOWER LIMB

Each of the two surfaces entering into the formation of the sacro-iliac articulation is covered with a layer of cartilage; these layers, though closely applied to one another, are not united except by fine transverse fibres in front. Occasionally, especially in elderly people, the rough and irregular articulating surfaces are separated by small spaces containing glairy fluid (Plate LII, Fig. 26). The sacrum and iliac bone are held together by the anterior and posterior sacro-iliac ligaments, and the articulation is further strengthened by the great and small sacro-sciatic ligaments.

As a rule, these articulating surfaces in ancient Egyptians were smooth and regular even in the skeletons of people who died at an advanced age. The majority of skeletons with spondylitis deformans had sacro-iliac articulating surfaces unworn by friction and with no traces of eburnation; this immunity is, doubtless, due to the absence of wear and tear in this articulation, for not only does very little movement take place between the bones, but almost the entire weight of the body rests on the posterior sacro-iliac ligament, from which the sacrum is in great part suspended, so to speak. The rough space above the auricular surface of the ilium, and the depressions on the back of the lateral mass of the sacrum to which the posterior sacro-iliac ligament is attached, were often distinctly rough in cases of spondylitis deformans, whereas the surfaces of attachment for the anterior sacro-iliac ligaments were usually normal. The surfaces for the attachment of the great sacro-sciatic ligament on the posterior-inferior iliac spine and the side of the sacrum and coccyx were generally quite normal, while the inner margin of the ischial tuberosity, the margin of the ischial ramus, and the obturator fascia often showed very marked pathological changes. The strain due to the weight of the body being borne, chiefly, by the sacro-iliac ligaments, the loss of power consequent on the involvement of these structures certainly affected the carriage of the trunk, in the standing position.

Two cases of severe disease of the left sacro-iliac articulations were observed. The first was discovered in a mummy of the XXIst Dynasty, and has been partly described by Elliot Smith, who wrote as follows:

In the case of an extremely emaciated old woman, called Nesi-Tet-Nab-Taris, a curious state of affairs was revealed. Large, open ante-mortem wounds, possibly bedsores, were found on the back, between the shoulders, and on each buttock. These had been made use of for the purpose of packing the back, and two square sheets of fine leather (gazelle skin?) had been applied to cover the upper wound and the whole buttock respectively.

These sheets had been sewn to the healthy skin beyond the sores and the edges hidden by strips of linen, which were smeared with a resinous paste. A large opening, probably an abscess or sinus, extended transversely from the left pudendal labium outward into the buttock; this had been sewn up with string.

A long ulcer on the back of the leg had been covered up by a sheet of linen soaked in a solution of resin.

Evidently this old woman had been long bedridden. Professor Elliot Smith obligingly gave me the pelvis and lower limbs, in the hope that histological investigation might throw light on the nature of the chronic disease from which she had suffered. The histological examination threw no light on the etiology of these sinuses, though we discovered that the peroneal arteries were completely calcified.

The remains of the pelvis and the lower limbs having been macerated, the following pathological alterations were discovered:

Right femur (Plate LII, Fig. 27).—Thick deposit of new bone round head of femur. Surface of great trochanter very rough, owing to deposits of whitish, spongy-looking bone, specially thick at upper extremity of diagonal line. Depression for the ligamentum teres irregular, and deeply pitted at bottom.

Left femur (Plate LII, Fig. 27).—Neck about 1 cm. shorter than that of right femur, owing to absorption; this process having taken place more rapidly at the back, the neck had partly collapsed and the head of the bone looked almost directly backwards. All round the head, especially anteriorly, new bone had been deposited. Great trochanter roughened by deposit of new spongy bone, thickest superiorly and anteriorly. Fossa for the ligamentum teres deeply pitted and much enlarged.

Pelvis.—Complete ankylosis between sacrum and right os innominatum. In right acetabulum, separation between articular and non-articular parts was almost obliterated by friction. The term ankylosis is badly chosen, for it cannot be shown that the sacro-iliac articulation was attacked at all, it being entirely surrounded by new bone. The two bones were bound together firmly by the completely ossified anterior and posterior sacro-iliac ligaments.

On the left side, no trace of inflammation, except on the ischial tuberosity, which was rougher than usual. In the acetabulum a layer of new bone existed at the junction of the articular and non-articular parts. The latter had been so much worn away by friction that it was of transparent thickness.

The bones of the leg were normal.

The second specimen showed, among other points of interest, the iliac bones firmly ankylosed to the sacrum.

The anterior sacro-iliac ligament was completely ossified as far as the lower border of the first sacral vertebra, and posteriorly the bones were united by two strong bridges of osseous tissue, separated by a small interval. The articulation appeared to be normal. The whole length of the external surface of the ischial ramus, especially near the inferior border, was covered with thick, rough, new bone, thinner, though still very noticeable, near the ramus of the pubis—the margins of the obturator foramen, the superior ramus of the pubis, and ilio-pectineal eminence were roughened by stalactites of inflammatory osseous tissue. The process, therefore, had attacked the sacro-iliac ligament and all the tendons at their points of attachment with the ischium and pubis.

The stalactite formations round the left obturator foramen were even more marked. The non-articular portion of the right acetabulum was normal, whereas a strong ridge of new bone, thickest on the outer side, lined the upper border of the articular portion.

The right ischial tuberosity, especially its external and inferior border, showed signs of very severe chronic inflammation, and the left acetabular cavity was much worn, without any formation of new bone.

It remains doubtful whether the sacro-iliac articulation was involved, in spite of the almost complete ossification of the anterior and posterior sacro-iliac ligaments, owing to the fact that here, as elsewhere, the disease was periarticular and not articular.

The pubic articulation, which is hardly movable in the normal, non-pregnant person, occasionally showed changes which may have been caused by osteo-arthritis. A curious lesion found in one Coptic body may be described here, although its etiology is uncertain.

The external surface of the right ramus of the pubis and part of the body were covered with a layer of new bone, which was smooth for the most part, except where it had a worm-eaten appearance. This plate of bone measured 40 by 45 mm., and was about 7.5 mm. thick in some places; it was sharply limited superiorly by a ridge and a deep groove, and there had evidently been some periostitis along the lower border of the ramus of the pubis, as far as its junction with the ramus of the ischium.

The articulating surfaces of the symphysis pubis were smooth and appeared healthy, and on each side of the joint on the internal surface there was a layer of new spongy bone, 5 mm. broad, and about 2.5 mm. thick on the right, and 1 mm. thick on the left side. The left innominate bone was otherwise healthy, and there was no trace of any suppuration round the pubis. An interesting point was that on both dorsal and lumbar vertebrae there was a small amount of lipping due to deposit of new bone along the upper and lower anterior borders of the bodies. The intervertebral discs and the ligaments were not ossified.

It is certain that, possibly owing to the lesions described, this person had long been bedridden, as a huge bedsore occupied the lumbar region, in which numerous micro-organisms were seen with the microscope.

Far more important than the changes in the sacro-iliac and pubic articulations were those on the points of attachment of the muscles arising from the iliac bones and pelvis. In a skeleton from Kom el Shougafa, for instance, the rami of the ischium and pubis, the tuberosities of the ischium, and especially the spaces between the inferior curved line and the upper border of the acetabulum were covered with small, round, osseous elevations (Plate LII, Fig. 28). Very often, the crest of the ilium was disfigured from end to end by jagged new bone, which testified to previous severe, chronic inflammation. Of course, this crest is always rugged, but in these cases important bone stalactites sprang from the internal and external lips and from the intermediate ridge. The attachment of the gluteus maximus was thus involved in the disease, and therefore extension, abduction, and rotation of the limb, the maintaining of the erect position and the regaining of it after stooping, were probably rendered difficult; let it be noted that the last is the most painful and difficult movement for sufferers from "muscular rheumatism" of the back. The attachments of the latissimus dorsi were also attacked, and as this muscle plays an important part in inspiration, walking, climbing, and in movements of the arms, the lesions of its attachments to the pelvic brim helped to make all these movements difficult and painful. Similarly, the disease involved the attachments of the abdominal obliquus externus and internus, which keep the abdominal cavity tense and act as expiratory muscles when the vertebral column is fixed; thus the changes seen at their attachments perhaps rendered the bending and the rotation of the thorax somewhat distressing, as is sometimes the case now in patients with chronic muscular rheumatism. Lesions of the tendon of the gluteus medius, where this muscle is attached to the pelvis, must have interfered with the abduction of the thigh and the maintenance of the erect position of the body.

From the posterior part of the iliac crest arise the quadratus lumborum and erector spinae, and the pathological changes in the attachments of these muscles must have caused the maintenance of the spine in the erect posture and the bending of the trunk backwards to be painful and distressing.

Very important were the lesions of the surfaces for the attachments of the tendon of the rectus femoris muscle on the anterior-inferior iliac spine, and of its reflected tendon just above the acetabulum (Plate LIII, Fig. 29). Both places were sometimes covered with small mammillated exostoses, developed partly in the periosteum, and doubtless in the tendinous muscular attachments as well. As this muscle, together with the psoas and iliacus, supports the pelvis and trunk upon the femur, or bends them forwards, lesions in this situation checked the maintenance of the erect attitude of the trunk, and probably also impaired the other actions of this muscle.

Disease of the rami of the pubis and ischium might involve the tendinous attachments of the obturator externus, adductor gracilis, and quadriceps in front; of the obturatur internus, levator prostatae, transversus perinei, erector penis, and compressor urethrae behind; of the pectineus, rectus abdominis, and pyramidalis near the angle of the pubis, and of the levator ani on the posterior surface. All the movements of the thigh, therefore, and especially progression, were to some extent checked by disease in that region, for many of these muscles assist in drawing the limb forward. Similarly, the maintenance of the body in an erect posture, flexion of the pelvis forwards upon the femur, movements of the thigh on the pelvis, of the pelvis on the thigh, of the leg on the thigh, and vice versa, were obstructed by the lesions described above.

The attachments of the hamstring muscles, semi-membranosus, semi-tendinosus, biceps, gemelli, coccygeus, and levator ani to the ischial tuberosity and its neighbourhood often suffered severely; in consequence, flexion of the knee, rotation of the tibia outwards by the biceps, semi-tendinosus and semi-membranosus, together with extension of the hip, were impeded, and doubtless occasioned great distress to the patient. The lesions of the attachments of the gemelli interfered with the support of the hip-joint posteriorly and with rotation and abduction of the limb. Forcible expiratory and other expulsive efforts were checked by the changes in the coccygeus, levator ani, and other muscles of the perineum; the lack of support to the pelvis must have caused unpleasant symptoms, such as difficult evacuation of the rectum.

In such cases, therefore, the movements of the back, lower and upper limbs, micturition, and defaecation were embarrassed and rendered painful by the implication of the attachments of the upper extremities of voluntary muscles; and it will be obvious presently that matters were often rendered worse by the implication of many of the inferior attachments of these same muscles.

The lesions of the hip-joint were perhaps the most important of all, because, even when slight, they interfered more than any other lesions with the maintainance of the erect posture and progression forwards or backwards.

The cotyloid ligament, a thick fibro-cartilaginous ring round the margin of the acetabulum, which, as the transverse ligament, bridges over the gap of the acetabular border, suffered less than one would have expected. Even with severe lesions of other parts of the articulation, the margin and immediate neighbourhood of the acetabulum were often smooth and to all appearance healthy. Sometimes, however, the margin of the acetabulum was topped by a ring of new bone, so fragile as to be usually more or less broken by post-mortem injuries; but occasionally this hyperostosis was sufficient to increase the depth of the joint (Plate LIII, Fig. 30). In cases still more severe, the inflammatory area extended to neighbouring parts—even, as we have seen, to the attachment of the reflected tendon of the rectus.

The transverse ligament was never completely ossified, though severe changes at its attachments were often recognisable; the osseous borders which the ligament unites often displayed distinct post-inflammatory hyperostosis, and it was unfortunate that the ligaments themselves had been destroyed by post-mortem changes. One important lesion was represented by a festoon of new bone formed by the thickening of the lower border of the articular portion of the joint, most marked at the point of attachment of the ligamentum teres (Plate LIII, Fig. 29). Further, while the pit for the ligamentum teres on the head of the femur is normally a small, smooth, round depression, in femora with lesions of chronic osteo-arthritis this pit was more or less completely obliterated by new bone, which, like melted wax (Plate LIII, Fig. 31), had filled it and then flowed over the neighbouring surfaces. The lesions at both ends of the ligament indicate that most probably the whole was ossified, and as flexion, abduction, or rotation of the hip must necessarily stretch this ligament, these movements must have been greatly impeded.

A more advanced lesion was the gradual wearing down of the lower brim of the articular portion of the acetabulum, until at one particular point the division between the articular and non-articular portions was obliterated. This point was almost opposite to the transverse ligament, but slightly posterior to it (Plate LIII, Fig. 32). The top of the head of the femur was always normal except for the changes in the fossa for the ligamentum teres. Eburnation was never seen.[1]

[1] NOTE BY J. G. WILLMORE.—In the late Sir Armand Ruffer's manuscript we found at this point a note to this effect: "Put here paragraph on Coxa Vara."

The limited time at my disposal unfortunately precluded us from making anything like a complete examination of the mass of material upon which Sir Armand based the conclusions given in this paper; but, as far as I have been able to determine, his results would seem to agree with the findings of Wood Jones, who stated (*Archaeological Survey of Nubia*, Bull. No. 2 [Cairo, 1908], p. 57) that many examples of coxa vara were found by him among skeletons exhumed from the cemeteries at Shellal, above the First Cataract.

Wood Jones drew attention to the absence of any of the cardinal signs of the bony manifestations of rickets in any single instance, out of the large number of skeletons of young people, of all ages up to puberty, which he had examined; at the same time later bone changes, in which it has been customary to invoke rickets as the causative factor, were by no means uncommon. He therefore suggested that the origin of these later bony changes lies in some factor other than rickets.

Sir Armand appears to have arrived at the same conclusion: an idea which is strengthened by the fact that the femora which I have been able to examine show merely shortening of their necks due to atrophy and absorption of the bone, without any of the deformity due to bending and twisting of the bone which is typical of coxa vara of definite rachitic origin (Plate LIII, Fig. 33).

The lesions in the attachments of certain parts of the capsule were serious, especially those already described at the point of origin of the upper extremity of the ilio-femoral ligament, on the lower anterior spinous process. The maintenance of the erect position puts a strain on the ilio-femoral ligament, and inflammatory lesions at the point where it is attached to the anterior intertrochanteric line were among the most common lesions. The whole length of this bony ridge was in some cases studded with small rough exostoses, and the lesions of this important ligament, by impeding the extension of the joint, produced a certain amount of pain and made the standing position almost impossible (Plate L, Fig. 10).

The upper attachments of the femoral ligament band opposite the outer head of the rectus, and the lower attachment to the upper and fore part of the great trochanter and neck of the femur often exhibited similar changes, which during life doubtless impeded movement, more especially adduction of the hip-joint. Whereas the upper attachment of the pubo-femoral band was generally intact, the lower end connected with the neck of the femur, level with and in front of the small trochanter, was frequently the seat of osteophytes which interfered with movement of the hip-joint, particularly with abduction of the limb.

Perhaps the most important lesion of the capsule was that affecting the bands of transverse fibres, which is about as wide as the middle finger, and arches like a collar round the neck of the bone. At this point, just below the neck of the femur, there was often a pad of bone, generally about 30 mm. long, 15 mm. wide, and perhaps 2 mm. thick, which represented this ossified ligament; and it was clear that the longitudinal as well as the transverse fibres of the capsule had been involved in the pathological processes.

To sum up: The pathological changes in the hip-joint were most obvious where the ligaments were attached, whereas evidently the acetabular cartilage was involved later. The head of the femur, where it was covered by cartilage, was never the seat of disease, except at its periphery and at the point of insertion of the ligamentum teres.

The extra-articular changes in the superior extremity of the femur come next in order. The surfaces of the great torchanter were often the seat of severe lesions. The whole trochanter, for instance, might be covered with rough new bone without any recognisable ligaments or tendinous framework; on the other hand, the structure of the tendons inserted in that situation was in some cases still so plainly visible that occasionally the whole, but more often only the anterior surface of the great trochanter, looked as if delicate tendinous fibres had been frozen on to it. The muscular attachments involved were those of the gluteus medius on the external surface, gemelli, pyriformis, obturator internus, and, above all, the tendon of the obturator externus in the digital fossa, which cavity was often filled with remnants of the ossified tendons of this last muscle. All these lesions certainly did not conduce to freedom of movement.

The upper part of the anterior intertrochanteric line to which the capsular ligament of the hip-joint is attached, and the lower part from which some of the fibres of the vastus internus originate, were often extensively altered. The posterior intertrochanteric line suffered less than the anterior, and indeed was rarely the seat of pathological changes; the small trochanter often escaped more or less completely.

The anterior part of the shaft below the anterior intertrochanteric line, and the lateral parts as far as the proximity of the knee-joint, were practically always normal, and they contrasted therefore with both extremities of the bone.

The two lines of attachment for the gluteus maximus, pectineus, and iliacus were often roughened by many thick, bony outgrowths which might extend to half the length of the shaft. This condition was not due to abnormal muscular development, as it was seen in femurs in which the other muscular attachments were, if anything, rather slighter than the average, but which showed distinct osteo-arthritic changes at their extremities.

A peculiar deformity of the femur is shown in Plate LIII, Fig. 34. Here the great trochanter and the intertrochanteric line are capped by an enormous growth of spongy bone measuring about 5 cm. in thickness, which is reflected in a thick layer round the junction of the neck of the bone with the shaft. The neck of the bone itself is practically normal. This enormous growth consists of loose, spongy bone, which, microscopically, shows nothing peculiar.

The lower extremity of the femur presents some slight signs of osteo-arthritis round the borders. The shaft of the femur is nowhere enlarged.

The diagnosis in this case must remain doubtful. I thought at first that the specimen was one of osteoma or osteosarcoma. Against this diagnosis it may be pointed out that the shaft of the femur itself appears to be quite normal, and the surface of the tumour, except over the great trochanter, is everywhere quite smooth. The interior of the growth is composed of normal, loose, osseous tissue.

Considering that this person had slight osteo-arthritic lesions of the lower extremity and of the head of the bone, it may be argued that the more striking lesions were also of the same nature. Assuming this to be possible, it is not a little strange that the lesions should be almost entirely limited to the part round the trochanters. Unfortunately, the other bones belonging to this skeleton could not be discovered, this lying loose in the ossarium.

Another interesting femur found in the same ossarium showed the head almost completely worn away, though signs of inflammation could still be seen along its upper and outer borders (Plate LIII, Fig. 35). The great trochanter had been badly smashed. In this instance, I do not think the possibility of the lesions having been tubercular can be excluded. Similar changes also existed all along the bony ridge to which the two vasti and the three adductor muscles were attached. It has been shown already that the upper attachments of these muscles to the os pubis were often the seat of pathological lesions, so that both ends of the muscles were involved; consequently, as one or more of these muscles take part in almost every movement of the lower limbs, walking, running, jumping, getting up from the kneeling or recumbent position, and other movements must have been greatly impeded.

The knee-joint was perhaps the articulation most frequently attacked by chronic osteo-arthritis, possibly on account of its size, of the number of ligaments entering into its composition, and of the fact that, more than any other large joint of the body, it is liable to traumatisms of all kinds.[1]

The part of the anterior lateral ligament passing over and intimately incorporated with the patella was very often the seat of chronic inflammation, which hardened in pathological ossification. The upper surface of the patella was then striated longitudinally, and the raised borders of these striae were prolonged into thin osteophytes, which in well-preserved specimens overhung the borders of the bones for a few millimetres. Lower down, where the anterior

[1] NOTE BY J. G. WILLMORE.—Another possible factor is that the knee-joints combine great mobility with the support of the weight of the trunk—compare the frequency with which gout attacks the joint of the great toe in modern people.

ligament and the lateral patellar ligament are connected with each side of the tubercle of the tibia, pathological changes were uncommon.

On the back of the outer condyle of the femur, a mass of new bone often indicated the point of insertion of the posterior ligament, and, similarly, the point of insertion of the ligament on the tendon of the semi-membranosus muscle was indicated in the same manner.

The lower end of the femur in many cases was disfigured by a thick rim of new bone which closely followed the borders of both condyles and greatly resembled the narrow brim of an old-fashioned billycock hat (Plate L, Fig. 8). The superior-anterior border of the external condyle was often prolonged upwards into a thick spur, an osteophyte which sometimes was nearly 5 mm. long, and which stood out prominently from the neighbouring tissues below. The borders of the intercondylar notch at the back of the joint did not escape, though the rim of new bone there was less thick and prominent than on the lateral or anterior edges of the articulation. In such cases, the attachments of the capsular ligament being ossified from end to end, the great part of the ligament was very probably ossified during life, and produced great difficulty in the movements of the knee-joint or even immobilised it. The imposing thickness of newly formed bone was proof of the chronic character of the disease, which doubtless had lasted for many years before death.

At the back of the external condyle of the femur, a thick patch of new bone sometimes marked the attachment of the anterior or external crucial ligament; a similar new formation in the depression in front of the spine of the tibia corresponded to the inferior attachment of this ligament; a tag of new bone, sometimes 15 mm. long, remained as evidence of the partial or complete ossification of this ligament. Similarly, the hinder part of the depression behind the spine of the tibia, the popliteal notch, and the inner condyle of the femur often presented the lesions typical of chronic periarticular disease, and there was no doubt that both crucial ligaments had been partly or wholly ossified. The ligaments of the knee, therefore, had undergone the same changes as those of the hip; and as most if not all of the joints had been attacked in some patients, the articular surfaces remaining normal, it follows that impairment of motion in, or even complete immobility of, the articulation sometimes resulted from periarticular lesions alone. The surfaces of attachment for the articular cartilages of the tibia were sometimes distorted by osseous proliferation, but as these lesions were seen only in those cases in which the periarticular alterations were intense, without any ossification of the cartilages, it follows that in all probability the disease did not attack the cartilages till very late. Sometimes an ivory-white, eburnated patch on one or both articulating surfaces of the tibia had resulted, and the eburnated surface was usually striated longitudinally, elongated from before backwards, and measured from 20 to 35 mm. in its longest, and about 15 to 20 mm. in its shortest transverse diameter. In the large majority of skeletons no new bone had been deposited on these surfaces of the femur or patella, which are normally protected by cartilages; the latter had been worn through the eburnation of the bone as a consequence (Plate LIII, Fig. 35).

Occasionally, the inflammation of the bony articulating surface led to its disfigurement by small round or oval patches of raised bone, studded with numerous small holes, the sites of enlarged blood vessels, which were not infrequently surrrounded by eburnated borders. These were evidently the vestiges of inflammatory reaction following on the wearing through of the cartilage. These patches, fairly common on the femur, were rare on the tibia.

The very important changes on the head of the tibia were similar to those on the femur. Contrary to expectation, the attachment of the ligamentum patellae was normal, even when periarticular lesions of the knee-joint were conspicuous; whereas the anterior parts of the internal and external tuberosities often suffered severely, fragments of the ossified ligaments, as much as 10 mm. long, sometimes remaining as evidence of the severity of the morbid process in the past. The surface of attachment for the semi-membranosus was often thickened by new bone, and as we have seen that in some cases the upper attachments of the muscles had been attacked also, the work of this muscle must have been impeded considerably; on the other hand, the attachments of the lower ends of the sartorius, semi-tendinosus, and gracilis were usually healthy.

The spine of the tibia, close to which the extremities of the semilunar cartilages are attached, and the rough depression behind it for the attachments of the anterior and posterior crucial ligaments, were often the seat of obvious lesions (Plate LIV, Fig. 37).

Very marked also were the changes in the neighbourhood of the tibio-fibular articulation. The borders of joints otherwise normal were rugged and thickened by new bone, and sometimes it was clear that a complete osseous capsule had surrounded the joint. The external surface of the styloid process of the fibula was usually most affected, and was covered with delicate, bony stalactites, as if fibres of the anterior-superior or posterior-superior ligaments had been frozen on to the process.

The crest, the internal cutaneous surface, the tibial attachments for the tibialis anticus and tibialis posticus were practically always normal. The inferior extremity of the tibia was but seldom seriously altered by lesions. The articular surface with the astragalus was always normal, the periarticular changes were never more than slight.

This immunity, however, did not extend to the lower tibio-fibular articulation, the borders of which were altered like those of the hip or knee-joint. A triangular patch of rough bone, with its base at the inferior extremity, often extended up the tibia for 2 or 3 inches, and opposite to it there was a similar patch on the fibula. The surfaces of attachment for the ligaments were frequently rough and aberrant in shape.

The oblique line to which the soleus is attached was the only part of the shaft of the tibia ever involved. It was often considerably thickened and protruded for 3 or 4 mm. with an external edge as much as 2 or 3 mm. broad.

The four borders of the fibula were often extremely rough and uneven, whereas the surfaces of attachment for the muscles of the big toe and foot remained smooth. It would seem, therefore, that the aponeuroses suffered, while the muscles escaped (Plate LIV, Fig. 38).

IV. LESIONS OF THE STERNUM, CLAVICLE, RIBS, AND UPPER LIMB

The sterno-clavicular articulation is formed by the sternal end of the clavicle, the upper and lateral part of the manubrium sterni, and the cartilage of the first rib, and allows limited movements in almost every direction—upwards, downwards, backwards, and forwards, as well as circumduction; the clavicle in its motion carries with it the scapula. The importance of this joint is great because it is the only point of articulation of the supporting arch of the shoulder with the trunk.[1] The result of these connections is that almost every movement of the shoulder produces a corresponding movement in the sterno-clavicular articulation, and, therefore, pressure on the interarticular fibro-cartilage. Elevation of the clavicle is principally limited by the costo-clavicular, depression by the interclavicular, ligament. The movements of the costo-clavicular part of the articulation are markedly increased in dyspnoea, and are limited by the anterior and posterior sterno-clavicular, the interarticular and costo-clavicular ligaments.

Complete ossification of adjoining surfaces was never found. The articulating surface of the clavicle was often greatly worn, and sometimes almost eburnated.

The attachments of the sterno-cleido-mastoid, pectoralis major and subclavius muscles, closely connected with the articulation in front, and the attachments of the sterno-hyoid and sterno-thyroid behind, were always normal. The interclavicular ligament also escaped as a rule, although the impression for the rhomboid ligament was often altered by chronic inflammation.

The borders of the small, flattened, oval facet of the acromial end of the clavicle were usually normal, while the articulating surface on the acromion and its periarticular borders and the attachment of the conoid and trapezoid ligaments were often thickened by bony deposits (Plate LIV, Fig. 39). In many instances the articulating surfaces looked as if they had been worm-eaten and were distinctly eburnated. Though the movements of the acromio-clavicular articulation were perhaps never entirely prevented by neighbouring lesions, it is certain that any pressure on this articulation, such as that produced by movements, must have caused intense pain.

The lesions of the costo-central and costo-transverse articulations have been already described. The only other frequent change in the rib was extreme roughening of the interior border near the angle, for about 3 inches in front and behind, but that this attrition was due to arthritis was not established.

[1] Gray, *Anatomy*.

It is strange that when most articulations, and especially the large articulations of the lower limbs, were attacked, the shoulder-joint in the large majority of Egyptian cases should have remained immune. Here the articular ligaments do not limit to the same extent the degree of movement by maintaining the articular surfaces in such close apposition as they do in the hip; and the looseness of the articulation may have been the cause of this comparative immunity.[1]

The lesions of the glenoid ligament, the fibro-cartilaginous rim attached to the margin of the glenoid cavity, consisted in the formation of a periarticular ring, and considering the close connection of the tendon of the biceps with this ligament, these lesions must have interfered with the action of the muscle.

The attachment of the capsular ligament to the scapula was seldom if ever attacked, whereas the anatomical neck was often surrounded by a slightly raised border of smooth new bone, never projecting for more than about 1 mm. nor exceeding 3 mm. in breadth. This new border was never disfigured by projecting osteophytes, and gave the impression of having been the result of a very mild chronic process.

Occasionally, the acromion process and the portion of the scapular spine from which the deltoid arises were much deformed by the comparatively large masses of bone deposited on them. The action of the deltoid, one of the most powerful muscles of the arm, was therefore interfered with.

The lesions of the humerus were most marked at the points of insertion of muscles closely connected with the shoulder-joint. New bone was deposited on the greater tuberosity to which the supraspinatus, infraspinatus, and teres minor are attached, on the lesser tuberosity, at the point of insertion of the subscapularis, and on the anterior and posterior bicipital ridges of the bicipital groove, where the pectoralis major, teres major, and latissimus dorsi are inserted (Plate LIV, Fig. 40). In many cases, therefore, although the articulating surfaces were perhaps intact, the movements of the arm and shoulder-joint may have been rendered painful, or may have become impeded, or even totally arrested, by lesions of ligaments and of tendons passing over the joint. The lesions in the shaft of the

[1] NOTE BY J. G. WILLMORE.—Further, the shoulder-joint has no weight to support.

humerus were limited, as a rule, to the bicipital groove and neighbouring parts. So in the humerus, as in the femur, tibia, and fibula, it is evident that the disease attacked the neighbourhood of the articulation, and the shaft of the bone escaped almost completely.

The changes in the shoulder-joint, therefore, were identical with those of all the joints studied so far, namely, apparent immunity of the articulating surfaces and involvement of the neighbouring attachments of ligaments and muscles.

The observations just related were made on skeletons from Upper and Lower Egypt. In Nubia,[1] on the other hand, the disease was by no means uncommon in the shoulder-joint, and here the deformity produced in the head of the humerus was often conspicuous. Hard, bony masses developed round the margins of the articular surface of the head of the bone, the articular surface itself became frequently displaced, and a considerable impairment of movement must have been the result of this deformity of the bone.

The lesions of the two articulations of the elbow may be described together.

In front, the upper and lateral borders of the coronoid depression were often covered by a ring of dense, almost eburnated, new bone, and the coronoid depression itself sometimes contained a mass of dense, often typically eburnated, new bone, which almost filled it. The same alterations existed in and around the radial depression, which was sometimes almost completely obliterated.

The internal borders of the trochlea and the articulation for the head of the radius were often lined with a thick border of new bone forming a ring round the articular surfaces, which, though less massive than that round the knee-joint, nevertheless must have caused considerable inconvenience (Plate LIV, Fig. 41). The olecranon depression was often disfigured by osteophytes, thickest at the apex of the triangle formed by that cavity, that is, on a level with the posterior ligament. Eburnation of the trochlear surface was rarely very marked, and the eburnated surface was streaked with parallel longitudinal lines resulting from the grinding of the articulating surfaces on one another.

The changes in the ulna were peculiar. The inner and outer borders of the lesser sigmoid cavity and of the coronoid process were

[1] Wood Jones, *Archaeological Survey of Nubia, 1907–8*, II, 275.

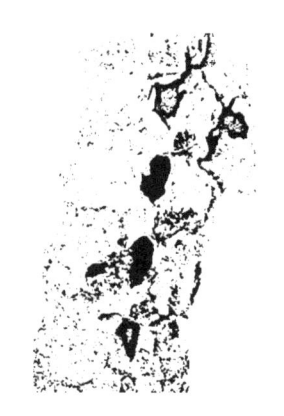

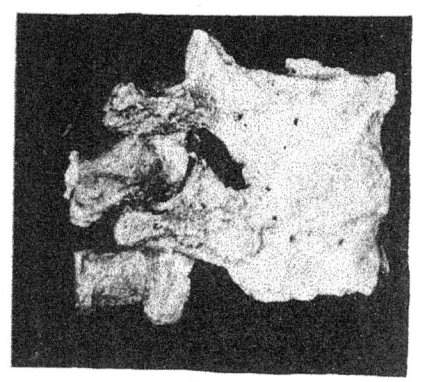

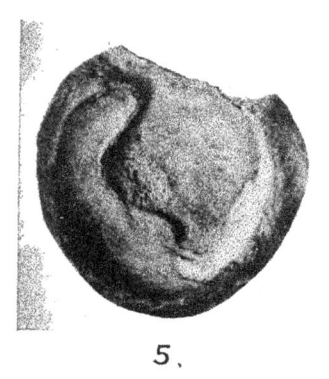

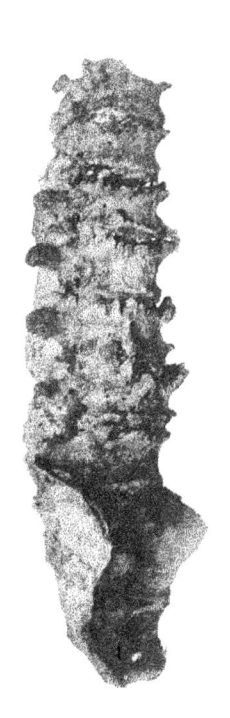

1.

2.

4.

3.

5.

7.

8.

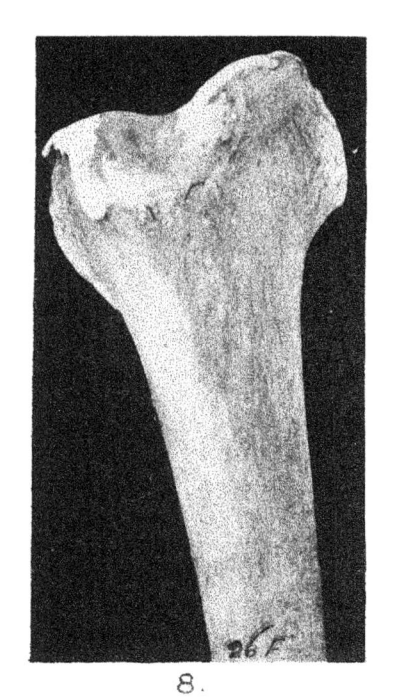

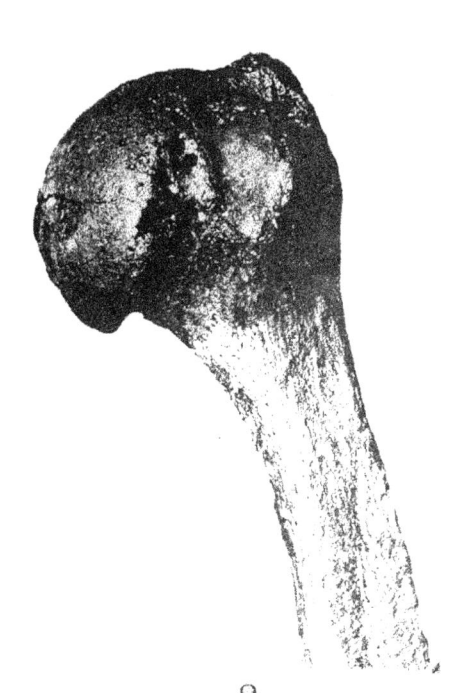

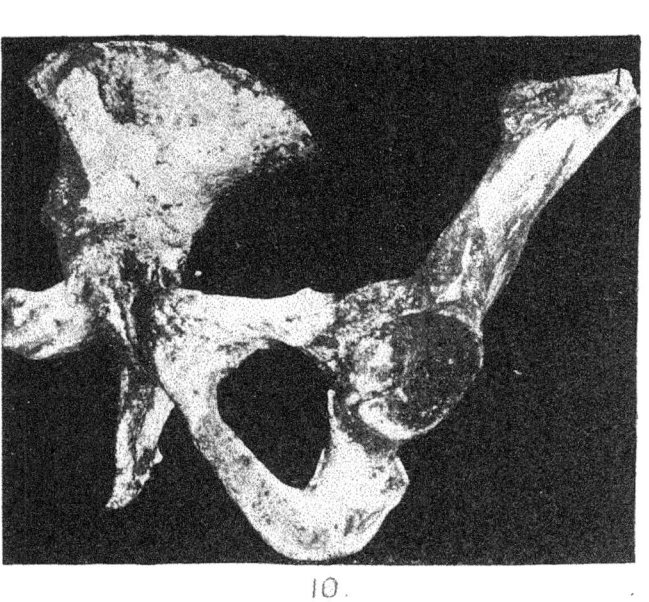

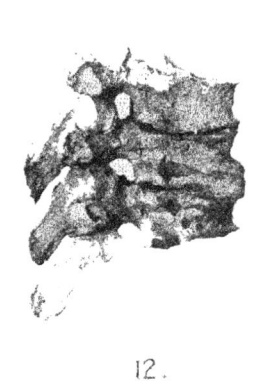

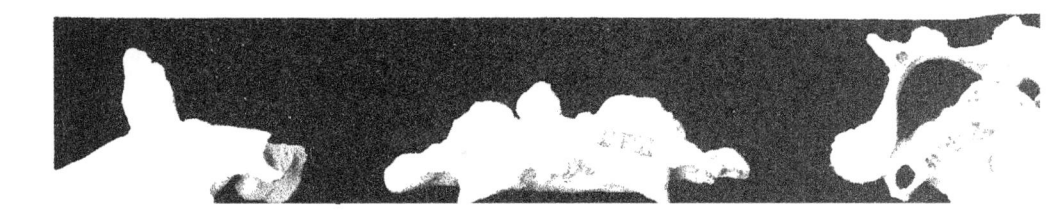

9.

10.

12.

PLATE LI

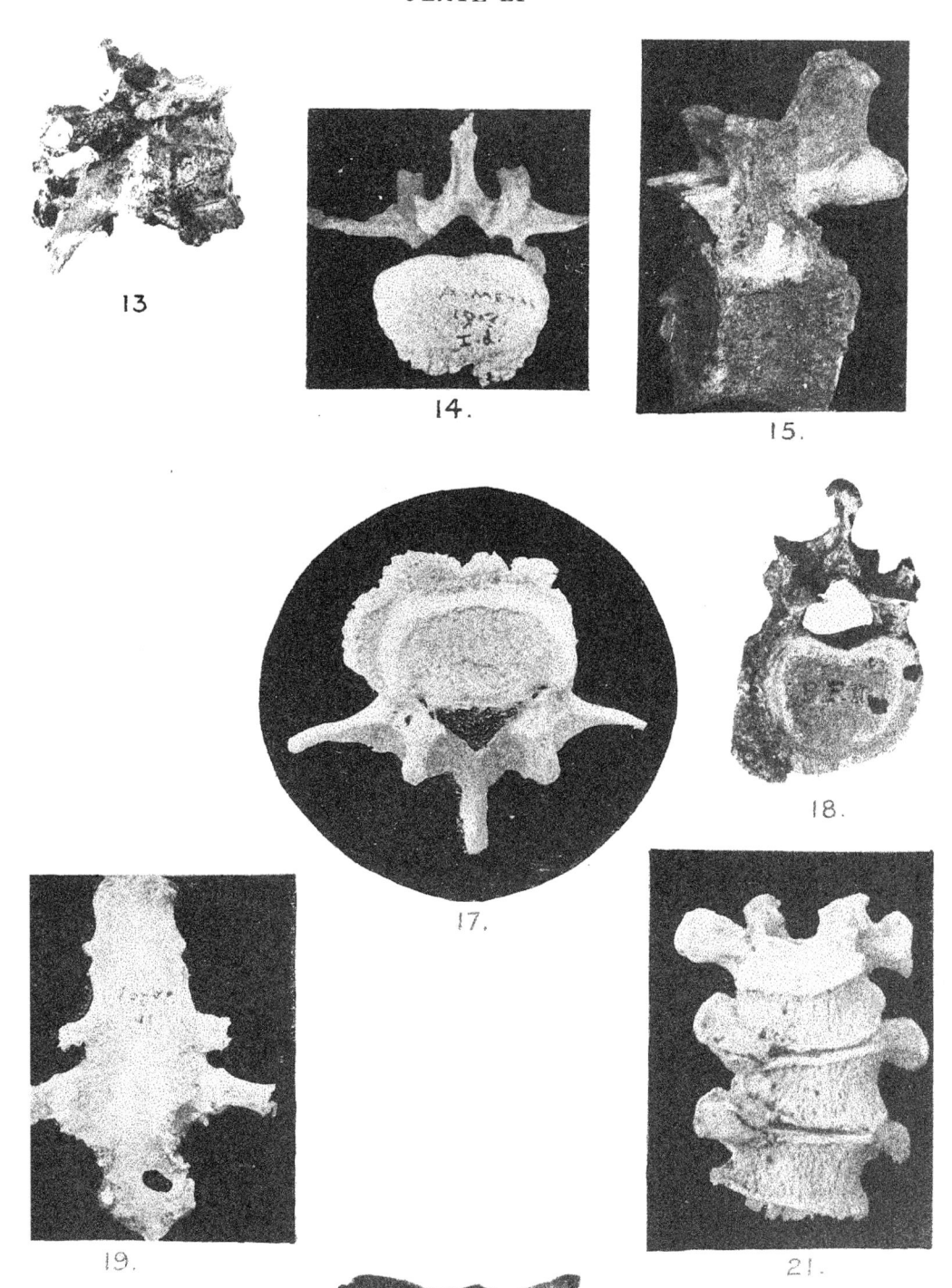

13

14.

15.

17.

18.

19.

21.

22.

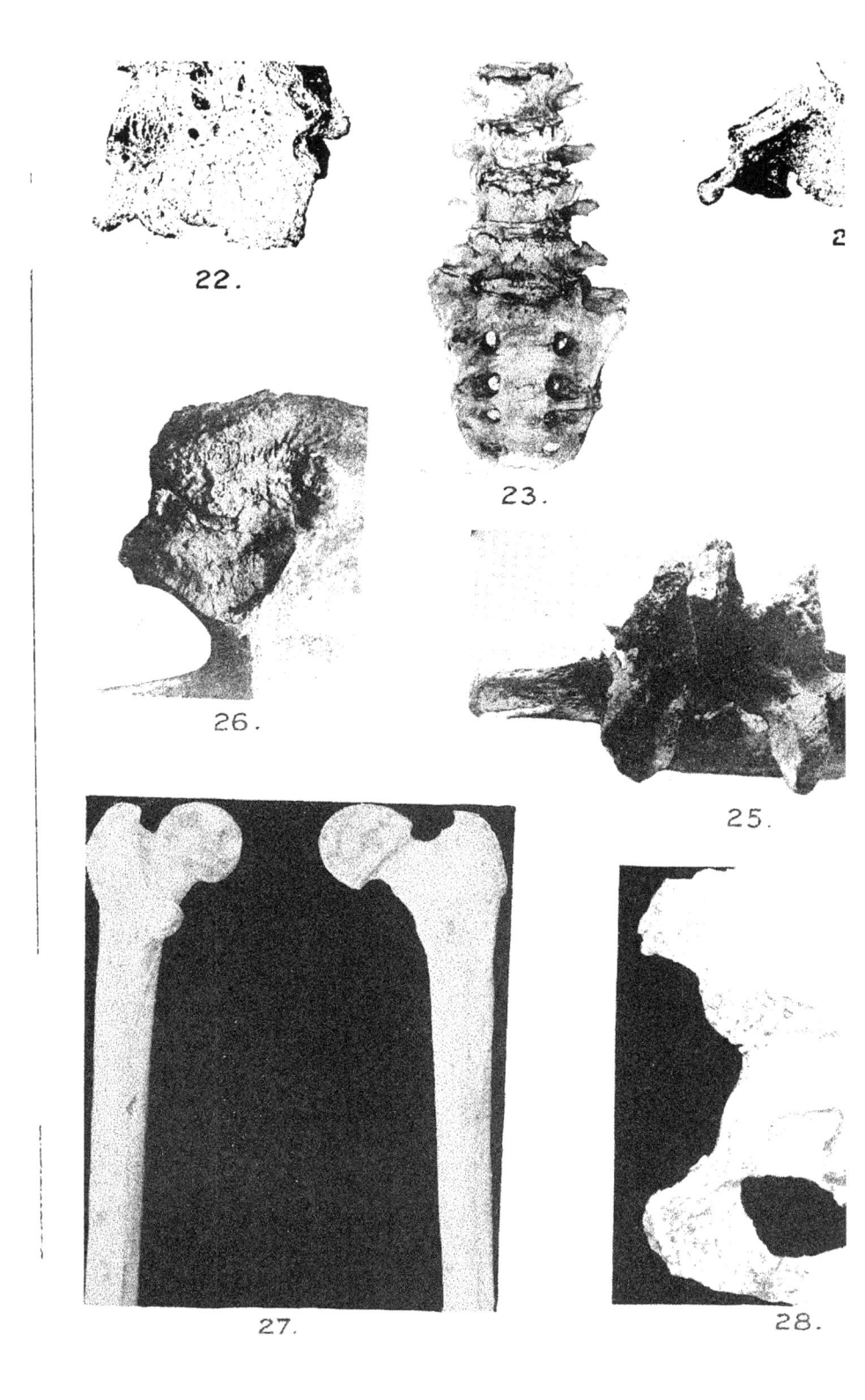

23.

24.

26.

25.

27.

28.

29.

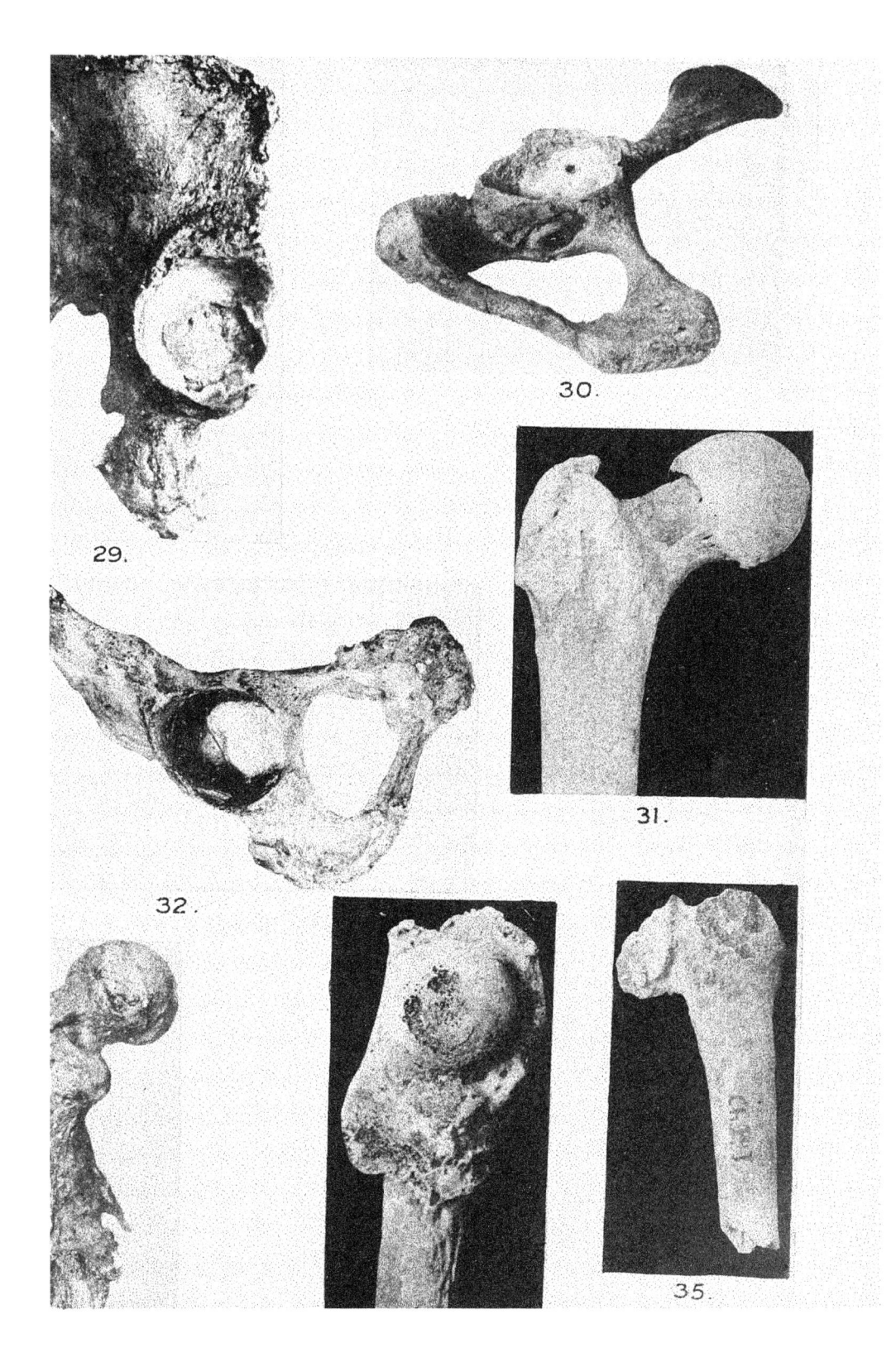

30.

31.

32.

35.

PLATE LIV

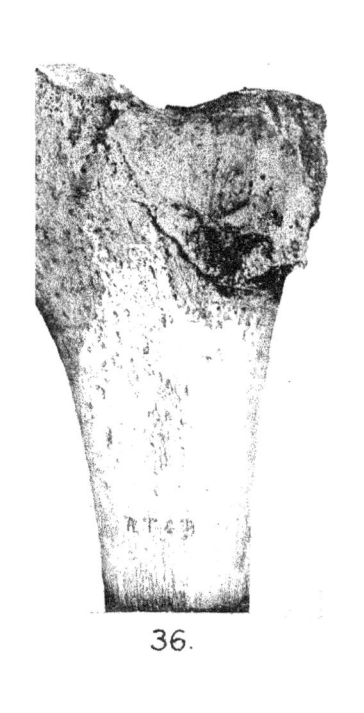

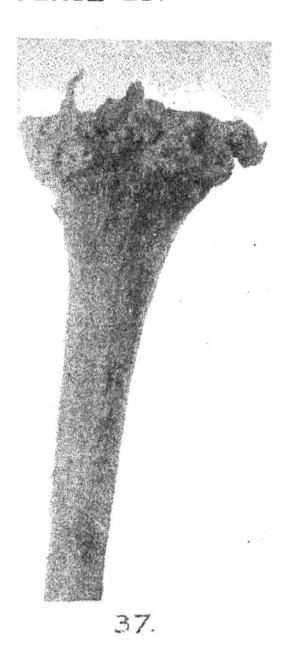

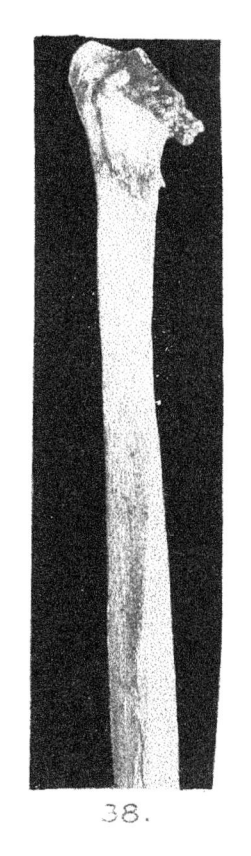

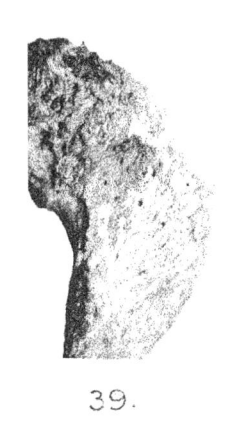

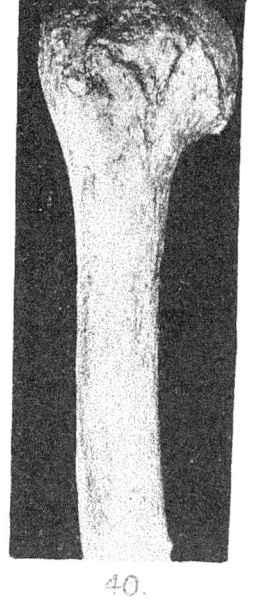

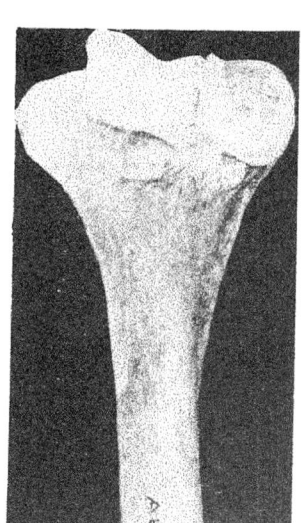

36.

37.

38.

39.

40.

often greatly thickened; on the other hand, the articulating surface of the greater sigmoid cavity almost always escaped and eburnation was rare.

The subcutaneous part of the posterior surface of the olecranon, covered by a bursa, was always normal, while the top of the olecranon was often capped by a thick layer of new bone, sometimes as much as 5 mm. thick, which had formed in the posterior articular ligament and in the tendon of the triceps. The attachment of the anconeus generally escaped, whereas that of the coronoid head of the flexor sublimis digitorum was often rough.

The border of the coronoid process of the sigmoid cavity did not escape, and the lesions were most marked on the triangular surface below it, that is, at the point of attachment of the brachialis anticus (Plate LIV, Fig. 42). In Nubian[1] skeletons, the roughening and deformity of the joint outweighed the process of eburnation, so commonly seen in typical modern examples of arthritis deformans.

The head of the radius escaped, except in a few cases in which eburnation was present, though but little bone was worn away. Sometimes the head was capped by new bone which was prolonged into a point at the ulna articulation.

Eburnation of the lesser sigmoid cavity was very rare, even though the borders of the cavity were surrounded by a delicate rim of smooth new bone, possibly an ossified orbicular ligament.

The upper part of the shaft of the radius was practically always normal except for hypertrophy and roughness of the bicipital tuberosity, which in many cases were doubtless due to powerful muscular development; when the remainder of the skeleton did not point to the presence of mighty muscles, this condition was probably pathological. The attachments of the interosseous membrane between the radius and ulna were always normal.

The pivot formed by the head of the ulna and the lower end of the radius was always healthy, except for some occasional slight thickening round the articular surfaces.

The surfaces of attachment for the anterior and posterior radioulnar ligaments also escaped as a rule.

(The Description of Plates XLIX–LIV will be found in the text)

[1] *Ibid.*

STUDY OF ABNORMALITIES AND PATHOLOGY OF ANCIENT EGYPTIAN TEETH

(*American Journal of Physical Anthropology*,
Vol. III [July, 1920], No. 3)

PREFATORY NOTE

My husband intended to publish almost simultaneously with this paper on Ancient Egyptian Teeth, another on Arthritis and Spondylitis, considering dental disease an important etiological factor in the causation of arthritis.

Owing to his untimely death, he left the latter work incomplete, and I have been unable to supply many missing links between the two papers, as I cannot prove to my satisfaction that certain diseased teeth, mandibles, etc., belong to the same skeletons which show marked arthritic lesions of various joints. However, with the kind assistance of Captain Willmore, R.A.M.C., I have finished the paper on arthritis to the best of my ability, and it has appeared in the *Journal of Pathology*.

A third paper was begun in connection with the present one, for on remarking the effect of the food of the people in producing attrition, caries, etc., Sir Armand made a study of the food of the ancient Egyptians.

These with three other papers which I shall endeavor to finish for him, and fourteen which he had already published, were destined to form parts of a book he intended to call "Studies in Palaeopathology."

ALICE RUFFER

I. INTRODUCTION

Mummery's[1] classical paper dating from over forty-five years ago, to which I shall refer repeatedly, was the only contribution of any permanent value regarding the incidence of dental disease in ancient Egyptians until the publication, by two members of the Archaeological Survey (A. S. N.) of Nubia, G. Elliot Smith and F. Wood Jones, of the report on the human remains found in Nubia.[2] Elliot Smith was responsible for the anthropological work, the field notes and the whole of the pathological section being Dr. Wood Jones's contribution. The independence of judgment of both observers is demonstrated by the fact that they do not always entirely agree regarding the conclusions to be drawn from their observations. Their memoir, published in 1910, is valuable, first

[1] J. R. Mummery, *Trans. Odont. Soc. Great Britain*, II (1870).

[2] *Archaeological Survey of Nubia, 1907–8*, Vol. II, "Report on the Human Remains," by G. Elliot Smith and F. Wood Jones, Cairo, 1910. This work will in future be referred to as *A. S. N.*

on account of the large number of skeletons examined, and second because all the material is dated—a most important point, as Egyptian or Nubian skeletons may belong to any period from over 4000 B.C. to the present time, a stretch of over six thousand years. The excavations in Nubia brought to light skeletons dating from some time before dynastic times, that is, before 3400 B.C., down to the Coptic and Christian times. The field notes are not the least valuable part of the work and have been carefully analyzed by me, and, indeed, except for some observations made[1] at Merawi and Faras, practically the whole of my remarks regarding dental disease in Nubia will be based on this memoir.

Interesting facts concerning dental disease in ancient Egypt are to be found in Elliot Smith's description of the royal mummies in the Museum of Cairo.[2] A most valuable collection was the series of skulls discovered by the Hearst expeditions of the University of California. These are repeatedly alluded to by Elliot Smith in several of his anthropological papers, but I am not aware that a full account of the pathological lesions of these skulls has ever been published; they are now in the United States, partly at the Museum of the University of California and partly at Harvard. The Museum of the Medical School in Cairo contained for a time a large number of these, and they, with additional ancient Egyptian crania collected by Elliot Smith, Derry, and others, were repeatedly examined by me. Skulls from the Naga el Deir, dating from the VIth to XIIth Dynasties, Coptic skulls from the same locality, and skulls from the pyramids of Gizeh belonging to the IVth and Vth Dynasties, were also studied. All this material proved most useful for forming an opinion as to the nature of the dental and other[3] lesions, but

[1] Marc Armand Ruffer, "Note on the Diseases of the Sudan and Nubia in Ancient Times," *Mitt. z. Gesch. d. Med. u. d. Naturw.*, XIII (1914), 453.

[2] G. Elliot Smith, *The Royal Mummies*, Cairo, 1912.

[3] Marc Armand Ruffer and Arnoldo Rietti, "On Osseous Lesions in Ancient Egyptians," *Jour. Path. and Bact.*, XVI (1912), 439; Marc Armand Ruffer, "Studies in Palaeopathology in Egypt," *ibid.*, XVIII, 149; "Pathological Notes on the Royal Mummies of the Cairo Museum," *Mitt. z. Gesch. d. Med. u. d. Naturw.*, XIII (1914), 239; "Note on the Diseases of the Sudan and Nubia in Ancient Times," *ibid.*, 453; (with Arnoldo Rietti) "Notes on Two Egyptian Mummies," *Bull. Soc. Archéol. d'Alexandrie*, No. 14, 3.

owing to the large number of teeth lost in the graves, it was practically useless for a statistical study regarding the incidence of any particular form of dental disease.

For part of the material on which this paper is based, my best thanks are due to the late Sir Gaston Maspero, to Professor W. M. Flinders Petrie and his collaborators, to Professor G. Elliot Smith, and to Professor E. Breccia, of the Museum of Alexandria.

At Chatby, near Alexandria, about two minutes' walk from the sea, lie the tombs of the Macedonian soldiers of Alexander the Great and Ptolemy I. In view of the constant growth of the town, which will soon extend over the whole of this region, the Municipal Commission ordered an archaeological survey of this site. The work was entrusted to Professor E. Breccia,[1] the curator of the Alexandria Museum, who gave us permission to examine most of the bones found in the necropolis, and to be present during some of the excavations. Owing to a lawsuit, the work has been suspended for a time, and this delay is specially unfortunate because the names on the tombs to be yet opened indicate that the crypts contain the skeletons of the prostitutes who accompanied the Greek army. Here, if anywhere, evidences of syphilis should be found, provided venereal disease existed at that period.

The bodies here had been placed in rock-hewn graves. The first grave was an ossarium measuring about 2 c.m., filled with sand and bones, and closed with a stone slab which had been sealed with mortar. The bones, after the bodies had undergone decomposition elsewhere, had been thrown into the ossarium, and little care had evidently been taken in their gathering, as among the human bones the femur of a horse was found. The other graves were horizontal shafts, 3.5 feet high, 6 feet deep, and about 3.5 feet wide, cut in the solid rock and closed in the same manner as the ossarium. Rarely, such a tomb contained but one body, lying on a layer of sand about 6 inches deep; as a rule, several skeletons, five, six, or even more, were present. Funeral urns filled with ashes or half-carbonized bones were discovered also. The Greeks of that period,

[1] This eminent archaeologist will soon publish a full account of his researches, which will throw much light on the habits of the Greek immigrants in Egypt.

therefore, were eclectic in their customs, some families burning, others burying their dead.

Unfortunately, the level of the land has sunk several feet since the last body was consigned to the grave. Hence some tombs were partially filled, others merely infiltrated with sea water, and the bones were often found lying in water, or in thick, wet mud. Such skeletons were in bad condition, and most of the smaller with some of the larger bones could not be found, even when the slush was removed carefully by hand.

Although, as might be expected, the bones were rather better preserved in dry than in wet graves, yet this was by no means the rule. The skeleton of a female, for instance, lying on a bed of dry sand, was so fragile that some bones were broken when their removal was attempted; on the other hand, bones lying in liquid mud were sometimes very hard, whereas others, in the same grave, broke as soon as touched.

Sometimes the soldiers had been buried with their wives and children; nothing, however, could be learned from the skeletons of the last named, as hardly a single bone was preserved sufficiently well for examination.

We shall not enter into anthropometric details, as the skeletons have been handed over to an anthropologist for examination. We may say, however, that a superficial examination sufficed to show that various races were represented. Of the thirty-two skulls examined, some had high-bridged noses, others remarkably flat ones. Some were brachycephalic, others markedly dolichocephalic; two skulls were evidently negroid. The variations in stature were great also, some men being tall, others short. These differences are not to be wondered at considering that, from the start, Alexander's army was distinctly a "mixed crew." It is stated, for instance, in Smith's *Classical Dictionary*, that of the 30,000 foot soldiers who left Greece with Alexander, only 12,000 were Greeks; the others were foreigners, chiefly Thracians. The inscriptions on the tombs were in Greek, but it is highly probable that the soldiers settled in Egypt had intercourse with and often married native women, just as their successors have done in modern times. The present Berberine, for instance, especially when coming from Korosko, often boasts that he is a descendant of a Turkish soldier and a native woman, and the name Turk, as used by him, includes Greek, Herzegovinian, Bosnian, Bulgarian, and Servian.

Another part of our material was derived from the catacombs of Kom el Shougafa, which are situated close to Pompey's Pillar at Alexandria, and, according to Professor Breccia, the bodies dated from the second century A.D. The tombs contained hundreds of skeletons, most of which, owing to the gradual infiltration of water, were in such a bad condition that they could not be examined. It has been supposed that these catacombs contained the skeletons of the Alexandrian youths who were massacred by order of Caracalla. A simple examination of the skeletons showed this supposition to be wrong, as the bones were those of men, women, and children. On the whole, the mode of burial was almost identical with that seen at Chatby. The first body had been placed on a layer of sand about 4 inches high, and later on the skeleton had been pushed aside to make room for the second occupant.

I was also fortunate enough in obtaining fragments of about forty Egyptian skulls buried at Ras el Tin and dating from the time of Cleopatra, but again, these were quite useless for statistical purposes; and I have examined five Coptic bodies coming from Upper Egypt and dating from the fifth century A.D., while other Coptic bodies were given me by Professor Breccia and came from Antinoë in Upper Egypt. The bodies of the latter had been originally placed in wooden coffins and buried in sand. When handed over to me, they were dressed in long linen shirts in which they had been buried, and from the embroideries adorning these garments I concluded that these persons had belonged to a wealthy class of the community.

For the purpose of this paper the chronology used in the *Archaeological Survey of Nubia*[1] has been adopted, the dates being those given by Breasted.[2]

1. Predynastic periods: early, middle, late. These three periods cannot be accurately dated, but they certainly extended before 3400 B.C.
2. Early dynastic period=the first three or four dynasties. (Approximately A group.) 3400–2750 B.C.

[1] G. A. Reisner, *Archaeological Survey of Nubia*, Vol. I, Arch. Rep., p. 6.
[2] *History of Egypt*, p. 597.

3. IVth–VIth Dynasties. (Approximately B group.) 2750–2475 B.C.
4. Middle Empire = VIIth–XVIth Dynasties. (Approximately C group.) 2475–1600 B.C. (?).
5. New Empire = XVIIth–XXth Dynasties. (Same as D group.) 1780–1200 B.C.
6. Late period = XXth–XXXth Dynasties. 1200–332 B.C.
7. Ptolemaic-Roman period. 332 B.C.—300 A.D.
8. Coptic period. 300 A.D.

II. DENTAL ANOMALIES

The description includes abnormalities in the number, position, and structure of deciduous and permanent teeth, which are of both medical as well as anthropological concern.

Irregularities of teeth have been attributed to modern civilization, and are said to be rare in ancient and even some modern races. None were found, for instance, in the large collection of skulls in the crypt of Hythe Church, England, but these, as a matter of fact, were comparatively modern, and of mixed origin, most dating from 450 A.D. The frequently quoted comparisons between ancient and modern Britons, or between ancient and modern Italians, are of little value, owing to the extensive crossing of races which has taken place, few modern Englishmen and Italians being descendants of ancient Britons and Romans.

The causes of irregularities of teeth in modern times are said to be: (1) premature removal; (2) persistence of deciduous teeth; (3) supernumerary teeth; (4) mouth-breathing; (5) habit of sucking thumbs, lips, tongue, or toes; (6) presence of a frenum of the tongue; and still others. The only factors which can be appreciated by examination of skeletal material are the first three.

Abnormalities of the dentition are certainly not peculiar to modern times either in France or in Egypt. The dentition of the *Homo Mousteriensis* was, as is well known, somewhat aberrant. The eruption of the right canine had been delayed, and the deciduous canine on the same side, already much worn, was still present. It has been maintained that the pathological process accompanying the retention of the left deciduous canine had left traces on the corresponding articulation, for the condyle did not fit the jaw exactly, and its shape differed from that of its fellow, being thicker in the sagittal direction and shortened in the transverse direction.

In England, abnormalities in the position of the teeth have been seen in prehistoric remains; at Halling and Caithness, for instance. The third lower molar of a skeleton from the brick-earth deposit at Halling, Kent, lay obliquely at the junction of the ramus and body of the jaw, due to want of room.[1] The left upper canine from a prehistoric skull at Caithness was thrust inwards out of its place.[2] Torsion of a canine tooth from the Bronze Age found at Adlerberg,[3] and also from a *Hökergrab*[4] at Reiherwerder, is on record. The roots of the molar teeth at St. Brelade's, Jersey, were conjoined or fused. Abnormalities in the position and structure of the teeth have been discovered in several ancient skulls of France. The incisors and canines of a mandible at Cro-Magnon were compressed laterally and slightly thrust forward, and the left third lower molar was smaller than the others and had two roots only.[5] A prehistoric skull found in the Carrière Hélie at Grenoble had an "atrophied" third molar.[6] A bifid canine was found at Grenelle,[7] and a cranium of La Magdaleine had a very small third molar with two double roots.[8] Ancient Danish jaws, according to Nielson, also sometimes had teeth aberrantly placed or with an abnormal structure.

These instances, gleaned from the limited literature at the writer's disposal, suffice to show that dental abnormalities were certainly not uncommon in ancient times. Doubtless the study of further records and the systematic examination of ancient skulls would add materially to their number.

[1] A. Keith, "Report on the Human and Animal Remains Found at Halling, Kent," *Jour. Anthr. Inst.*, XLIV (1914), 234.

[2] S. Laing, "Prehistoric Remains of Caithness; with Notes on the Human Remains by Th. Huxley," *Jour. Anthr. Soc.*, London, III (1865), xx f.

[3] P. Bartels, "Über Schädel und Skelettreste der früheren Bronzezeit aus der Umgebung von Worms am Rhein," *Prähist. Zeitschr.*, Vol. IV (1912), Nos. 1–2.

[4] Busse, "Gräber mit Hökerbestattung und Flachgräber auf den grossen Reiherwerder im Tegeler See," *Prähist. Zeitschr.*, II (1910), 60–78.

[5] Quatrefage et Hamy, *Crania ethnica*, p. 49.

[6] *Ibid.*, p. 120.

[7] *Ibid.*, p. 86.   [8] *Ibid.*, p. 55.

ABNORMALITIES OF DENTITION IN ANCIENT EGYPTIANS

The supernumerary teeth of modern peoples are often like normal teeth in shape and character. They are more frequent in the upper than in the lower jaw. They resemble a lateral incisor most often, a premolar less frequently, molar rarely, and a canine very exceptionally. The last point, however, calls for a qualification: small conical supernumeraries are not uncommon, but they are more like the deciduous canines, or like the ancestral conical teeth, which they possibly represent, than like the permanent canines.[1] They occur most commonly in the upper incisor region. Two supernumerary teeth are occasionally met with in the premolar region, and a supernumerary tooth not infrequently erupts near, mostly posterior to, the third molar. Supernumerary first and second molars have never been recorded.

Supernumerary teeth have been reported before in ancient Egyptian skulls.

A very curious case dates from the XIIth Dynasty.[2] The two left maxillary incisors of a youngish man were joined together and formed a large tusk, which certainly did not add to the bearer's good looks during life, and an accessory incisor tooth had perforated the palate behind this extraordinary structure.

A young Nubian woman[3] of the New Empire period, with normal teeth, had a supernumerary tooth, situated 3 mm. within the nasal margin, and unconnected with the normal alveolar cavities. It was conical in shape, visible from the front, measured 5 mm. in its antero-posterior diameter, and its visible portion was covered with enamel. In the second case, an adult woman from the same grave and a possible relation of the first, the supernumerary tooth had appeared in the palate to the left of the middle line behind the first incisor, and just externally to the anterior palatine foramen.

Supernumerary incisors were seemingly rare in the ancient Nubians, and the writer has found but one case on record. In this

[1] A. Hrdlička, "Physiological and Medical Observations among the Indians," etc., *Bur. Am. Ethnol., Bull. 34*, Washington, 1908, p. 124.

[2] M. A. Murray, "The Tomb of Two Brothers," *The Manchester Museum Handbooks*, Pl. II, Fig. 4.

[3] *A. S. N.*, p. 230.

person, the tooth had erupted immediately to the inner side of the left maxillary second incisor.[1] Similarly, only one instance of a supernumerary canine has been described, and this was situated just behind the left maxillary canine of no less a personage than Queen Nefer buried at Dahshur.[2] Supernumerary premolars were found in two Nubian negroes only, who, as they occupied neighboring graves, may also have been relations. Each had a supernumerary tooth near the posterior normal premolar; otherwise the jaws were normal with no signs of crowding. The abnormality most often found in the molar region of Nubians was the presence of one or two supernumerary molars.

As to Egypt proper, a supernumerary central upper incisor, and a small supernumerary intercalated between the second and third right lower molars, were found by the writer in one out of 156 Egyptian predynastic maxillae and 35 mandibles. The fourth molars will be discussed with the abnormalities of the molar region. In a skull from Faras, dating from about 300 B.C., the teeth had all fallen out after death, but the alveolus of a supernumerary was plainly visible to the outer side of the normal first molar. Neither among the Macedonian soldiers, nor among the Copts, nor among the ancient population of Alexandria were any supernumerary teeth discovered. Attention has been drawn to certain "accessory dental masses,"[3] which were seen somewhat frequently in Nubia, most of them in the alveolar margin posterior to the normal second molars. These have been considered as rudimentary teeth, or perhaps more correctly as the remains of the roots of deciduous teeth.[4]

The preceding data, while somewhat fragmentary and not fit for exact comparisons, indicate that while supernumerary teeth did occur among the Egyptians and Nubians, they were not very frequent.

Deficiency in the number of teeth may be studied next.

In modern people the missing elements are almost restricted to the third molars,[5] the upper lateral incisors, and the second man-

---

[1] *Ibid.*, p. 170.
[2] J. de Morgan, *Fouilles de Dahshur* (1894), p. 49.
[3] *A. S. N.*, p. 238. [4] F. Dixon, *Proc. B. A. A. S.*, 1908.
[5] L. E. Colyer, in Smale and Colyer's *Diseases and Injuries of the Teeth*, 1901.

dibular premolars. Cases where many, most, or even all the teeth are absent are not unknown; but these are pathological cases, and the condition may be associated with great abundance of hair, malformation, and other pathological conditions.

Reduction in the number of teeth not due to disease or interference was rare in ancient Nubia. In a middle Nubian Christian there were only one upper bicuspid and two upper molar teeth on each side (lower jaw?). Another Nubian skull showed a similar condition. An Egyptian predynastic skull from Naga el Deir had no left lateral upper incisor, and the corresponding right incisor was very small; besides which the right first molar was distinctly twisted. A skull from the same period had no left upper central incisor, in spite of an exceedingly roomy palate. A similar abnormality has been noticed in an ancient Egyptian animal. A monkey, *Papio anubis*, from Thebes,[1] had three maxillary incisors instead of four, one being missing on the left side. This deficiency was probably congenital, as there was no alveolus, and the median line of the premaxillary was displaced to the left, causing marked asymmetry. Petrie,[2] in his excavations of Hyksos and Israelite cities, found a female human jaw which had only one molar on each side and was peculiarly wide and short (2.4 cm. wide and only 1.2 cm. from back to front, forming a semicircle).

Absence of the first left mandibular incisor must have been fairly common in Lower Egypt, as four such cases have been observed in ancient Alexandrian skulls.

Gaps, or diastemae, between the teeth sometimes occurred in ancient Nubians. In an adult man[3] of the early dynastic period, a space of 4 mm. existed between each upper lateral incisor and the canine; his jaws were large and his teeth excellent; another adult man[4] of the same period showed a gap of 3 mm. in the same position, and another of 3 mm. between the left lower canine and the first premolar. An Egyptian predynastic skull from Naga el Deir had a large gap between the central incisors.

Retained deciduous teeth occurred at all periods in Nubia. The left maxillary deciduous canine of a predynastic young Nubian

[1] Lortet, *La faune momifiée de l'Égypte*, Série II, p. 11.
[2] *Hyksos and Israelite Cities*.   [3] *A. S. N.*, p. 208.   [4] *Ibid.*, p. 180.

woman of the middle period, for instance, was retained directly to the outer side of the permanent canine,[1] the retention being combined with malposition of the teeth. The left upper second deciduous incisor of an adult male of the early dynastic period was retained upon the palatal side. In a woman of the Byzantine period, the permanent upper canine was displaced towards the palate, and the retained deciduous canine occupied exactly the normal position. A Nubian woman of the predynastic period showed exactly the same condition on the left side. Retained teeth were rare in predynastic and later Egyptians, but Petrie[2] mentions the case of a predynastic adult with erupted wisdom teeth whose permanent canines had been retained.

There is no evidence to show that retardation of the eruption of the permanent teeth was at all common in Egypt. Still, except in Nubia, crowding and malposition of teeth were not rare. Crowding of the teeth was observed by the author in 7 out of 156 Egyptian predynastic skulls. The left canine and the two premolars of one skull were so pressed together as to overlap; in four other cases, the crowding was limited to the front teeth, incisors, and canines, and in one the crowding was evidently due to the size of the incisors which had not permitted the canines to assume their normal place.

Various malformations of teeth were observed, but as a rule they affected the roots chiefly. The roots of the first molar of a predynastic skull in the Cairo Museum, for example, were fused together into a mass filling the greatly distended alveolus. Fusion of two or three roots was not rare in Alexandrian skulls, though it was seldom as marked as in the preceding case, and in Egyptian predynastic skulls abnormalities of the roots were possibly fairly common. The right mandibular canine (predynastic) had two roots in two cases, and in another skull of the same epoch both maxillary second premolars also had two roots.[3]

Occasionally abnormalities of the cusps were seen. A second upper molar had five cusps; both first molars of one mandible had

[1] *A. S. N.*, p. 165.   [2] *Tarkhan, I*, and *Memphis, V*, 11.

[3] It is not possible to ascertain abnormalities of the roots without taking out the teeth. This could not be done, but the observations are based on teeth which had accidentally dropped out, and are therefore valueless for statistics.

six cusps, and two mandibular first molars from two different skulls had the same number. All these belonged to the Egyptian predynastic period.

The Egyptian teeth, as a rule, were very regularly planted except in cases of overcrowding; usually the "bite" was good and marked overbites were rare.

At Ras el Tin, overbites were present in three skulls. The maxillary and mandibular incisors and canines of the first skull did not meet. A similar defect was present in the skull of a young adult whose teeth were otherwise perfect. Lastly, a skull with molars still unerupted had overlapping central mandibular incisors.

A curious malformation was observed in the skull of a young person. The right upper canine was inclined almost directly forwards, and the neighboring premolar being in its normal position, the roots of the premolar and canine, necessarily crossing, touched one another, with chronic periostitis at the point of contact as the result. The alveolar walls of the other teeth had suffered severely from chronic rarefying periostitis, the posterior root of the maxillary right second molar, for instance, being almost completely bare. The maxillary right first molar and right second incisor had been lost during life, and there was no germ of a maxillary right third molar.

Anomalies in the region of the third molars were often met with. Pits in the alveolar process behind the third molar were seen very commonly in ancient negroid Nubians,[1] and also in predynastic and dynastic skulls. These pits were sometimes superficial, or formed a cavity several millimeters in depth, and it has been suggested that their frequency was connected with the roominess of the jaw. It is not unlikely that some of these alveoli actually contained teeth.

Fourth molar teeth were found in Nubia in a few cases only.[2] An adult negroid man had fourth molars as large as normal molars, and in a negroid woman of the Byzantine period, a well-formed and large fourth molar had erupted upon the right side of the upper jaw. Upon the left side there was a deep groove, like an empty alveolar cavity, which corresponded to the fully developed tooth upon the opposite side. In another case of the anomaly, the condition was

[1] *A. S. N.*, p. 165.   [2] *Ibid.*, p. 237.

associated with a peculiar dentition: the right mandibular third molar was just visible, the corresponding left tooth was absent, and the maxillary third molar was still retained in the alveoli. On the whole it may be said that less than 1 per cent of predynastic and dynastic Egyptians had a fourth molar, and no case was met with in Alexandria.

Absence of the third molars on one or both sides was present in a Nubian skull from the middle predynastic times, which had also a retained deciduous left maxillary canine, situated just to the outer side of the permanent canine. In 156 predynastic skulls examined by the author, one or both third molars were absent in 19, namely: the right upper in 5, the left upper in 3, both uppers in 7, the right lower in 1, the left lower in 2, and both lowers in 1. The jaws were roomy in some of these cases, so that lack of room could not be generally adduced as a reason for this anomaly. Unilateral absence of one third molar occurred in no less than 7 per cent of all the adult Alexandrian skulls dating from about 300 B.C., although the jaws were large and the teeth not crowded.

Anomalies in size and position of the third molars were not at all rare in Egyptian predynastic people.

The upper third molars were noticeably smaller than the other molars in 45 Egyptian predynastic skulls of 156, and in 19 out of 35 mandibles. In 45 the smallness was bilateral.

The following anomalies were also present: case 1, left lower third molar, one root only; case 2, left lower third molar, two roots only; case 3, 4, 5, and 6, left lower third molar, root very small, not more than a peg; case 7, left lower third molar, two roots only. In one upper jaw the third molars were probably impacted.

The following anomalies were met with in 112 skulls from Thebes.[1] First, adult female: The third upper molar was twisted on account of want of room, so that its masticating surface was turned outwards. The same alteration, though to a slighter extent, was seen in nine other upper jaws. In 4 cases, the mandibular third molar was twisted inwards and forwards. Secondly, in several cases (exact number not stated) the alveolar border was prolonged so as to leave room for a possible fourth molar. Thirdly,

[1] Hermann Stahr, *Die Rassenfrage im antiken Ägypten*, Berlin, 1907.

in the following cases one or more third molars were absent: (*a*) one rudimentary left lower third molar only had erupted; (*b*) male adult, no upper third molars; (*c*) young male, no germs for upper third molar; (*d*) male adult, no third molars; (*e*) adult female, no upper third molars; (*f*) adult female, no lower third molars.

Abnormalities in size were very common also. In 11 cases, the second molars were smaller than the third molars; in 7 cases the third molars were larger than the first and second molars; whereas in three skulls some of the third molars were larger, and the others smaller than the other molars.

At Ras el Tin also, in skulls dating from the time of Cleopatra, several abnormalities of the third molars were observed. The right maxillary third molars were absent in three adults, and the corresponding teeth on the other side in three others. Moreover, malpositions of these teeth were common. In two cases, the right third lower molar was planted at the base and on the inside of the ascending ramus, so that the tooth was invisible when the mandible was looked at from the side. The left third lower molar of another skull, though firmly planted, was almost horizontal. A similar curious deformation, not due to an accident, was that of a left third lower molar which was almost horizontal, being implanted at the base of, and at right angles to, the ascending ramus. The tooth had not been used at all for mastication, for its crown, in contrast to those of the other teeth, showed no sign of attrition. The same malformation existed in still another mandible. Lastly, the upper third molars of three middle-aged persons were noticeably smaller than the corresponding second molars.

In the Macedonians buried at Chatby, the small size of many third molars was striking.

NODULES

Enamel nodules or pearls are small enamel excrescences or droplets, occasionally met with on the roots of teeth. They are generally found upon multirooted teeth, being situated a little below the neck and often at the junction of two roots. On section they are seen to consist of a cone of dentine covered with a rather thick layer of enamel. Only one such nodule was seen in the Egyptians, but as many of the molar teeth were lost, this cannot be taken as a proof of the rarity of this condition.

Dental anomalies lead at times to trouble, as illustrated by the following case. The anterior left part of the upper jaw of a Nubian Christian was in a state of very acute inflammation starting from the alveolar cavities of the front teeth. A large part of the alveolar margin was necrosed, the septic process had spread in various directions, and the large anterior abscess cavity, communicating freely with the antrum of Highmore, also opened on the palate by a large sinus. The process had spread up the nasal duct, and to the inner wall of the left orbit. A sinus opened upon the surface of the superior maxilla behind and upon the first left premolar tooth. An irregular mass representing the conjoined roots of the front teeth occupied the large abscess cavity. The root of the anterior premolar and the roots of the two teeth immediately anterior to it were joined together into one solid mass, and all had been the site of an acute septic dental disease.

III. WEAR

The intensity of attrition is said to depend largely on the nature of the food, the density of the tooth substance, and lastly on the character of the bite. All the teeth are involved, as a rule, and when a few teeth only are worn this anomalous condition is almost always due to an irregularity of the dentition.

The change proceeds slowly until the enamel has been worn away and much more speedily afterwards. As the upper incisor and canine teeth of normal persons bite somewhat in front of the lower teeth, attrition is usually more conspicuous on the lingual side of the former and on the labial side of the latter. Moreover, the slope of the upper and lower teeth towards one another produces a corresponding slant in the masticating surfaces, which increases as the attrition gets more pronounced; the worn-down crowns of the upper incisors, for instance, are usually inclined obliquely towards the lingual side, whereas those of the lower incisors tend to slope in the opposite direction.

Nowadays attrition is a characteristic of people living on raw, fibrous, vegetable food (Egyptian fellaheen), of old people, and of

ABNORMALITIES OF ANCIENT EGYPTIAN TEETH 283

deciduous teeth in their last stages, and great individual differences exist both in its mode and degree. Should the food consist of hard seeds, roots, or tough meat, attrition is most marked on the lingual side of the upper, and the labial side of the lower teeth. In people living on rich, nitrogenous food, the pulp is generally replaced by secondary dentine and the tooth is often worn down to the neck, without the formation of an alveolar abscess; whereas, when the food is deficient, inflammation, abscesses, and extensive resorption of the alveoli are common.

There are generally recognized four degrees of attrition.[1] In the first degree the enamel is abraded without obliteration of the cusps or exposure of the dentine. The second is characterized by disappearance of the cusps and partial exposure of the dentine. When the height of the tooth is reduced still further the third stage is reached, characterized by a complete dentine exposure, and in the fourth stage, the wear extends to the neck, the crown having entirely disappeared. It is, however, often difficult to place a tooth in any of these divisions, as different parts of the masticating surface of one tooth may exhibit more or less intense stages of attrition. A first molar, for instance, may be worn down to the gums on the labial or lingual side, but the rest of its crown may be almost normal. In this paper no use will be made of any classification.

Ancient peoples, like uncivilized modern ones, used their teeth for many purposes, which may account for some severe lesions, in which connection may be recalled the professional attrition of the teeth of cigar-makers, seamstresses, pipe-smokers, or that produced by the clasps of artificial teeth.

Attrition was very common in the teeth of ancient peoples of Europe, Asia, and Africa. The human teeth found in the Thames mud at Tilbury, for instance, showed this change to a very marked extent. The lesions in the teeth of the Tilbury skull have been observed in other ancient British crania, e.g., in the earliest skull lately found in Kent. The severity of the attrition in the prehistoric teeth found at Caithness and elsewhere varies somewhat, it is said, according to period. The teeth of the skull found in the

[1] P. Broca, "Instructions relatives à l'étude anthropologique du système dentaire," *Bull. Soc. Anthr.*, Paris, II (1879), 149.

brick-earth deposit of Halling, Kent, had been ground until only half the crown remained, and it has been mentioned that both in the Tilbury and Halling skulls, the teeth were not lost through the modern disease of caries, but by exposure of the pulp cavities with the consequent formation of abscesses at the root of the teeth. Certain it is that in late Palaeolithic and early Neolithic times tooth wear and alveolar abscesses were not uncommon.[1]

The teeth of the Bronze Age are stated not to be worn as deeply as those of the Saxon or Middle English period. A very characteristic first- to second-degree attrition disfigures the teeth of the Heidelberg as well as the Neanderthal jaws, and a wear of a more pronounced nature is seen in the jaws of Gibraltar and Chapelle-aux-Saints.

In the teeth of ancient Germans, attrition beyond a certain age was the rule. The prehistoric skulls from Reiherwerder[2] and Halberstadt[3]—to mention only those more lately discovered— show a marked degree of wear. Similar lesions are noticeable in the teeth of ancient Frenchmen. The teeth of the skeleton of Chancelade, for instance, dating from near the end of the Quaternary period, are worn down, while numberless other examples of attrition are mentioned in French memoirs. Wear is also well marked in the teeth of the Most or Brux skull of Bohemia, in the Ochoz jaw of Moravia, in the older individuals of the Maska's Moravian mammoth-hunters, and in still other old specimens from the central and other parts of Europe. The teeth of prehistoric children even show attrition in some instances, and the same is well marked in young adults from La Chaumière,[4] Cro-Magnon, Montréjeau, Barma Grande,[5] etc. The skulls from Swiss pile dwellings show like alterations.[6]

[1] W. H. Cook, "On the Discovery of a Human Skeleton in a Brick-Earth Deposit in the Valley of the River Medway at Halling, Kent"; A. Keith, "Report on the Human and Animal Remains Found at Halling, Kent," *Jour. Anthr. Inst.*, XLIV (1914).

[2] Hans Virchow, "Die Schädel von Reiherwerder," *Prähist. Zeitschr.*, II (1910), 78.

[3] A. Schliz, "Untersuchungsbericht über drei Schädel aus dem Halberstädter Museum," *Prähist. Zeitschr.*, IV (1912), 377.

[4] Quatrefage et Hamy, *Crania ethnica*, pp. 49, 114; also French anthropological periodicals.

[5] R. Verneau, *L'homme de la Barma Grande*, 1893.

[6] Marcel Baudouin, "De l'usure des dents chez l'homme du paléolithique inférieur et moyen," *Arch. Prov. d. Chirur.*, XXI, 66.

The teeth of ancient Egyptians were frequently worn down in a characteristic fashion. The most prominent parts of the crown, the cusps, were the first to vanish, the masticating surfaces being ground flat. This stage, however, was seen in ancient Egyptians only exceptionally, as even in young adults attrition had usually passed this stage. At this early period, in the maxilla, a thin groove, not more than 1 mm. wide and 5 mm. deep, formed along the whole length of the cutting surface of the incisors; and the crown of the canine was hollowed into an irregular, roughly lozenge-shaped cavity, similar to that which had formed by that time on the labial side of the crown of the neighboring premolar. Very often, also, the lingual border of the canine was worn down somewhat obliquely, even when the enamel was apparently intact.

At that stage, two shallow cavities, separated by a bridge of strong, normal dentine, had formed on the masticating surfaces of upper premolars, the bow- or half-moon-shaped cavity on the lingual side being always the deeper of the two, with its convex border towards the proximal side. The other, shallower cavity was irregularly lozenge-shaped.

The masticating surfaces of the first upper molars with few exceptions were the chief sufferers, and the cavities produced by attrition were very irregular and not easily described, as may be seen from the appended photographs. (Plates LV–LXII.) The cavity first formed was deeper near the lingual and proximal borders close to the second premolar, and the attrition of these teeth was conspicuous even before the second molar tooth had erupted. Later on, the changes in the second molar teeth might still be slight when the attrition of the first molars was already far advanced. The masticating surfaces of this tooth were ground flat or a small, bow-shaped cavity occupied the lingual side, with another just showing close to it, and at this stage the third molar tooth was still practically normal.

A more advanced degree of wear was characterized by the formation of a large cavity in the masticating surfaces of all the teeth. In the incisors, the single cavity previously described became deeper; in the other teeth, the bridge of dentine separating the two cavities previously formed was worn away and the cavities coalesced, but the attrition of the first molars was always more marked than that of the other teeth.

The changes in the lower teeth resembled those in the upper teeth, save that the cavities formed in the crowns were deeper on the labial side.

As attrition proceeded, the dentine surrounding the cavities gradually disappeared, the crown was worn deeper and deeper, until the masticating surfaces were just above the level of the gums. The pulp cavity was then often widely open and unprotected, and at the same time the masticating surfaces, sloping more and more, formed an acute angle with the fangs.

The attrition of the posterior half or two-thirds of the masticating surface of the third molar was often peculiar in so far that the worn surface looked directly backwards and more or less downwards. The same irregularity was often seen in the second molar when the third molar had fallen out, and was conspicuous in any tooth which had no immediate neighbor behind it. Other irregularities in attrition, caused by irregularities in the dentition, need not be discussed here, as they were of no special significance. The general health of the teeth was not necessarily affected by attrition, and in some ancient Egyptians, the teeth, although worn down to the roots, were healthy otherwise. This, however, was the exception rather than the rule, for, as will be shown later, alveolar and perialveolar abscesses were often unmistakably caused by infection through teeth opened by attrition.

In Egypt and Nubia attrition of the teeth has been the rule from the earliest times to the present. Predynastic Nubian teeth were levelled down uniformly, whereas in more modern times,[1] it is said, a deep cavity forms in the centers of the crowns, and hence a distinction is made between the mode of attrition in ancient and that in more modern Nubians. The distinction cannot be proved, as the formation of a central cavity is only one of the stages of attrition, but, nevertheless, the study of several hundreds of skulls did suggest that the teeth were ground down evenly in some cases, whereas in others attrition was characterized by the formation of deep cavities, surrounded by a ring of strong dentine.

[1] *A. S. N.*, p. 279.

At Merawi in Nubia most of the teeth were ground down, and although attrition had evidently progressed rapidly in early youth, yet it was never as marked as in predynastic skulls or in those of modern Egyptians. The change had apparently taken place in old people at a much slower rate than in the young, and probably it had sometimes stopped altogether in the old.

In Egypt the teeth of people of the Ancient, Middle, and New Empires, of Greek, Roman, and early Coptic times, were all more or less affected by attrition. The change was conspicuous in people of every class—in the cemeteries of common folks, in the priests of Deir el Bahri, in the rich Alexandrians of Greek and Roman times, and even in some royal personages. The teeth of Ramses II, for instance, show marked attrition.[1]

Universal though attrition was, its severity appeared to vary. It was perhaps most marked in Upper Egypt, including Nubia, and in very ancient predynastic times, and least conspicuous in Lower Egypt among the Greek, Roman, and Egyptian populations of Alexandria. Whereas, for instance, the teeth of even young subjects from predynastic Egypt and Nubia were much worn, those from the young people buried at Kom el Shougafa, Ras el Tin, and Chatby and its neighborhood were often almost, if not quite, normal. The crowns of the teeth of Nubian or upper Egyptian adults from predynastic times were often level with the gums, whereas this was never observed in Alexandrians, not even among old people.

The degree of attrition has been used by anthropologists as a guide in the estimation of age, but there are several points which must be remembered before definite conclusions can be drawn in this respect, the most important of which is that the condition is sometimes very pronounced in young people. The attrition of the teeth of the *Homo Aurignacensis* was more pronounced in the second molar than in the third, and the lesion therefore had been produced in the period between the eruption of the second and that of the third molar. Similarly, the permanent teeth of young subjects at Cro-Magnon, Montréjeau, and La Chaumière were worn before the

[1] "Observations relevées sur quelques momies royales d'Égypte," *Bull. Soc. Anthr.*, Paris, IX (1886), 578–90.

eruption of the third molars, and the cusps of the deciduous premolars of Neolithic people from Vendrest in the Vendée were worn at five years of age, the lesion being very pronounced in six-year-old children. The attrition of the posterior premolars, affecting the external cusps chiefly, began a little later in life. In ancient Germany, also, early attrition was the rule. At Adlerberg, for instance, the molars of the two young people of the Bronze Age were much worn, although the third molars had not yet emerged. Among the ancient Nubians and Sudanese, the process started early in life and the rapidity of its progress could be estimated approximately. In several mandibles examined by one at Faras and Merawi, in which the canines were just showing through, the first lower molars were already much worn. In about three years, therefore, most of the mischief had been done. Similarly, the crown of the second premolar was ground down very deeply in the interval between its eruption and that of the third molars. Further, the lesions may be not more advanced in the teeth of old people than in those who die young. The teeth of modern Egyptians are sometimes worn to the gums before the age of twenty-five, but I have seen Egyptians more than fifty years old with teeth showing little trace of wear. This may be due to the character of the food, but the impression gained from the examination of hundreds of skulls is that attrition in these people proceeded very rapidly up to the age of twenty-five or so, and then became almost completely arrested. This is not in accord with observations on other peoples.

The reason for the severe attrition of ancient Egyptian teeth was doubtless due to the food. The Egyptians were nicknamed "eaters of bread," and to them as to the Hebrews, bread was synonymous with food. It was made from spelt, bearded wheat, or barley. Cereals were cultivated from early times, though opinions may differ as to which at different periods was most used for breadmaking. Flour was prepared already in the predynastic period by grinding grain between two stones or pounding it in a mortar. At a later period a handmill, and later still a mill driven by machinery replaced the more primitive apparatus. The specimens of old Egyptian bread which I have examined consist of a very coarse paste usually containing a large amount of husks and some straw even, together with coarse fragments of unbroken wheat or barley grain. Undoubtedly this bread did not improve the masticating surfaces, even if it did contain plenty of fibrous material to clean the interstices of the teeth. One cannot help wondering whether the barley and wheat were cleaner than the native cereals contaminated with sand and earth now sold in Egyptian markets; in any case, the pounding in a mortar or the grinding between stones necessarily detached many fine stone particles, which mixed with the dough escaped detection, but which chewed every day certainly did not improve the crowns of the teeth.

The contents of the intestines of dried predynastic bodies and of mummies from dynastic to Coptic periods, prove the considerable quantity of coarse vegetable material—barley husks chiefly—that was eaten, and this observation together with the composition of the samples of bread examined by the writer explains the attrition of the dental crowns. The teeth of soldiers, for instance, must have been severely tried by their daily ration of four pounds of bread.

The teeth were not improved by the mastication of the roots of marshy plants, which, raw or cooked, the poorer Egyptians—and possibly the richer—ate in large quantities. Indeed, many of the children of the poorer class were brought up on them. The chief fruit eaten by the Egyptian consisted of grapes, figs, dates, dates from the dûm palm, pomegranates, melons, *Balanites Aegyptiaca*, *Paliurus*, carobs, olives, apricots (?), and the seeds of marshy plants. With the exception of dates, the *Paliurus*, and the seeds of aquatic plants, the fruit eaten had but little or no effect on the teeth, for although the rich had extensive fruit gardens, Egypt has never been a great fruit-growing country and the Egyptians of the poorer classes, like the present fellah, probably tasted little fruit except dates and melons. It may be remarked that dates are not infrequently very stringy.

Attrition was intensified by the consumption of raw vegetables. Lentils, beans, artichokes, asparagus, beetroot, and cabbages doubtless were cooked before being served up; but, on the other hand, onions, cucumbers, garlic, radishes, turnips, etc., were eaten raw with bread, as is done now. The six small cucumbers which at the proper season an Egyptian fellah takes for his breakfast, make fine exercise for his masticating apparatus and doubtless provoke a good flow of saliva, but they do not improve the crowns of his teeth.

The diet certainly was not wholly vegetarian, for the predynastic refuse heaps of El Toukh have given up remnants of many animals that had served for food. Also, cattle were kept as far back as Egyptian civilization can be traced, and many wild animals and birds were either hunted or kept in captivity and artificially fattened. The Nile and its canals were inexhaustible reservoirs of fish; salted and pickled fish was a favorite article of food and exported to foreign countries. It would have been interesting to know how the meat was cooked, whether it was eaten well done or underdone, and whether, in fact, it helped in wearing down the teeth. The diet sheets which have come down to us point to a mixed diet having been the rule with people in government employment and with the better class. Under Menhuhotep III[1] each soldier of an expeditionary corps into the desert received two jars of water and twenty small biscuit-like loaves. In the XIXth Dynasty, under Seti I,[2] "His Majesty increased that which was furnished to the army in ointment, ox-flesh, fish, and plentiful vegetables without limit. Every man among them had four debens [about four pounds] of bread daily, two bundles of vegetables, a roast of flesh, and two linen garments monthly." The king's messengers had "good bread, ox-flesh, wine, sweet oil, fat, honey, figs, fish, and vegetables every day."

At Silsileh,[3] every one of the thousand workmen employed in the sandstone quarries received daily nearly four pounds of bread, two bundles of vegetables, and a roast of meat. The king's bodyguard[4] was given in addition "to each five minae in weight of baked bread, two minae of beef, and four arysters of wine."

The following inscription copied from the tomb of Beha in the XVIIIth Dynasty[5] refers to the diet of children: "The children were—great and small—sixty. . . . . They all consumed 120 ephahs of durra, the milk of 3 cows, 52 goats, and 9 she-asses, a hin of balsam, and 2 jars of oil." According to this, bread of durra,

[1] Hammamat inscriptions of Henu.
[2] Assuan inscription.
[3] Breasted, *History of Egypt*, p. 414.
[4] Herodotus ii. 163.
[5] Brugsch, *Egypt under the Pharaohs*, p. 121.

milk, and oil were the children's diet. The children of well-to-do people who went to school carried their daily food, bread, and oil with them, but the poorer people's children were not so spoilt: "They give[1] them very simple cooked foods which can be grilled before the fire, roots, and roots of plants growing in marshes, sometimes raw and sometimes roasted.' The Alexandrians, of course, ate the native dishes and all the luxurious dishes of Rome and Greece.

The attrition of the Egyptian teeth, the contents of the refuse heaps, the intestinal contents, the offerings of food in tombs, the mural decorations, and the literary evidence, all point to a mixed diet, of which coarse bread and vegetables formed the chief constituents. To explain the attrition it is not necessary to assume, as has been done, that the Egyptians ate earth or that the food was contaminated with sand.

IV. CARIES

Carious human teeth from ancient remains have been discovered in so many places that it is legitimate to doubt whether there was ever an epoch when the human species was not cursed by toothache.

The population of England has certainly suffered from it for thousands of years. Of 69 skulls from Wiltshire tumuli,[2] dating from the Stone Age, 2 had carious teeth. The people buried in the tumuli, a pastoral and agricultural race, lived by the chase and "their habits were barbarous." Nine cases of caries, namely 4 on occluding and 5 on approximal surfaces, were found in 44 skulls of a similar group inhabiting more northern districts of England. In the people of a later race (Bronze period), the agricultural population referred to by Caesar in his *Commentaries*, there were 6 cases of caries in 32 skulls, 5 on approximal and 1 on occluding surfaces. The teeth of Romans in England were not infrequently carious; of 143 skulls, about 32 showed signs of caries, and in one instance the disease was extensive. In 76 skulls of the Anglo-Saxon period, caries was present in 15.

The painful ailment was common in the inhabitants of ancient France. At least two skulls from Aurignac,[3] several crania of the Furfooz, La Truchère, and Aurignac races,[4] a skull from the cavern

[1] Diodorus Siculus i. 93.
[2] J. R. Mummery, *loc. cit.*
[3] Quatrefage et Hamy, *op. cit.*, p. 104.
[4] *Ibid.*

of Engilhoul,[1] a prehistoric skull from the Carrière Hélie at Grenoble,[2] skulls from dolmens (Billancourt, Moulin-Quignon),[3] all these had carious teeth, sometimes associated with extensive lesions.

It is estimated, but on what appears to me insufficient data, that only about 1.5 per cent of the people found in the Neolithic ossarium of Bagoges-en-Pareds had carious teeth. At Vendrest, in the Vendée, of 1,948 teeth collected in a Neolithic ossarium, 49 molars and 11 premolars were carious, but no incisors or canines. The dental pulp of 36 was attacked; in 25 there was slight caries of the neck only; and in 1 the caries was limited to the masticating surface of a wisdom tooth. Of 317 deciduous teeth, 2 molars showed slight caries in the neighborhood of the neck. From these observations the conclusion was drawn that caries was neither common nor severe in that period. A Neolithic burial[4] contained a carious tooth pierced for suspension.

Carious teeth have been discovered in the grotto of Mayrannes (Bronze Age),[5] in dolmens of the Gard, of Saint-Vallier de Thoy (Reviere), in the grottos of Albarée (Alpes Maritimes), in the grotto of La Marthe, and at Carzy-la-Rouet. The Roman settlers in Gaul suffered, for the right upper second premolar and second molar of a Roman skull were carious, and the left lower second premolar and all the molars had been shed prematurely.

Caries worried the ancient Germans also. A skull from the 6th to 10th century B.C., unearthed at Reiherwerder, had 4 carious teeth out of the 5 remaining; and the disease had probably been extensive, for the absorption of the alveoli proved that the missing teeth had been lost during life. Other examples were discovered in the Ruhr Valley, where several teeth from 32—or possibly 34—cavern burials[6] were carious. Human teeth dating from the La Tène

[1] E. T. Hamy, "Note sur les ossements humains fossiles de la seconde caverne d'Engilhoul près Liège," *Bull. Soc. Anthr.*, Paris, VI (1871), 370–86.

[2] Quatrefages et Hamy, *op. cit.*, p. 20.

[3] *Ibid.*, Pl. XCVII-3, p. 112.

[4] Camus, *L'homme préhistorique*, VI (1908), 326.

[5] Ch. Cotta, "La carie dentaire et l'alimentation dans la Provence préhistorique," *L'homme préhistorique*, III (1905), 74.

[6] Carthaus, "Über die Ausgrabungen in der Valedahöhle unweit Velmede im oberen Ruhrtale," *Prähist. Zeitschr.*, III (1911), 137.

period from Zeiningen[1] and Worms am Rhein,[2] showed similar changes. Ancient Denmark,[3] Sweden, Norway, and Italy[4] were certainly not free from the disease.

From the earliest to the present times, caries had attacked human teeth in Nubia, Upper and Lower Egypt, and yet, from the data at our command, it is almost impossible to form an opinion regarding the incidence of the ailment during successive centuries. One observer whose opinion certainly carries great weight expresses himself as follows:[5]

Both in Nubia and Egypt the ordinary form of caries is exceedingly rare in predynastic and protodynastic people, and among the poorer classes it never became at all common until modern times. . . . . Dental caries became common as soon as people learned luxury. In the cemetery of the time of the Ancient Empire, excavated by the Hearst expedition at the Giza pyramids, more than five hundred skeletons of aristocrats of the time of the pyramid-builders were brought to light, and in these bodies I found that tartar formation, dental caries, and alveolar abscesses were at least as common as they are in modern Europe today. And at every subsequent period of Egyptian history one finds the same thing—the wide prevalence of every form of dental disease among the wealthy people of luxurious diet, and the relative immunity from it among the poorer people who lived mainly on a coarse, uncooked diet.

Among the Biga people of Nubia in whom dental caries appeared to be very prevalent, everything points to the fact that the people buried at Biga were not leading the life of their neighbours. The abundance of clothes and the number of wine-jars suggest a life of luxury—and gout is not engendered by the ordinary fare of Nubia. This all means that dental caries in the early Christians of Biga was due to the operation of the same factors which are supposed to be causally related to it elsewhere, namely, an improper diet. This conclusion is borne out by the extreme rarity of dental caries in children throughout these Egyptian and Nubian cemeteries, because they lived on the food supplied by nature and not that provided by the chemist.

That the frequency of caries in Nubia and Egypt increased gradually from predynastic to Christian times and later is undoubtedly the first impression produced by the examination of ancient

[1] Hölder, "Untersuchungen über die Skelettfunde in den vorrömischen Hügelgräbern Württembergs und Hohenzollerns, *Fundberichte aus Schwaben*, II (1895).

[2] P. Bartels, "Über Schädel und Skelettreste der früheren Bronzezeit aus der Umgebung von Worms am Rhein," *Prähist. Zeitschr.*, IV (1912).

[3] H. A. Nielsen, *Danemark Arch. f. Gesch. d. Med.*, IV, 377.

[4] Quatrefages et Hamy, *op. cit.*, Pl. XCI, Fig. 3.

[5] Elliot Smith, *A. S. N.*, II., 281.

Egyptian skulls, and yet no observer has brought forward any satisfactory statistical evidence to support it. An estimation of the incidence of caries in any given community based on the examination of skulls is very difficult always, and not infrequently well-nigh impossible. Many teeth invariably disappear during excavations, and there is every reason to suppose that some of these teeth were carious, although they never figure as such in statistics. The incidence of caries, therefore, is always estimated too low.

An attempt was made to estimate the number of cases of caries in the large collection of skulls in the Museum of the Medical School of Cairo, which contained a large number of predynastic skulls, others dating from the IVth to the XIIth Dynasties, others again from the time of the pyramid-builders at Gizeh, and from Ptolemaic and Coptic times. The result was worth nothing; firstly, because it was impossible to diagnose why a missing tooth had been lost during life, and secondly on account of the enormous number of teeth which had fallen out after death. In the case of the skulls from Gizeh and the dynastic skulls, not even an approximate idea regarding the incidence of caries could be formed.

The field notes on cemeteries in Nubia prove that the disease existed in predynastic times, and among the archaic Nubians. Some of the lesions connected with caries in Nubians from the middle of the Ancient Empire were very severe. The skull of an old man, for instance, had extremely carious teeth, with alveolar abscesses at the roots of eight upper and eight lower teeth.[1] In other skulls of the same epoch, caries was limited to one or two teeth.

No less severe were occasionally the lesions in more modern times, in the later B group, for instance.[2] The front teeth of a man from this period were much worn, the stumps of the upper teeth and upper right second premolar were carious, and all the lower teeth behind the premolars had been lost during life, with the exception of the carious stumps of the right molars. A Nubian woman from the Middle Empire, with teeth very much worn and carious, had extensive inflammation of the left mandible spreading from the alveoli. During the Roman, Christian, and Byzantine periods in

[1] *A. S. N.*, p. 75.   [2] *Ibid.*, p. 118.

ABNORMALITIES OF ANCIENT EGYPTIAN TEETH 295

Nubia the disease was active and the coexistent lesions sometimes very severe. The skull of a middle-aged Christian woman[1] was disfigured by a dental abscess round the roots of the right upper second premolar and of the first molar, which opened on the palate and the face, and there were also small abscesses round other carious teeth. A very old woman[2] had lost all her teeth except one carious upper stump and four similar fragments in the lower jaw. Other skulls had evidently lost most of their teeth from the disease, as several of the remaining teeth were carious.

The teeth of prehistoric skulls from Naga el Deir in Egypt were not infrequently carious, but, as a rule, there were not more than two or at most three carious teeth in any one skull or mandible. Lesions secondary to caries were usually absent, and in one case only was secondary disease of the maxilla noted.

I attempted to tabulate the cases of dental disease in Nubia according to the notes of the Archaeological Survey, and the table so prepared certainly showed a rise in the number of cases of caries and dental disease after Ptolemaic times. Of 72 skulls of the B group, for instance, 20 per cent had lost some teeth and four had carious teeth, whereas of 165 skulls dating from a time after the Ptolemaic period 74 per cent had missing and 28 per cent had carious teeth. At first sight only one conclusion appears possible, namely, that dental disease and especially caries increased in frequency in the two thousand odd years between the B group and the beginning of the Christian era.

On examining the notes more closely, however, the incidence of dental disease and caries was found to have remained practically stationary for a long period and then to have risen suddenly to an unprecedented level after Ptolemaic times. When seeking an explanation for this startling fact one was led to wonder, as Wood Jones had done, whether this extraordinary rise was not due to any immigration of people who accommodated themselves badly to their new conditions of life and their new food.

The facts are as follows: The predynastic and the A group of dynastic people in Nubia were the old Egyptian race with little admixture of negro. The percentage of black blood increased

[1] *Ibid.*, p. 42.   [2] *Ibid.*, p. 52.

slightly in the people of the B period and still more in the C group. The New Empire saw a considerable influx of Egyptians until, later on,[1] the Nubian element again increased. Groups of negroid people then began to make their appearance (Group E). These have been met with in Ptolemaic and even in some Roman cemeteries of Nubia, and some possibly emigrated or were brought as slaves into Egypt. The race inhabiting Nubia, therefore, was fairly pure at first, but gradually became more and more mixed. The intermixture increased still more after the Ptolemaic period, especially among the Biga people who, as had been noted, suffered much from dental disease, as 43 out of 86 skulls had missing teeth and 16 had caries. Most of the Biga people, among whom the incidence of caries was highest, were immigrants, perhaps from Asia Minor, who intermarried with Nubian women together with a few Egyptians and many Sudanese. It is considered probable that at the time of their deaths these immigrants had not been settled in the neighborhood for more than thirty-five to forty years. A comparison between a race of immigrants and dynastic or predynastic Nubians must lead to fallacious conclusions because the age, habits, and perhaps the cookery of the two classes of people were probably very different.

It is not necessary to assume that the increase in caries and dental disease among the Biga people was the just punishment for a more luxurious mode of living. The food, to judge from the attrition of the teeth which is noted in several observations, was fairly coarse, for attrition is not the characteristic result of soft food, the alleged cause of caries. Those people probably drank wine, but wine was used in Egypt and Nubia from the earliest times, vineyards existed in both countries, and Nubian beer had a great name long before the Christian epoch, indeed, it is mentioned in so ancient a book as the *Liturgy of Funerary Offerings*. Neither is the fact that one case of gout was discovered a proof of luxurious living. There is such a thing as poor man's gout. Uric-acid calculi have been taken from Egyptian bodies dating from the IIId Dynasty and possibly earlier times, and indeed occur among herbivorous animals. When these foreign immigrants were excluded, the inci-

[1] *A. S. N.*, p. 36.

dence of dental disease was seen to vary considerably in different cemeteries during Ptolemaic and Christian times.

The author's study of the predynastic skulls in Egypt showed that caries and dental disease were present from very early times. The results of the examination of these skulls are as follows: *Maxillae:* Out of 156 specimens, the number with missing or carious teeth was 54, or 35 per cent; the number with carious teeth, 32, or 20 per cent. *Mandibles:* 95 specimens; number with missing or carious teeth, 21, or 20 per cent; number with carious teeth, 15, or 15 per cent. A little less than one-half of the maxillae of prehistoric Egyptians and four-fifths of the mandibles had not lost any teeth and showed no decay, which is a remarkably good record.

These figures taken by themselves, however, would give a wrong impression regarding the prevalence of the dental disease in predynastic times, for 60 per cent at least of all maxillae and mandibles were scarred with lesions of chronic suppurative periodontitis. Forty-five skulls had abscesses connected with the maxillary teeth, of which 12 were associated with caries, 10 with missing teeth, 5 with both defects, and in 28 skulls with abscesses no teeth were missing and there was no caries. Eighty-two upper jaws out of 156, or 53 per cent, therefore, had gross pathological lesions of or connected with the teeth. Of the 95 mandibles, 12 had dental abscesses. These abscesses were associated with missing teeth in two cases, and with carious teeth in two others. Twenty-nine per cent, therefore, showed gross lesions of dental disease.[1]

The following data give the incidence of carious and missing teeth according to their position:

Upper: M 1, M 3, M 2, I, Pm 2, Pm 1, C, I 2;
Lower: M 2, M 3, M 1, Pm 2, Pm 1, I, I2 C.

These figures prove clearly that the molars, the first molars especially, were in the old Egyptians the teeth most prone to caries, and this observation agrees with the results of modern statistics regarding the incidence of caries in individual teeth, statistics nearly always derived from records of extractions.

[1] The cases of chronic suppurative periodontitis without abscesses are not counted.

Statistics from Vienna based on examination, and not on extractions, do not give the same results, and according to them the liability of individual maxillary teeth to caries stands in the following order:

I 1, M 1, I 2, Pm 1, M 2, Pm 2, C, M 3;

and in the mandible:

M 1, M 2, Pm 2, Pm 1, M 3, C, I 2, I 1.

On the whole, our data correspond fairly well with the statistics that have been based on the extraction of teeth, which are:

Maxillary: M 1, M 3, M 2, I 1, Pm 2, Pm 2, Pm 1, C, I 2;
Mandible: M 2, M 3, M 1, Pm 2, Pm 1, I 2, C, and I 1.

The following were the results obtained by the author's examination of skulls in the predynastic to Ist Dynasty cemeteries of Tourah near Cairo:[1]

Of 29 skulls 3 belonged to children not more than sixteen years of age. Seven of the remaining skulls were more or less broken and parts of the dentition were missing; in 2 others some teeth were broken away in the first specimen and the teeth had dropped out after death in the second. There was no caries in any skull: a very striking fact, for, even making allowances for the number of skulls more or less damaged, and for the youth of many of the cases, a series of 17 skulls free from caries could not easily be discovered anywhere in collections of modern skulls. On the other hand, lesions of periodontal disease, abscesses, loosening of teeth, etc., were present in 10 of the complete skulls and 1 skull had lost many teeth post mortem.

Caries was present also in some of the predynastic skulls at Dahshur,[2] and in one of them the only remains of the teeth consisted of a few worn and carious stumps. In the same locality[3] the princess Nourhotep, who was about forty-five years old at the time of her death, had two carious first molars, and the alveoli of these were inflamed.

---

[1] D. E. Derry, in Hermann Junker, "Bericht über die Grabungen auf dem Friedhof in Turah," *Denkschr. Ac. Wiss.*, Wien, LVI (1912).

[2] De Morgan, *Les origines de l'Égypte*, p. 280.   [3] *Ibid.*, p. 148.

An examination of skulls from the XXVth to XXVIth Dynasties at Merawi, in the Sudan, and of crania dating from the Meroitic kingdom of Faras, revealed the presence of caries in 12 per cent of the skulls only. Owing to the pressure of time, however, the examination at the graveside was rather superficial, and the crowns of a large number of teeth had been broken off, while numerous teeth had been lost after death. Of the 36 skulls and fragments of mandibles from Faras and Merawi which were taken to Alexandria for examination all but 2 had one or more carious teeth. The crowns, as a rule, were not affected, the carious hole being in the neck of the tooth.

Of 110 ancient though not accurately dated skulls from Thebes,[1] 12 only had carious teeth, and in 2 cases only a very small part of the tooth was affected. It must be noted, however, that many of these skulls also had lost a number of teeth during life, of which some may have been carious.

Several aristocrats, whose mummies are now in the Cairo Museum, were martyrs to caries during life. All the maxillary teeth of a woman, for instance (Princess Maritamon, XIIth–XIIIth Dynasties, about 1900 B.C.), were carious with the exception of the canine and the third molar, and the first and second molars were reduced to mere stumps. An aged court lady (XVIIIth Dynasty, about 1400 B.C.) had a carious upper first molar, and alveolar abscesses at the root of the neighboring molar.

Nineteen hundred years ago, caries also was by no means rare in the Egyptian population of Alexandria, and it attacked children and young adults also. A child with complete deciduous dentition had deep caries of the first upper right molar and neighboring premolar, the crowns of these teeth being completely destroyed, and traces of suppuration were to be seen round the maxillary molars on both sides. A young adult, with wisdom teeth still unerupted, showed caries of both first upper molars on the approximal side. The right second upper molar of another young woman was so deeply carious that the whole had disappeared.

Some cases of caries in adults were very severe. A male, for instance, between forty and fifty years old, had lost the left upper

[1] Hermann Stahr, *Die Rassenfrage im antiken Ägypten.*

first molar and neighboring premolar during life, the alveolus of the latter showing an external fistulous opening about 2 mm. wide. The dental canal of the right second upper premolar had been opened by attrition, as the right first upper molar was also carious on its approximal side. Both teeth were covered with thick tartar, and, the buccal border having been completely absorbed, both alveoli communicated with the mouth by a wide aperture. Attrition, caries, and rarefying periostitis had all helped to produce these lesions.

The Copts of Antinoë must often had suffered acutely from toothache, as may be seen from the following notes on the teeth of these people:

1. Adult man, probably about forty-five years old, had lost the right first upper molar and second premolar, together with the left first upper molar. In the mandible the right second premolar and first molar together with the left molar had been shed during life. The left lower second premolar was carious on distal side.

2. Adult woman, probably about twenty-six years old. The lower third molars were present, whereas the corresponding upper teeth had not emerged. The right lower first molars and left molars and premolars were shed during life. There was extensive caries of the posterior part of the left lower second molar extending almost to the fang, and of the right second and third molars at the point of contact. The crowns showed but slight attrition.

3. Man, adult, but not aged, probably about thirty years old. Teeth missing—upper, all right premolars and molars, left second premolar and third molars; lower—right second molar, left molars and premolars. Second right upper incisor carious; region occupied by left first and second upper molars hollowed out into a cavity with deeply pitted floor, measuring 15 mm. from before backwards and 12 mm. from side to side; outer wall of the alveolus of the first molar completely gone.

Very startling is the statement[1] that in Nubia caries was not met with in the deciduous teeth of children of the archaic period— that it did not make its appearance until the Christian era, and that, even in Christian children, the disease was very rarely seen. The observation, though interesting, does not justify the conclusions which have been based on it. In the first place, many of the infantile skulls that have been discovered were those of newly born children or babies, in whom for obvious reasons caries could not have

[1] A. S. N., p. 279.

occurred, and in Egypt as in Nubia the number of children's skeletons which have been studied is so small as to be, in my opinion, almost useless for forming an estimate regarding the incidence of infantile caries, or of any other infantile disease. In Nubian adolescents and adults extensive lesions, directly or indirectly due to caries, were not rare, especially in Christian times. A Coptic boy of Nubia,[1] seventeen years old, had a large abscess cavity at the root of the right upper second molar on the outer side; the right second lower bicuspid also was carious, and the right and second molars together with their alveoli had disappeared; the left second lower molar was represented by a carious stump only. A young woman from the Roman period had worn and carious teeth. A young Christian woman had lost seven teeth during life, and the right upper second incisors together with the right lower second premolar were carious; 'another young Christian woman had caries of several upper teeth; and several more young early Christians suffered extensively from caries.

The teeth of the Macedonian soldiers buried at Chatby were not often attacked with caries and in no case was this found to have been very severe. Here also, however, the same difficulty presented itself in estimating the exact percentage of dental disease, owing to the fact that many of the teeth had dropped out after death and could not be found, and therefore only the teeth of which the alveoli showed partial or complete absorption were considered as having been lost through disease.

V. OTHER LESIONS

Alveolar and perialveolar abscesses have been frequently observed in ancient skulls in England, Germany, and France, and have been usually attributed to infection through dental canals opened by attrition. In England, for instance, many teeth of a skeleton from Halling (Kent), dating from late Palaeolithic or early Neolithic times, had been lost apparently through exposure of the pulp cavities, which had led to the formation of abscesses at the roots.[2] At Zairingen in Germany, a skull from the grotto of Ale had an abscess, apparently due to the opening up by attrition of the dental

[1] *Ibid.*, p. 48.   [2] A. Keith, *Jour. Anthr. Inst.*, XLIV (1914).

pulp of the left upper third molar. Many similar cases have been discovered in French ossaria—in the Vendée, for instance—and in Denmark, Sweden, Norway, Australia, and elsewhere.

Dental abscesses were common in every cemetery of Nubia and Egypt. An ancient Nubian,[1] for instance, had several alveolar abscesses supposed to have resulted from infection through pulp cavities opened by attrition, and most of the upper as well as lower teeth had been lost. Another predynastic man[2] had only a few teeth left which were greatly worn and had abscess cavities at their roots; the right side of his face showed "abundant inflammatory disease" probably connected with the teeth. Again, well-worn teeth with five abscesses at their roots were found in an archaic Nubian[3] who died some time between the ages of twenty-five and forty; a young Christian woman[4] also had an abscess at the roots of the left upper third molar, and the pus had perforated into the antrum.

Of 100 maxillary abscesses in predynastic people, 22 were round the first molars; 17 were round the second molars; 15 were round the median incisor; 11 were round the posterior premolars; 10 were round the anterior premolars; 9 were round the canines; 9 round the third molars; 6 round the lateral incisors; and the position of 1 was doubtful.

Of 35 mandibular abscesses in the same people, 13 were round the first molars; 6 were round the canines; 5 were round the second molars; 4 were round the median incisors; 3 were round the posterior premolars; 3 were round the third molars; and 1 was round the anterior premolars.

The abscesses were often multiple. Thus the jaw of a Nubian female was riddled with dental abscesses, and in another such purulent collections had developed round the second and third molars on both sides.

In Egypt, numerous dental abscesses have been found in Theban skulls from various periods. At Tourah,[5] on the northern borders of Lower Egypt, single or multiple abscesses, due either to exposure

---

[1] *A. S. N.*, p. 117.
[2] *Ibid.*, p. 127.
[3] *Ibid.*
[4] *Ibid.*
[5] Derry, *loc. cit.*

of the pulp cavity through attrition or to alveolar inflammation, were met with, both in predynastic and dynastic skeletons.

A very remarkable case of possible infection through such an abscess has been put on record. An old woman from the IIId Dynasty cemetery at Tourah had upper teeth worn down to stumps and on each side a huge hole near the site of the first molar, communicating with the antrum. All the molars and most of the other teeth were gone and their alveoli absorbed, leaving behind traces of the former presence of alveolar abscesses. The lower teeth were much worn, and an alveolar abscess had formed at the root of the left first molar. The right first molar communicated with a huge hole on the right side of the mandible, and a necrotic process attacking this bone had eaten away almost the whole of the right half of the lower jaw, the disease extending along the bone and across the symphysis nearly to the left canine tooth. The hole in the mandible was oval, 6 mm. in length, commenced at the junction of the right ramus with the body, and the bare roots of the teeth protruded through the roof of the immense abscess cavity. In the pelvis, an apparently similar necrosis had destroyed practically the whole of the iliac portion of the left innominate bone, spreading to the sacrum and destroying its left auricular surface and much of the bone below it. The acetabulum was intact, but the disease had spread into the iliac segment of the cavity. The only part of the ilium left was the anterior three-fourths of the crest, the antero-superior spina, and a small arch of bone behind the spine. On the right side the ilium was intact, but here the disease had destroyed the ischial tuberosity completely, and had travelled some way up the ascending ramus.[1]

A very interesting case came from Heliopolis.[2] In this skull, one of a typical Egyptian adult, there had been a severe abscess, probably due to the exposure of the pulp cavity of the upper central incisor. All the incisors were very much worn and the roots of both left incisors opened into the abscess cavity which had perforated on to the face, the palate, and into the floor of the nose on both sides

[1] The writer has not seen the specimen and can therefore not give a definite opinion, but the diagnosis of cancer of the jaw with metastases in the pelvis does not appear to him improbable.

[2] Petrie and Mackey, *Heliopolis, Kafr, Amar, and Sharufa*, p. 47.

of the septum. The left second molar was carious also, and its crown had gone. In the mandible there were primary carious spots on the second bicuspid and first molar.

Many people from Merawi and Faras hada bscesses secondary to caries or periodontitis. The second mandibular premolar of one skull, for instance, was deeply carious on its lingual side, and the first molar, which had been lost during life, had perhaps been carious also, for the rough, spongy state of the alveolus bore witness to considerable inflammation in its neighborhood. An abscess had formed round one of these teeth, probably round the first molar, and the pus had worked its way firstly from one alveolus to the other, through a sinus large enough to admit a large probe, and secondly into the mouth on the labial side of the second premolar.

In the times of Cleopatra, the Egyptian inhabitants of Alexandria often suffered from dental abscesses due to various causes. Sometimes the abscesses were doubtless due to the entrance of micro-organisms through an open dental canal, but very often this was not the probable cause. An abscess round the fang of the left mandibular second premolar of one case, for example, had evidently not been the result of attrition as the dental canal was entirely closed; nevertheless the pus had ultimately worked its way into the buccal cavity by a fistulous opening 5 mm. wide.

The etiology of these abscesses was often somewhat obscure, as in the case of an old Christian woman[1] with numerous maxillary alveolar abscesses, whose right maxillary third molar was retained and ankylosed to the bone, the right temporo-mandibular joint being at the same time "disorganized" by arthritis. The abscess in this case may possibly have been the result of inflammation produced by the retained third molar. If the infection had spread from the exposed pulp to the apex of the root through the apical canal, signs of softening of the pulp chamber should have been evident, whereas in many cases no trace of such previous softening existed. On the contrary, except in teeth obviously carious, the pulp, though freely exposed, appeared hard and healthy, this state of things giving no support to the theory that the micro-organisms had penetrated through the apical canal.

[1] *A. S. N.*, p. 92.

The pathological processes involved in the production of abscesses in some skulls were sometimes very complex, as when dental abscesses co-existed with attrition and chronic suppurative periodontitis. In such cases it was impossible to say whether the infective agents had entered through the apical canal or through the space opened up by suppuration between the tooth and the alveolar wall. In an Alexandrian skull, the tips of the anterior fangs of the left mandibular second molar dipped into two small abscesses, each about the size of a very small pea; the crown was somewhat worn and the dental canal firmly closed. The alveolar wall on the buccal side had been almost completely absorbed and a depression round the roots of the left third molar suggested that these also had been bathed in pus. In this case rarefying suppurative periostitis had evidently opened the way for the infective agent.

The pathological processes which resulted in the formation of another mandibular dental abscess were still more complex. In this case both left premolars and the first molar had been lost during life and the left second molar was carious. An oval opening with smooth borders, measuring 12 by 8 mm., occupied on the alveolar border the position of the roots of the absent premolars. An aperture artificially made by me through the external wall of the mandible led to a smooth-walled cavity measuring 3.5 by 2 cm., in which the roots of the second incisor, first molar, and the anterior fang of the second molar protruded. During life, therefore, all these roots and those of the absent premolars had been bathed in pus, and the premolars and first molars had evidently either fallen out or been removed some time before death, a wide fistula remaining behind. The alveolar walls of the second and third molars had been partly absorbed and the teeth were thickly encrusted with tartar.

An old person, with teeth somewhat worn, had carious right molars. The right first and second premolars had been lost just before, or had dropped out after, death, though not before their alveoli had been converted by long continued suppuration into a cavity measuring 17 by 12 mm., and the buccal alveolar wall had been absorbed, with the exception of the posterior third which was perforated by a small opening on the buccal side. Almost the entire roots of the carious first molar, and to a less extent those of the neighboring molars were exposed, and all these teeth were covered with thick tartar. The path followed by the infective agents, therefore, whether through a carious tooth or a suppurating alveolar border, was not at all certain. The aetiology of many of these suppurations, especially in the maxillae of young people, remained obscure, for no obvious disease was found either in the tooth itself or its neighborhood.

Non-infectious periodontitis due to mechanical causes such as blows, etc., was rare in ancient Egypt, for no cases are on record; nor were there any reasons to suppose that intoxication by arsenic, mercury, or phosphorus played any part in the causation of dental disease. The majority of alveolar and perialveolar abscesses was evidently, if not due to, at any rate associated with, chronic suppurative periodontitis.

The name of pyorrhoea marginalis is given to a group of well-defined clinical symptoms, and anatomically it has all the characteristics of chronic, suppurating, marginal periodontitis. The disease is now considered by many to be caused by an amoeba, the presence of which in Egypt has lately been demonstrated by Dr. Crendiropoulo, my assistant.[1] In modern Alexandria it attacks the English, French, Italians, Greeks, Egyptians, Jews, Berberine, and negroes, people of the most different habits, diatheses, ages, and conditions, with truly international impartiality. The author has seen it in two members of the same household; the first, an Egyptian cook whose tartar-covered teeth had never been brushed; the second a fair Englishwoman, with spotless dentition, who had never had an illness except infantile measles.

The differences between the periodontitis caused by caries and other local lesions, and the periodontitis of pyorrhoea marginalis, are mainly clinical; the first being limited to a few teeth and coming to an end when the diseased teeth or lesion are removed, the other being a chronic disease, usually spreading from tooth to tooth which remain healthy. Suppurating chronic periodontitis occurred in ancient times both in Europe and Africa. In Europe the fossil

---

[1] While the amoebae are constantly found in this disease they are not considered by most authorities to be in any way concerned with the causation. (J. H. M.)

man of La Chapelle-aux-Saints[1] is said to have suffered from pyorrhoea. He lived in the Mousterian period, and was therefore certainly a hunter, though possibly also an agriculturist.

According to Baudouin, who described fully the pathological alterations of this skull, the alveolus of the left upper canine is diminished in depth and its cavity has a spongy appearance, doubtless owing to the long-standing inflammation which led to the loss of this tooth. The alveolus of the left first upper premolar also is shallower than normal. The alveoli of the right lower incisors, canine, and first premolar form large irregular cavities due to the partial absorption of their walls. The alveolus of the second molar is in a better state of preservation and slopes forwards. All the molars were lost long before death, and the alveoli, having been absorbed, are depressed and concave. The alveoli of the left incisors and canine are well preserved, the pathological signs are but slight and their diminished depth alone attracts attention. The alveolar border behind the second molar having been absorbed, the mandible is atrophied correspondingly. The third molar, on the other hand, was lost probably only just before death.

It is very probable that the loss of his molars in the La Chapelle man was the result of pyorrhoea alveolaris, though it may also have been caused by caries. With regard to the other alveolar lesions in this skull which have been described as being due to pyorrhoea, their causation, in my opinion,[2] is by no means clear.

The diagnosis of pyorrhoea alveolaris was made in the case of a Neolithic skull also,[3] in which all the left mandibular molars, the second maxillary premolars, and all the molars had been lost through disease during life; but here again caries may have been the active agent. Such cases of almost total destruction of teeth by caries occur nowadays in Egypt. I have, for instance, observed for eighteen years a man who during that period has lost from caries all the upper teeth with the exception of the second left molar, and

[1] Marcel Baudouin, "La polyarthrite alvéolaire depuis la quaternaire jusqu'à l'époque romaine," *Gaz. Méd.*, Paris, 1913, p. 397.

[2] My opinion is based on an excellent cast of this skull only, and is therefore provisional.

[3] Marcel Baudouin, *loc. cit.*

all the lower teeth with the exception of the incisors, canines, and the third molars, and who yet had never a sign of pyorrhoea. It is possible, therefore, that both the above subjects had lost their teeth through caries. The writer has observed similar lesions in a considerable number of ancient skulls.[1]

The typical lesions of chronic periodontitis marginalis were conspicuous in several skulls from Merawi, the fangs of many of the teeth being bare and looking as if they had been pushed out of their sockets. This early stage was the result of the absorption of the alveoli and consequent exposure of the roots. In a more advanced stage, the alveolar walls had completely disappeared, and consequently the fangs were exposed for a considerable length, while in a still more advanced condition the alveoli were almost completely absorbed and the teeth, on the point of being shed, remained attached to the skull by the tips of the roots only. It was most probably also this disease which was responsible for some edentulous ancient Sudanese skulls with alveolar borders completely destroyed.

Skulls from Faras in Nubia, from the time of the Meroitic kingdom, showed the same typical lesions. This is specially interesting because the disease exists now at Faras as it did two thousand years ago, and when I was collecting ancient pathological specimens there I was consulted by many members of the present population who had lost most of their teeth from pyorrhoea and were fast shedding the remaining few. The disease is spread all over Egypt and exists even in remote localities, far away from all civilization. In the desert of Sinai, on the gulf of Akaba, I found seven men, the whole garrison of a small isolated fort, who had the typical symptoms of pyorrhoea alveolaris, and were in a wretched state of health in consequence.

The most striking pathological lesions in ancient Coptic skulls were perhaps suppurative periodontitis. In one case, for instance, suppuration had completely exposed two molar teeth, and the pathological process had extended along the alveolar borders of the

---

[1] It is rather strange that the report in the *A. S. N.* does not mention the presence of this disease in Nubia, though there are plain indications that it was not uncommon there.

maxillae and mandibles, leaving the teeth bare and most of them very loose. Such lesions were extremely common at that period of Egyptian history.

Interesting as were the Coptic cases and those from Merawi and Faras, chronic suppurative periodontitis of the ancient Egyptians was best studied on Egyptian predynastic skulls, in which the lesions were most typical. In these, the first lesions were usually situated on the buccal side of the anterior or posterior root of the first molar, the alveolar wall being partly absorbed and the root thus laid bare for some distance. The remaining alveolar border was often riddled with small holes with smooth walls and borders; evidently the effect of unequal destruction of bone by a chronic inflammatory suppurative process. A more advanced stage was reached when this process had extended between the roots of the first molar and into the spaces between this tooth and its neighbors on one or both sides, and had thus given rise to a honeycombed surface. Owing to the continued absorption of the alveolar wall, the whole root was laid bare, even when, as sometimes happened, the lesions remained limited to the root. Absorption was nearly always most marked on the buccal side of the first molar or of any other tooth that was attacked.

The suppuration causing the disappearance of the alveolar wall and the loosening of the tooth appeared to follow one of two courses, which, though sometimes combined, were nevertheless fairly distinct. In the first, most often observed in the molar region, the absorption of the alveolar wall starting on the free border gradually extended towards the apex of the alveolus, and the whole or nearly the whole alveolar wall was absorbed, often without the formation of an abscess. In the other, the disease extended to the bottom of the alveolus without marked changes being noticeable in the upper part of the alveolar wall, but the bone protecting the tip of the root was absorbed, and the pus found its way into the mouth through this perforation near the extremity of the alveolus. Repeated examination gave the impression that the first process is typical of an acute form of disease, for the inflammatory lesions in the neighborhood were severe. The second indicated a more chronic form, in which the infective material, having penetrated between the tooth and the alveolus, had produced a small purulent collection round the apex of the root. The surface of the maxilla or mandible behind the tip of the fang was excavated somewhat, but not pitted, and exhibited no obvious signs of inflammation, its smooth surface somewhat resembling a stone worn down by the prolonged action of water. The apex of the fang never adhered to the neighboring bone, and the tooth is usually tightly held by what remains of the alveolus. The irregular pitting caused by the inflammatory process often extended bilaterally along the alveolar borders of several or all the maxillary or mandibular teeth, or of both. As a rule, however, the pathological process had attacked two or three teeth only and had extended to the others later on, for when several alveoli had been absorbed during life in a skull with lesions of suppurative periodontitis, the disease clearly had existed long before death, and after causing the loss of several teeth it had spread to the alveoli found diseased at the time of death.

The teeth, even when the walls of the alveoli had been almost completely destroyed, were healthy as a rule, except for the usual deep attrition of ancient Egyptian teeth, and very often, though not always, for more or less thick deposits of tartar. Sometimes, however, the root was shortened owing to absorption of its tip which was then smooth and rounded—blunted, so to speak. Very rarely the roots, although smooth, were somewhat uneven as if a slow process of ulceration had been acting. The crown itself was normal except for the changes due to attrition. In a late stage the alveolar septa were absorbed and the teeth might then lie in a cavity, which during life was doubtless purulent. As the septa between two or more neighboring teeth also disappeared, the alveoli of several teeth ran together, especially in the molar regions, and a huge cavity was thus formed by the coalescence of several alveoli.

The ultimate result of the process in the Egyptian skulls was often loss of the teeth, but sometimes before this occurred some, especially the premolars and molars, were forced out of position, owing to their attachment having been loosened by the absorption of the alveolus and the accompanying suppuration. The teeth had easily yielded to the presence of masticating or other movements, and had been ultimately pushed into a position at an angle with the other teeth. The tips of the roots of the "dislocated" teeth were thus directed towards the buccal side, and the roots were often bare for most or all of their lengths even. Such teeth were not infrequently firmly fixed in their new position, so firmly, indeed, that their removal from the skull was not at all easy, and sometimes the life of the bearer had been prolonged long enough for a new masticating surface to have formed on the lateral aspect of the fang lying at right angles to the other teeth.

This process, then, was essentially chronic, spreading from tooth to tooth and often ending in the loss of one, several, or even all the teeth. Very probably the edentulous maxillae and mandibles discovered in many ancient graveyards had been rendered so by this disease, but on the other hand, there can be no doubt that in the large majority of cases the disease improved locally or generally before the death of the patient. More than 60 per cent of predynastic, dynastic, Roman, and Coptic Egyptians had one or several teeth with exposed fangs, sometimes for as much as two-thirds of their length, and yet the alveolar borders, somewhat thickened, were smooth and even and the teeth themselves were healthy and *firmly fixed in their sockets*. This condition was a sign that the disease had become dormant after producing more or less severe lesions. In many cases there was no reason to doubt that the disease had been cured with the loss of one or several teeth.

The etiology of this condition in ancient Egyptians is by no means clear. The examination of the predynastic and dynastic Egyptian skulls from Naga el Deir, for instance, might lead to the conclusion that tartar had played a considerable rôle. Deposits of tartar on Egyptian teeth were common at all periods from predynastic to Coptic times, being laid down in layers round the tooth, and being always thickest at the margin of the gum. The teeth of other ancients besides Egyptians were sometimes thickly covered with it. Herodotus[1] relates that, after the battle of Plataea, there was found a skull in which "the upper jaw had teeth growing in a piece, all in one bone, both the front teeth and the grinders." The son of Prusias, king of Bithynia, and the king Pyrrhus are said to have been thus affected. Similar cases have been described in

[1] ix. 83.

modern times, where several or all the teeth even were imbedded in solid tartar.

Its presence is said to predispose to pyorrhoea and to hasten its progress by penetrating between the gum and the tooth, or between the alveolus and the tooth and thus loosening the latter. It is impossible to decide from the examination of a skull's teeth whether the tartar was deposited before or after the inception of pyorrhoea, but what the examination does show is that, very often, the deposit is confined to the necks of the teeth. It would appear, therefore, that tartar did not in those days play the important part which it is said to play now, and that in many cases its deposit on the root was of little if any pathogenic importance. The tartar was in many cases rather soft, white, and was fairly easily detached with the sharp end of a knife. This kind was most often seen in Roman, Coptic, and Greek skulls, whereas the brown variety was more common in predynastic Egyptian skulls. The enamel underneath was perfect.

Severe chronic suppurative periodontitis is so often associated with marked attrition of the teeth that the question arises whether the periodontal disease may not be caused, or at any rate rendered worse, by the latter. The answer to this question without clinical observations is well-nigh impossible. When the periodontitis and the subsequent suppuration and perforation into the mouth were most marked at the apex of the root, it is fair to assume that the infecting micro-organism entered by the dental canal, even if, as was usually the case, the pulp was unaltered. On the other hand, when the lesions were most marked at the alveolar borders, the probability was great that attrition had played no part. In many cases, probably, the micro-organisms causing chronic suppurative periodontitis were carried mechanically from the alveolar margin to the crown of the tooth and thus reached the bottom of the alveolus through an open dental canal.

VI. CORRELATION OF PATHOLOGICAL PROCESSES

Reading through the field notes of the Archaeological Survey of Nubia, the frequent coincidence of dental disease and of spondylitis deformans, or other chronic articular lesions, immediately attracts notice. These notes, it may be added, are all the more valuable because both observers were unprejudiced as to any theory regarding a possible correlation between lesions of the teeth and chronic joint disease.

Without going into the detail cases, a perusal of the records of the Survey makes it plain that spondylitis deformans and chronic osteo-arthritis coexisted in many cases and at all periods of Nubian history, and that often lesions of both were very severe.

The connection between chronic arthritis and dental disease is not disproved by the fact that in many cases of joint disease the dentition was stated to be healthy, for two reasons. The first is that in almost all cases of spondylitis the teeth were greatly worn, the pulp cavity was exposed, and thus a path for septic absorption was open. The second is that no mention is made of suppurative periodontitis which certainly did exist, as severe and multiple abscesses at the roots of the teeth were often mentioned and attributed to infection spreading down to the roots through the medullary canal opened by attrition. Undoubtedly infection often entered through this open path.

The author's opportunities of studying both diseases clinically have not been many, but the few observations on modern male Europeans and Egyptians in Egypt do not lead him to think that spondylitis is always caused by dental disease, e.g., pyorrhoea alveolaris. The few cases of chronic spondylitis (some of which have lasted for years) of which he obtained a good clinical history, had suffered from severe gonorrhoea, and several had not a trace of pyorrhoea. Moreover, pyorrhoea alveolaris is extremely common in Egypt now, whereas cases of severe chronic spondylitis are certainly not many. It is clear, however, that further investigations in these lines are desirable.

VII. SYPHILIS, RICKETS

Neither syphilitic nor rickety teeth were discovered, and this observation confirms the evidence derived from the study of skeletons, for no syphilitic bone dating from ancient times in Egypt has been unearthed so far, and rachitis was very rare indeed if it existed.

Sometimes the teeth were transversely striated, which was perhaps caused by some constitutional disturbance.

No lesions have been found pointing to the immoderate use of the toothbrush, and indeed there is no definite observation proving that ancient Egyptians used this instrument of torture. The teeth found in Alexandria and some of those from Faras and Merawi were remarkably clean and white, as a rule, and this may have been due to the use of some cleaning instrument during life; on the other hand, the predynastic, dynastic, and Coptic teeth were often covered with a thick layer of tartar.

VIII. DENTISTRY

The writer's studies have not revealed any facts showing that the Egyptians practised operative dentistry, in fact, the evidence rather points to the conclusion that even extraction was very seldom performed. It is not rare to find in Egyptian cemeteries diseased teeth almost dropping out of abscess cavities, or carious teeth which have caused extensive disease, and yet the patient was allowed to die without the relief that would have been afforded by a very simple operation. It is difficult to believe that extractions were not practised at times, but the evidence on that point is nil.

No tooth filled with gold or any other metal has been found. The only set of artificial teeth that has been discovered comes from a Roman grave and is deposited in the Alexandria Museum. Clearly it could have been of but little use in chewing and was probably tied in for aesthetic purposes only.

A similar set of teeth comes[1] from a grave of old Sidon, and two copper coins, an iron ring, a vase of most graceful outline, a scarab, and twelve very small statuettes of majolica representing Egyptian divinities, were found in the same grave. It consisted of four lower incisors (not "maxillary" as Gaillardot stated), and two canines held together by strong gold wire. Guerini pointed out that teeth strung together in the same manner are now being used in India.

[1] In Renan's *Mission de Phénicie*. See also Guerini, *History of Dentistry*, p. 29.

IX. CONCLUSIONS

1. Among ancient Egyptians, anomalies in position, structure, and number of the teeth were rare and did not seem to become more common as modern times were approached.

2. Attrition was, as it is now, very marked, and played probably a considerable part in favoring the entrance of the micro-organisms of suppuration, but not of those producing caries.

3. Dental caries occurred at all periods of Egyptian history. It is impossible to say for certain without more extensive statistics whether caries was much less common in ancient than in modern times, but the data from Tourah undoubtedly point to a very small percentage of caries in the predynastic period. Nothing definite is known regarding the incidence of caries in children.

4. Alveolar and perialveolar abscesses were common at all times in Egypt, and were evidently produced by the same processes as they are now. Attrition played some part in the etiology of these abscesses, but the majority were secondary to chronic suppurative periodontitis, and a few to caries.

5. Chronic suppurative periodontitis was a common disease in ancient Egypt, and the most frequent cause of the loss of teeth.

6. Spondylitis and osteo-arthritis were in numerous Nubians and Egyptians with diseased dentition, but a definite connection between the two affections has not been established.

7. No syphilitic or rachitic teeth have been found in the Egyptians up to and including the Coptic period.

8. There is no evidence to show that the toothbrush was in common use, and no such instrument has been found in Egyptian tomb deposits, but the Alexandrians and the people from Merawi and Faras appear to have used some cleaning instrument.

9. The severity of many of the lesions found post mortem—lesions which were undoubtedly very painful and could have been easily relieved—show that dentists did not interfere operatively in many if any cases.

10. A set of false teeth has been found dating from Roman times. This, however, like the one found at Sidon, was perhaps imported from Italy or Greece.

No one realizes more than the writer how incomplete this paper is, especially as regards statistics concerning the incidence of dental disease at various periods of Egyptian history, and the reason for this important lacuna is that the material which has been examined is unsuitable for statistical study. Satisfactory statistics of dental disease will be obtained only when large cemeteries containing bodies of several periods are excavated with due regard to pathological study; but up to the present, except in a very few cases, archaeologists have been more concerned about the objects found around skeletons than about the skeletons themselves.

DESCRIPTION OF PLATES LV-LXII

PLATE LV

Fig. 1.—Predynastic, Naga el Deir. Abnormalities of roots of molars.

Fig. 2.—Predynastic. Attrition of molars and premolars, crowding of incisors.

Fig. 3.—Ancient Nubian. Young adult. Accessory dental unit situated to lingual side of interval between right posterior premolar and first molar.

Fig. 4.—Predynastic. Great and oblique attrition of incisors and canines. Roots of premolars fused, labial wall of alveolus has disappeared, partly owing to post-mortem injury; there is, however, evidence of suppuration on the distal side of the posterior premolar. The molars disappeared long before death.

Fig. 5.—XIth Dynasty (from Murray's "The Tomb of Two Brothers"). Well-marked attrition; a supernumerary incisor; a bifid incisor.

Fig. 6.—Nubia. Supernumerary tooth at (a). (A. S. N.)

PLATE LVI

Fig. 1.—From Ras el Tin, Roman period. Alveolus of a tooth which was irregularly placed. Most teeth lost after death. Right canine and anterior premolar broken probably after death. Molar regions show signs of severe dental and perialveolar disease.

Fig. 2.—Predynastic, Naga el Deir. Alveoli of second molar and posterior premolar absorbed. Crowns of canine and anterior premolar show great attrition, especially on buccal side, whereas in the first molar the center of the crown is the part worn down most deeply. Canine covered with tartar at the neck. Some absorption of the alveoli of all the teeth, most marked round the root of first premolar which is bare for its whole length, and the wall opposite the tip of the root is smooth and rounded. Alveoli round roots of first molar also partly absorbed; that of second premolar almost completely absorbed, doubtless owing to long previous suppuration. Malposition of third molar.

Fig. 3.—Cleopatra's period. Faulty implantation of third molar. Alveolus of second molar completely absorbed.

Fig. 4.—Pyramid period (?). Some malposition of third lower molar; corresponding maxillary tooth is much smaller than its neighbor. Mandibular molars somewhat bare, alveolar borders showing signs of inflammation; second lower premolar bare and with distinct pitting of alveolar border. Roots of third upper molar bare, absorption of alveolar walls of first and second molars due to pathological process which, judging from the smoothness of the borders, was healing at the time of death.

Fig. 5.—From Ras el Tin, Roman period. Second left molar shows small oblong enamel nodule. Some absorption of alveolar wall of same tooth.

Fig. 6.—A Gizeh pyramid-builder. Third molar lower abnormally situated, corresponding upper tooth much smaller than its neighbor. Second molar lost during life, alveolus almost completely absorbed. Part of anterior root of first molar bare, but process of absorption appears to have stopped before death. Roots of anterior premolar and canine bare for about two-thirds of their lengths. Alveolar border of the three upper molars partly absorbed, leaving considerable part of roots completely bare. Borders of premolars and canine show marked signs of perialveolar inflammation.

PLATE LVII

Fig. 1.—From a pan grave at Ballalish. Early attrition of teeth. Third molar almost normal; second worn flat without formation of cavities; in first molar attrition more advanced, a cavity has formed on the proximal lingual and another, smaller, on distal lingual side. In first right molar similar cavities have coalesced. Remaining teeth show slight attrition, most marked in the first premolars in which three small cavities are forming.

Fig. 2.—From a pan grave at Ballalish. Early stage of attrition of all teeth. Incisors show narrow central groove in the biting edge. Attrition of first molar characteristic: right tooth worn into four distinct cavities, of which the two on the buccal side are coalescing. On left the two buccal and the distal cavities have united into one, the fourth being still separate. Second molars are slightly worn with formation of cavities near proximal surface. Third molar practically normal.

Fig. 3.—From a pan grave at Ballalish. Early attrition in a young adult, not marked near lingual border of first molar. Cavities in first and third molars.

Fig. 4.—Predynastic, Naga el Deir. Advanced, somewhat irregular attrition.

Fig. 5.—Cleopatra's period. Second molar lost before death, roots of all remaining teeth partly bare. Posterior premolar reduced to a carious stump at apex of which there is an abscess cavity, which communicates with alveolar cavity of proximal root of first molar.

FIG. 6.—Gizeh pyramid. Crown of first molar completely destroyed by caries, leaving two carious stumps. Tip of the posterior root almost completely absorbed. Alveolar wall had disappeared during life, bone underneath partly eaten away. Anterior root of the same tooth is almost completely bare. Roots of second and anterior root of third molar also bare, but some of the injury to alveolar wall probably post mortem. Perialveolar lesions of other teeth are slight, but all along alveolar border and for some distance below signs of chronic inflammation.

PLATE LVIII

FIG. 1.—Cleopatra's period. Maxilla of an elderly person. Crowns of remaining teeth show great attrition, especially left premolars and first left molar. Beginning caries of this tooth on its approximal border. Caries of left second molar posteriorly. First right premolar broken after death. All right molars lost during life. Hole seen at (x) made after death.

FIG. 2.—Predynastic, Naga el Deir. Lesions of chronic suppurating periodontitis along whole length of alveolar border. Roots of incisors and canine bare for some distance, and alveolar border over lateral incisor pitted. First premolar's root bare and tip of alveolar wall absorbed, only a narrow bridge of bone being left. The tooth is much worn. Second premolar shows similar changes, and bone about tip of the root and all round deeply pitted as result of suppuration. Almost whole of alveolar wall of first molar absorbed, and remainder carried by chronic periodontitis. Alveolar margin round two remaining molars somewhat pitted. All teeth show yellow tartar.

FIG. 3.—Coptic. Advanced oblique attrition; signs of alveolar suppuration.

FIG. 4.—Predynastic, Naga el Deir. Advanced attrition; incisors and canines deeply worn on lingual side. Dental canal of all premolars opened. Marked signs of chronic suppuration round the side of first right molar which has been shed during life and the alveolus of which is partly obliterated, and round second premolar on same side the buccal wall of whose alveolus has been absorbed; the tooth has been "dislocated," so that its root lies almost at a right angle to those of other teeth. The tooth had become firmly fixed in that position, for a small flat surface, evidently the result of mastication, had formed on the side of the root. Lesions of chronic periodontitis exist all along the alveolar borders of both remaining right molars, canines, and incisors. Left second premolar with first and second molars were shed during life as a result of process resembling that noticeable on the right side.

FIG. 5.—XIIth–XVIth Dynasties. Interior root of first molar contained in a smooth-walled cavity, result of previous inflammation and suppuration (suppurative periodontitis), tip of root surrounded by layer of new bone. Superficial periostitis below first molar.

ABNORMALITIES OF ANCIENT EGYPTIAN TEETH

PLATE LIX

FIG. 1.—Coptic skull. Advanced caries of first right molar. A sinus had formed and pus had perforated through palate. The sinus leading from tooth to palate was still plain.

FIG. 2.—Macedonian period, Chatby. Attrition of teeth which are planted somewhat irregularly. Large accumulation of tartar at junction of root of first right molar with the crown; tooth dislocated towards the labial side owing to intense suppurative periodontitis; small perforation in the crown of the tooth accidental.

FIG. 3.—Predynastic, Naga el Deir. Advanced and irregular attrition. An abscess about posterior root of first right molar.

FIG. 4.—Coptic period. Alveolus of left anterior premolar completely absorbed, a thin bridge of bone superiorly being all that remains of it; pus had evidently burrowed into the neighboring parts of the mandible; alveolus itself of normal size. In neighboring teeth same process has been going on, for the roots are partly bare, and at apex of root of posterior premolar a sinus has been formed. Other side was equally badly afflicted and upper jaw of same skull is almost edentulous, and had been so for some time before death, for the alveoli had been so completely absorbed that not a trace is left. The suppurating process, therefore, had attacked the whole mouth and had lasted for years before the patient finally succumbed.

FIG. 5.—Roman period, Kom el Shougafa. Roots almost completely bare.

PLATE LX

FIG. 1.—Coptic skull. All roots exposed. Lower third molar lost during life, its alveolus completely absorbed. Second molar has deep carious cavity on buccal side of root. Alveoli of second and first molars completely absorbed on the buccal side, probably owing to long-continued suppuration. Roots of the other teeth also bare.

FIG. 2.—Predynastic, Naga el Deir. Third molar fell out during life, and there are signs of perialveolar inflammation at (*a*). Roots of second molar completely bare, lying in open cavities which doubtless were filled with pus during life. Signs of chronic periodontitis all along the alveolar border.

FIG. 3.—From a pan grave, Ballalish. Deep-seated abscess connected with alveolus of lateral incisor, perforating through the palate into mouth.

FIG. 4.—Cleopatra's period, Ras el Tin. First molar wholly bare, owing to chronic rarefying periostitis. Roots of premolars partly bare; second and third molars nearly normal.

FIG. 5.—Cleopatra's period, Ras el Tin. Both left premolars and first molar lost during life and left lateral incisor carious. An oval opening with smooth borders, 12 by 8 mm. in outer wall of the jaw in alveolar border, in premolar region. An aperture artificially made through the external wall of the mandible leads into a smooth-walled cavity, 36 by 2 mm., in which roots of canine, lateral incisor, and anterior root of second molar are exposed. During life, therefore, these roots lay in extensive abscess cavity which, after the premolars and first molars had been lost, communicated by a wide opening with the mouth.

Fig. 6.—Predynastic, Naga el Deir. Molars and premolars with advanced lesions of periodontitis, most marked round first and second molars. Many little pits due to the inflammatory process seen along whole length of alveolar border.

PLATE LXI

Fig. 1.—Predynastic, Naga el Deir. Incisors lost, crowns of canine and first molar broken, probably post mortem. Crowns of premolars and first molar markedly and obliquely worn. Root of second molar bare for considerable length, and near its tip there is a deep cavity which connects with alveoli of second and first molars.

Fig. 2.—Predynastic, Naga el Deir. The third molar was evidently very small. Root of second molar somewhat exposed and crown distinctly worn. One root of first molar bare for almost its whole length. Distinct pitting round the roots of the premolars which are bare.

Fig. 3.—Predynastic, Naga el Deir. Crown of first molar deeply worn, root surrounded by open space which during life was doubtless filled with pus. Signs of inflammation all round this root and for some distance along the palate. Second molar's root partly bare, crown worn. Third molar was probably small.

Fig. 4.—Predynastic. Abscess cavity at base of first premolar which was shed before death. Crown of second premolar broken post mortem, its alveolar wall completely absorbed, and alveolus evidently communicated with abscess cavity of first premolar. The upper part of abscess wall especially near alveolar border shows signs of active pathological process, whereas lower part of wall is smooth, rounded as if pathological process had been quiescent there. Tip of root of second premolar is rounded off as if part had been absorbed.

Fig. 5.—Cleopatra's period, Ras el Tin. Right incisor and canine lost after death, second and third molars during life. Whole left molar and premolar region is changed into a huge cavity with spongy wall, owing to absorption of alveolar and interalveolar septa.

Fig. 6.—Meroitic kingdom, Faras. Middle-aged person. Completely edentulous upper jaw.

Fig. 7.—Predynastic, Naga el Deir. Advanced suppurative periodontitis. All the teeth were shed during life and the alveoli with their borders show signs of inflammation and suppuration.

PLATE LV

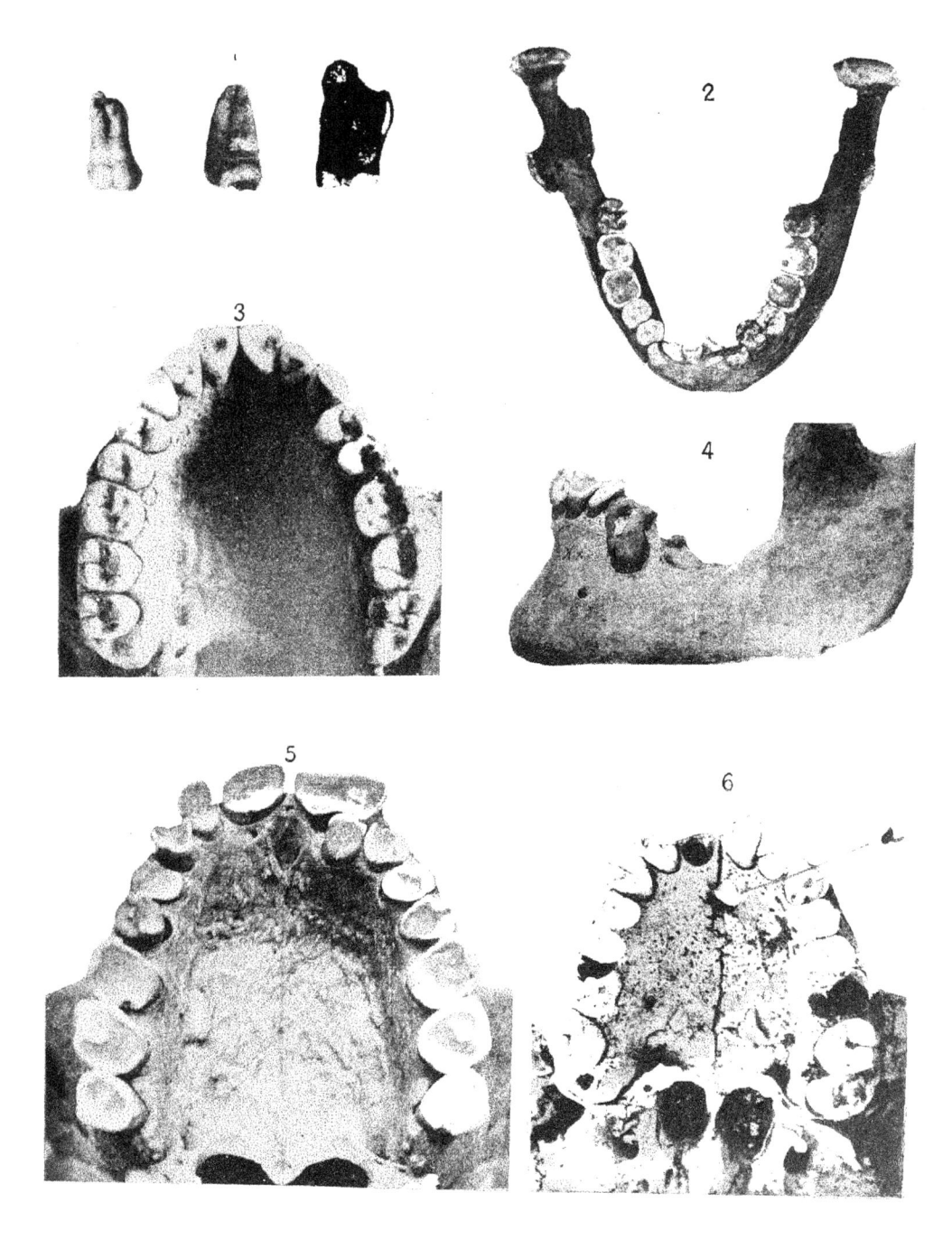

PTATE LVI

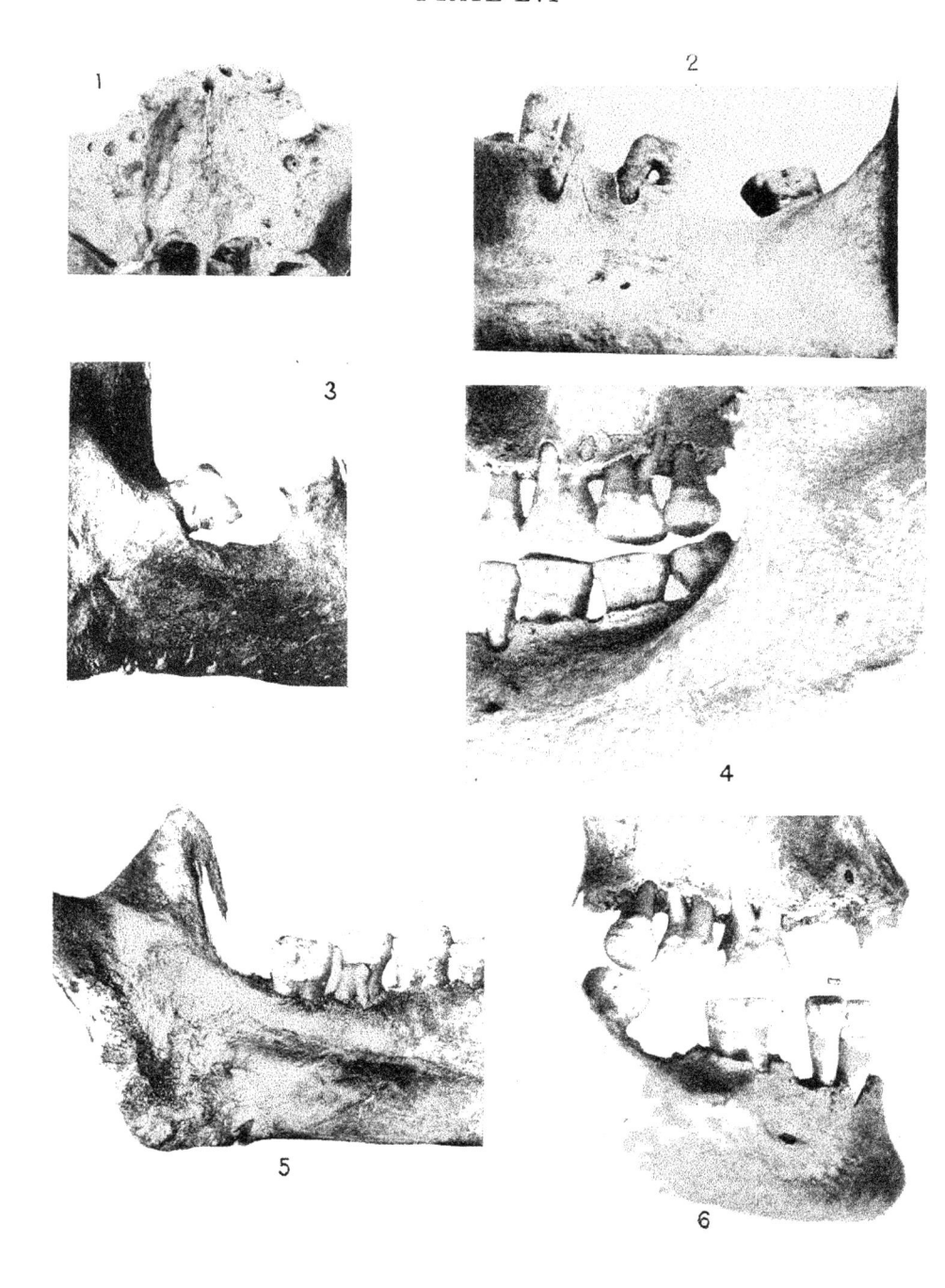

PLATE LVII

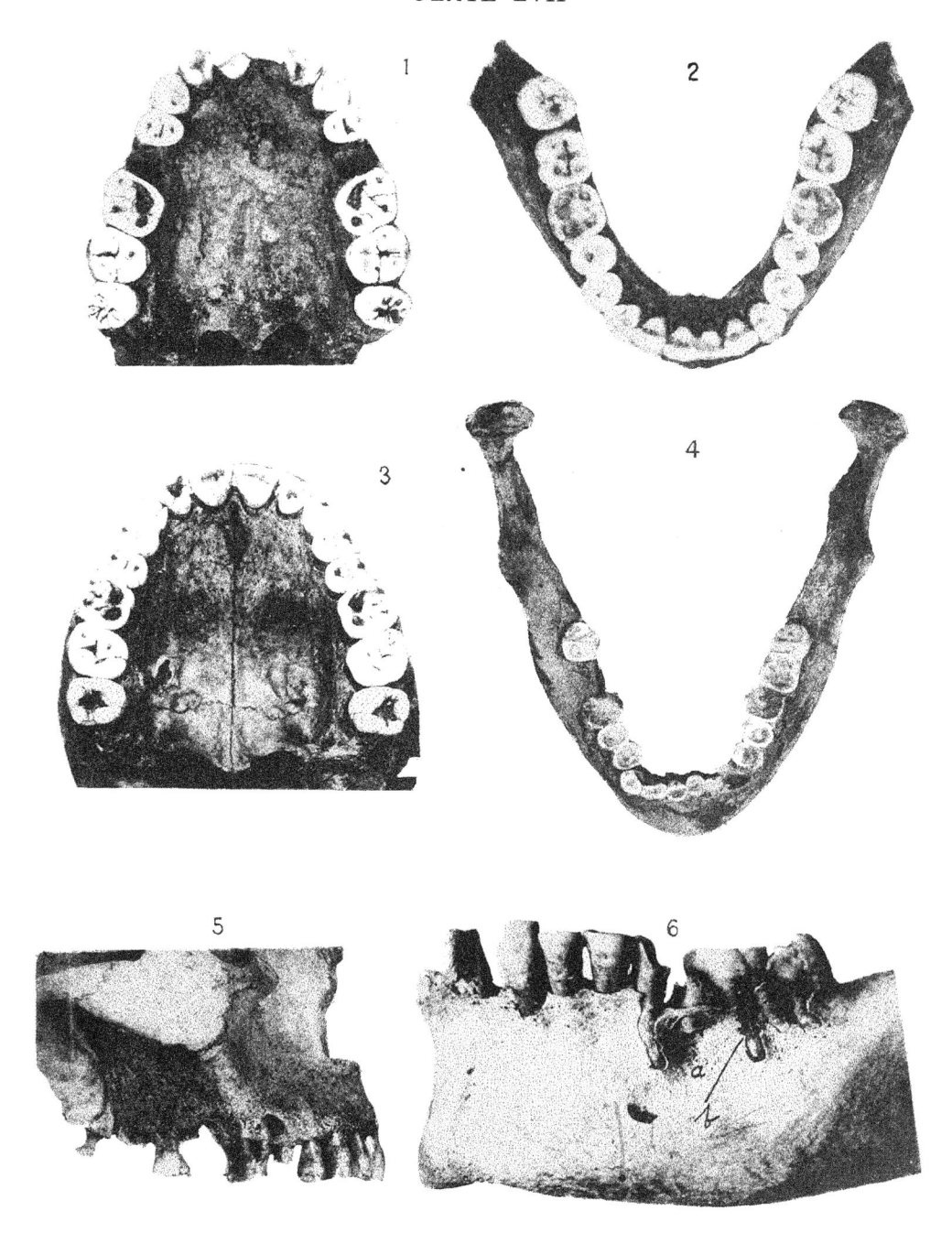

PLATE LVIII

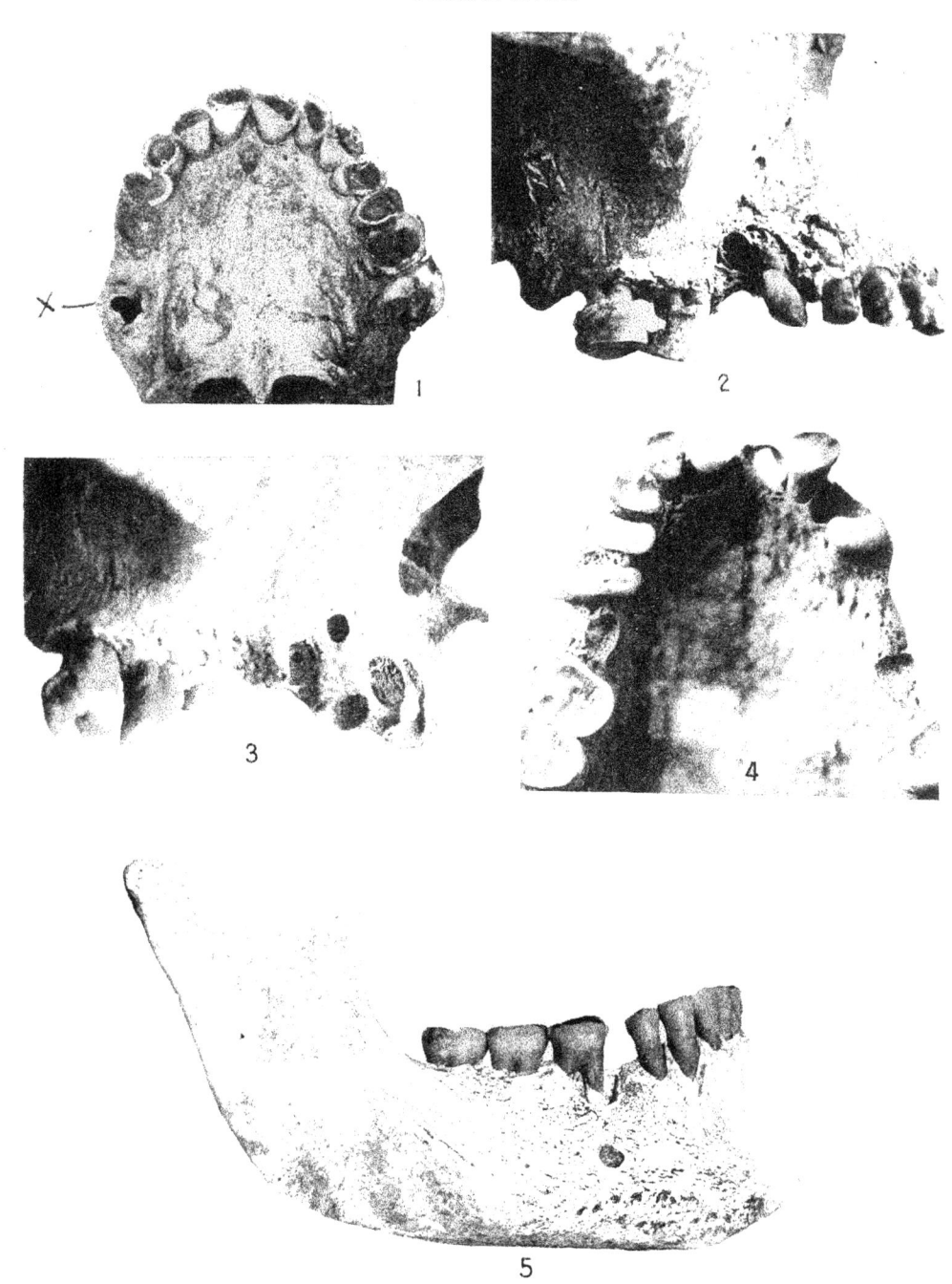

PLATE LIX

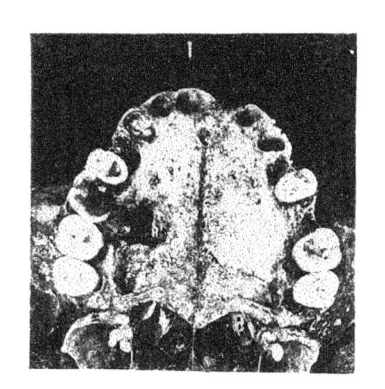

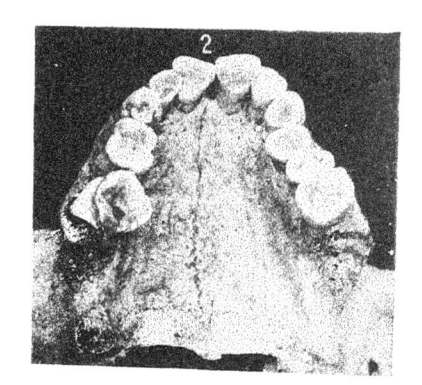

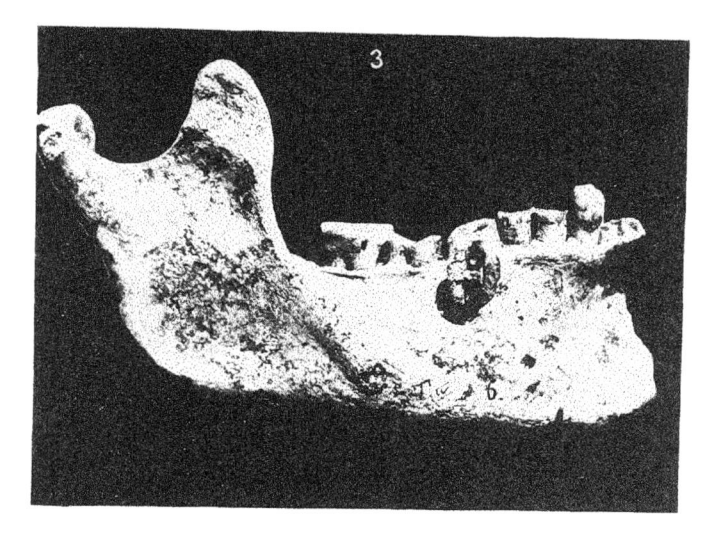

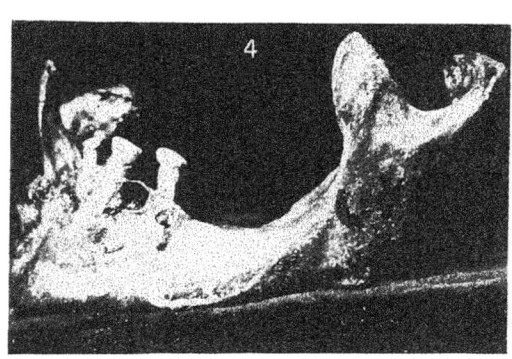

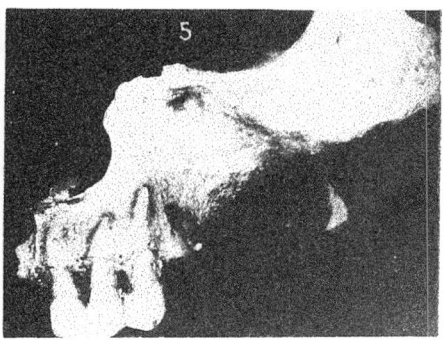

PLATE LX

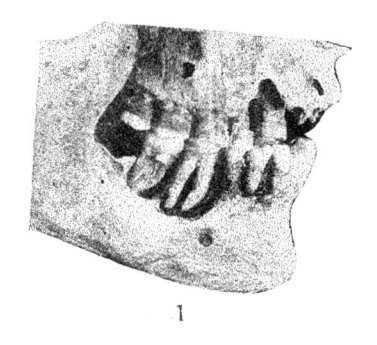

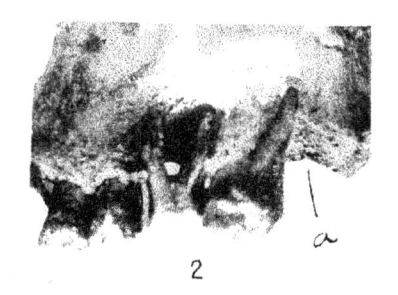

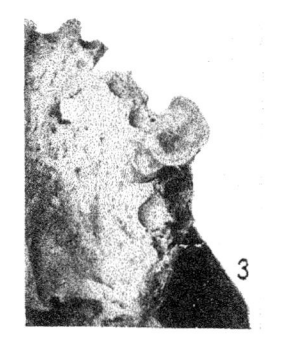

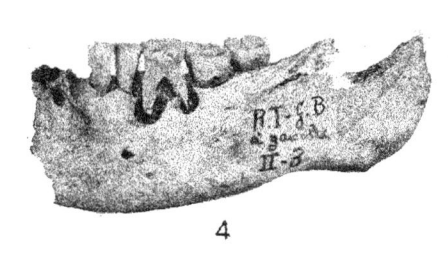

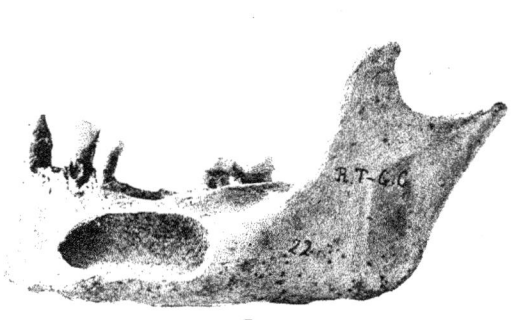

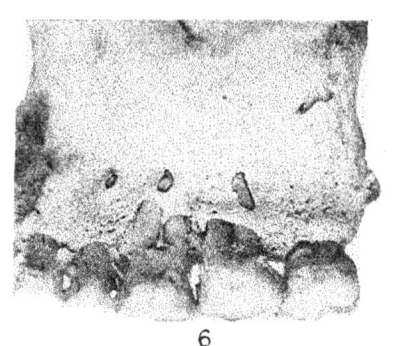

PLATE LXI

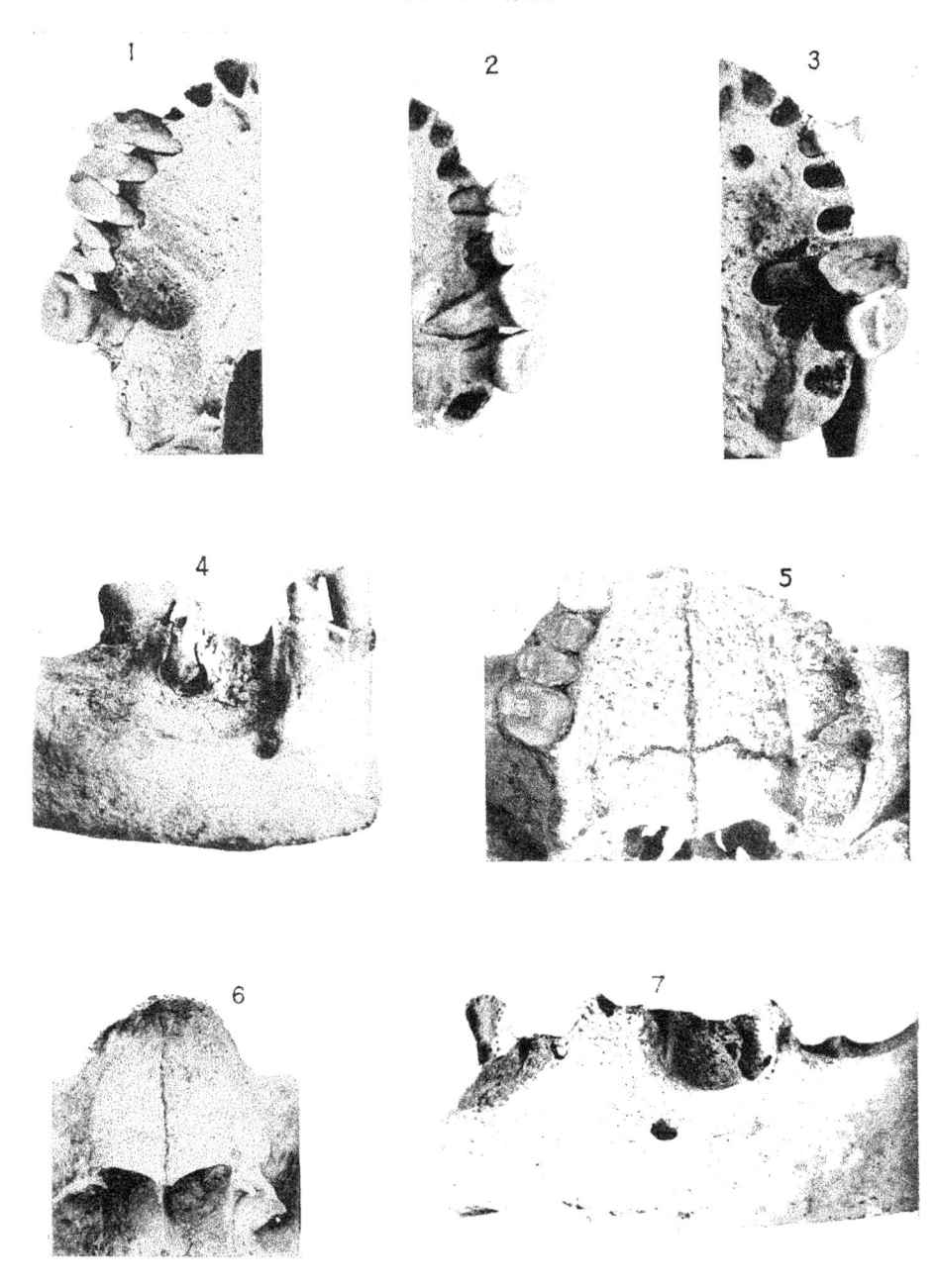

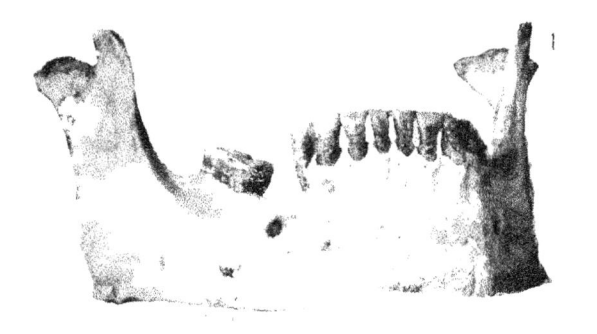

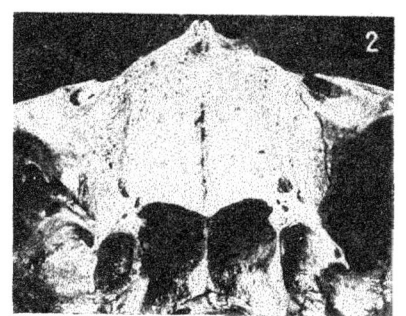

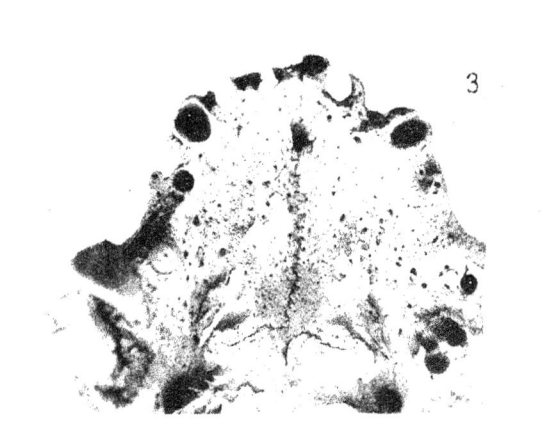

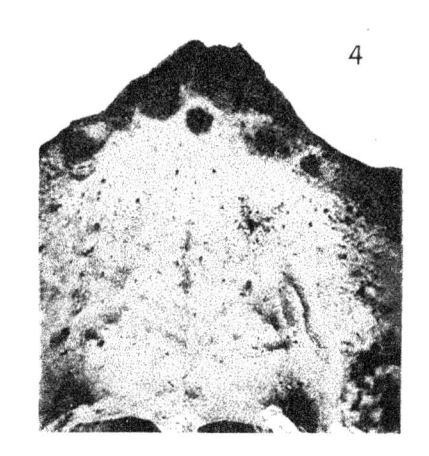

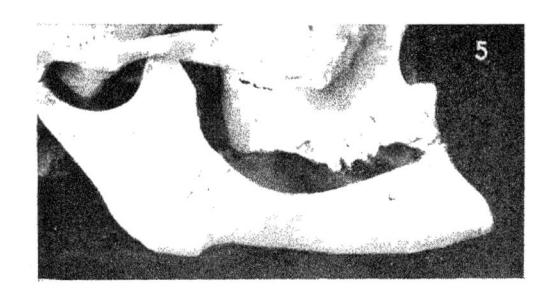

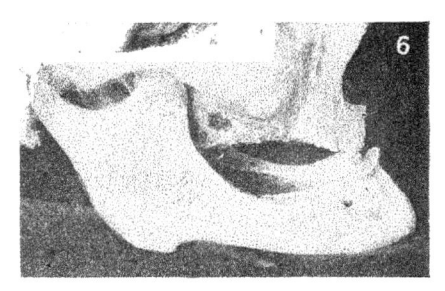

PLATE LXII

PLATE LXII

FIG. 1.—Coptic period. Transverse striation of teeth.

FIG. 2.—Coptic period. Old woman. Completely edentulous upper jaw. Alveolar process has entirely disappeared.

FIG. 3.—Predynastic, Naga el Deir. Most teeth lost during life, possibly owing to chronic periodontitis. Enlarged blood-vessel canals all over the palate.

FIG. 4.—Predynastic, Naga el Deir. Edentulous maxilla with alveolar borders almost completely absorbed. Foramina of blood vessels on palate enlarged.

FIG. 5.—Meroitic kingdom. Middle-aged man. Completely edentulous mandible and almost completely edentulous upper jaw.

FIG. 6.—Meroitic kingdom. Edentulous skull.

ON THE PHYSICAL EFFECTS OF CONSANGUINEOUS MARRIAGES IN THE ROYAL FAMILIES OF ANCIENT EGYPT

(*Proceedings of the Royal Society of Medicine, Section of the History of Medicine*, XII [1919], 145-90)

The question of the effect on the offspring of marriage between blood relations is still an open one. Whereas the view that the children of consanguineous marriages are likely to be weak and to be the bearers of some congenital defect is widely held, some students of heredity maintain that the facts on which this view is based are not convincing; and it must be admitted that, from the same data, divergent conclusions have been drawn. Thus the Veddahs of Ceylon systematically practise consanguineous marriage, and some years ago a lurid picture was drawn of the evil effects of these unions. The race, it was asserted, was becoming extinct, the people were stupid, sullen, and degenerated, children had disappeared from the villages, in which adults only were to be seen, and so on. Yet these fears were groundless, for the Veddahs have remained a very simple, harmless, and monogamous tribe.

In Europe the marriage of first cousins is not uncommon, but the effect of such unions on the offspring is still a matter for controversy, and some medical men categorically deny its dangers. Again the evidence is conflicting. At the Institution for Deaf-mutes in Paris, for instance, the percentage of deaf-mutes born from consanguineous marriages was 28.35 per cent, whereas in similar Scotch and English institutions it amounted to 5.17 per cent only.

The investigations of George Darwin did not reveal any distinct connexion between infertility, deaf-mutism, insanity or idiocy and consanguineous marriages; but this observer thought that the vitality of the children of first cousins was somewhat below normal, and that the death-rate was slightly higher than in the offspring of other unions. Observations made in France and in Denmark do not seem to prove the peril of such unions, and the facts collected in non-European countries are not convincing. When, for instance, the enormous mortality among Persian children is attributed to consanguineous marriages, the fact that in certain Eastern towns the death-rate in children less than one year old amounts to 30 per cent should be first accounted for.

Nevertheless, the majority of modern people exhibit in their legislation a conviction of the perils of consanguineous marriage, and believe that all kinds of evils threaten the offspring of such unions. It is strange, however, that this idea appears to be entirely modern, for although some ancient peoples were opposed to incestuous marriages, there is no reason to believe that this prohibition was due to a belief in evil results to the offspring.

Marriage[1] with a half-sister, not uterine, occurred in Athens, in late times. The Greeks and Romans of the classical period looked upon incest as a crime, though voices occasionally inquired the reason for this opinion, and the fable of Myrrha,[2] who conceived an incestuous passion for her father, is well known. The heroine pointedly asks why incest should be a crime among men when it is the rule among animals. "Defend me," she cries, "from a crime so great! *if indeed this be a crime.* It is not considered shameful for the heifer to mate with her sire; his own daughter becomes the mate of the horse; the he-goat, too, consorts with the flocks of which he is the father; and the bird conceives by him from whose seed she herself is conceived. Happy they to whom these things are allowed! The case of man has provided harsh laws, and what Nature permits, malignant ordinances forbid." Myrrha goes on to envy the fate of the nations which allow incestuous relationships.

Consanguineous marriages were not uncommon in early Hebrew records: Sarah was Abraham's[3] half-sister; during Jacob's life marriages between first cousins were allowed; Moses[4] sprang from a marriage between a nephew and his paternal aunt; and even in David's time[5] a marriage between half-brother and sister was allowed.

In Egypt, from very early times, marriages between brother and sister were fashionable, whereas incestuous unions between father

---

[1] Robertson Smith, *Kinship and Marriage*, p. 191.
[2] Ovid *Metamorphoses* x. 8.
[3] Gen. 20:12.   [4] Num. 26:59.   [5] II Sam. 13:13.

and daughter, or mother and son, were very rare, if indeed they ever took place. The Egyptian gods themselves had set the example of incest; Keb, the earth-god, and Nut, the sky-goddess, had four children—two sons, Osiris and Set, and two daughters, Isis and Nephthys—and children were taught that Osiris married Isis and Set took Nephthys to wife. Isis' lament at the loss of Osiris leaves one in no doubt as to the relationship between the two: "Come to her who loves thee, who loves thee, Wennoffre, thou blessed one. Come to thy sister, come to thy wife, thou whose heart is still. Come to her who is mistress of thy house. I am thy sister, born of the same mother, thou shalt not be far from me. . . . . Thou lovest none beside me, my brother, my brother."

The royal families followed this lead. Throne and property being inherited through the woman, mother or wife, as legal head of the house, it was very doubtful, says Petrie, "whether a king could reign, except as the husband of the heiress of the kingdom." As the king was the ruler, while the queen, though the heiress to the throne, had no executive power, the only way to keep the regal power in the family was for the nearest male descendant of a king to marry the heiress, who was very often his sister. In considering this relationship, as described in Egyptian records, caution is however necessary. The word "sister," often a euphemism for mistress or concubine, also meant sometimes the wife of a temporary marriage, or was even used as a term of endearment. The confusion has been increased by the fact that "Royal Sister" was one of the queen's titles, which did not imply that Her Majesty stood in that relationship to her consort. Therefore, in this study, I shall consider a king and queen to have been brother and sister only when there is sure evidence that they were so related.

The marriages of brothers and sisters were frequent among common people also as late as Greek, Roman, and early Christian times. Diodorus Siculus,[1] at the beginning of our era, mentions such marriages among Egyptians. An Amherst papyrus[2] contains an application from a woman asking that her son Artemon might be admitted to the list of privileged persons wholly or partially exempt

[1] Diodorus Siculus i. 1.
[2] Grenfell and Hunt, *Amherst Papyri*, p. 90, No. 75.

EFFECTS OF CONSANGUINEOUS MARRIAGES

from the poll-tax. The basis of the claim is that the ancestors of the boy on both sides were descendants from a gymnasiarch, and that therefore the boy himself had the right to be included among those "of the gymnasium." The genealogy of Artemon reveals, on the mother's side at least, three successive cases of intermarriage between brother and sister.

The custom persisted during the early Christian era. A papyrus,[1] dating from A.D. 108, gives a marriage contract between a certain Apollonios, a Persian τῆς ἐπιγονῆς, and his sister Tapeutis; another Persian married his sister Marouti, and a third married his sister Erieus. Wessely[2] published several genealogical tables of Egyptian families from which it appears that in four well-to-do families incestuous marriages were in the majority, and it has been stated[3] that, under the emperor Commodus, two-thirds of the citizens of Arsinoë had married their sisters.

As consanguineous unions were so common, the evil results should have been numerous and have attracted popular notice. Yet, as far as I know, no such observations are recorded in Egyptian literature. In what follows we shall select for illustration only those royal families the physical and mental characters of the individuals of which are known.

EIGHTEENTH-DYNASTY KINGS

Queen Aahotep I, the heiress of the royal line of Hierakonpolis, married first a man (name unknown) who was certainly her brother, for on the stele of Abydos, put up in honour of his (and his wife's) grandmother, Tetishera, her son Ahmose I exclaims: "I it is who have remembered the mother of my mother and the mother of my father, Tetishera."[4] The queen's second husband was Seqenenra, who was a relative, and perhaps a brother. The mummy of this slim and remarkably muscular king, who died fighting the Hyksos, measured 1.702 m. in length, and the cranium is 0.195 m. long and 0.131 m. broad. The portrait of Queen Aahotep I, on the lid of

---

[1] J. Nietzold, *Die Ehe in Ägypten*, p. 13.
[2] *Ibid.*   [3] Erman, *Life in Ancient Egypt*, p. 153.
[4] Petrie, *A History of Egypt*, I, 225.

her coffin in Cairo, is that of a well-nourished young person with good features. She had eleven children by her two husbands.[1]

Ahmose I, who was thus the son of an incestuous union, married his sister or half-sister, Nefertari (Figs. 1 and 2), whose wooden statuette at Turin represents a buxom, well-formed woman, with no obvious sign of degeneration. After reigning for twenty-five years with Ahmose I, she acted as adviser to her son, Amenhotep I, and must have been fairly advanced in years at the time of her death. She was "the first of those queens by divine right who, scorning the inaction of the harem, took on themselves the right to fulfil the active duties of a sovereign."[2] After her death the people raised her to divine rank; she, together with her son, Amenhotep I, sprung from the marriage with her brother, were regarded as specially "gracious and helpful." Her name was put on the same plane as those of the great gods, and she was worshipped for six hundred years after her death.

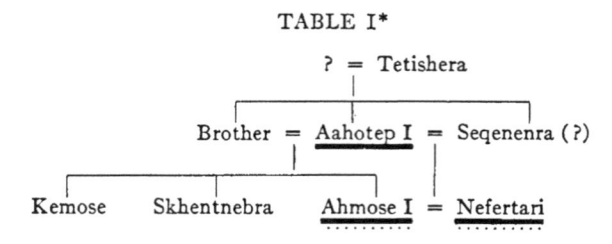

TABLE I*

```
              ? = Tetishera
                   |
        ┌──────────┴──────────┐
   Brother = Aahotep I = Seqenenra (?)
                   |
        ┌──────┬───┴────┬──────────┐
     Kemose  Skhentnebra  Ahmose I = Nefertari
```

* [In this and the following tables I have underlined the descendants of consanguineous marriages with a full line, and the rulers (who succeeded to the throne for the most part by right of marriage with their sister-wives) with a dotted line.—ALICE RUFFER.]

Ahmose I, her brother and husband, ascended the throne about 1580 B.C., when Egypt was endeavouring to throw off the yoke of foreign conquerors, the hated Hyksos, who for nearly two hundred years had ruled the country. During his brilliant reign of twenty-four years this great king drove the aliens out of Egypt, and by carefully protecting the frontier made a new invasion extremely difficult. He thus made Egypt a strong military state and established the dynasty on a firm footing. His successors conquered Syria and held it for several generations in spite of the repeated risings of local

[1] Petrie, *Abydos*, III, Plate LII. [2] *Ibid.*

chiefs. Ahmose also began the restoration of the buildings of Upper Egypt, which had fallen into decay under the Hyksos rule. He died at the age of fifty-five. His mummy measures 1.63 m. in length. The face, like that of all the rulers of the earlier Eighteenth Dynasty, is comparatively small, the nose prominent, though in the dried body this organ looks small and narrow; the face is ovoid, the chin narrow, the superciliary ridge fairly marked, and the upper teeth are prominent as in the women of the family and in Thutmose II. The length of the head (including wrappings) is 0.207 m., and the breadth (without wrappings), 0.156 m.

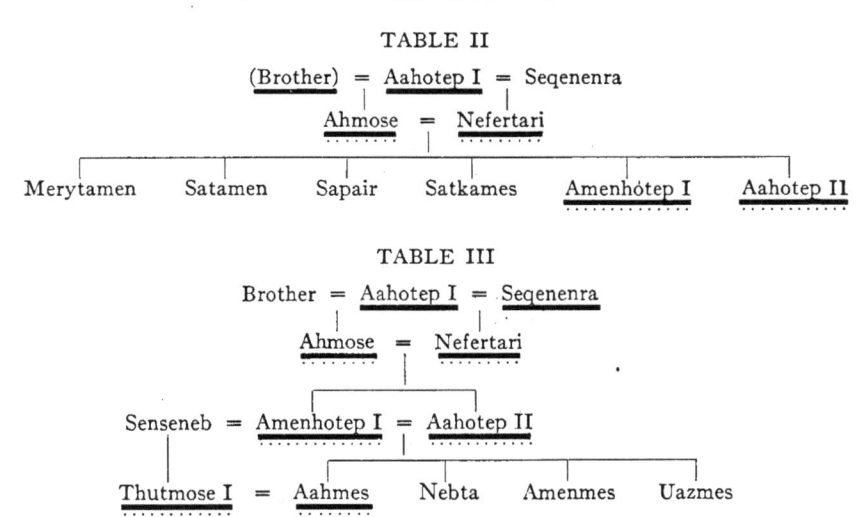

TABLE II

```
        (Brother) = Aahotep I = Seqenenra
                        |
                  Ahmose = Nefertari
                        |
   ┌─────────┬─────────┬─────────┬─────────┬─────────┐
Merytamen  Satamen  Sapair  Satkames  Amenhotep I  Aahotep II
```

TABLE III

```
        Brother = Aahotep I = Seqenenra
                        |
                  Ahmose = Nefertari
                        |
          Senseneb = Amenhotep I = Aahotep II
                        |
        ┌──────────┬─────────┬─────────┬─────────┐
   Thutmose I = Aahmes   Nebta   Amenmes   Uazmes
```

Amenhotep I, son of Ahmose I, reconquered Nubia, repelled an attack of the Libyans, invaded Syria, and reached the Euphrates. He added to the temple of Karnak and to those on the opposite bank of the Nile. The divine honours which were paid to him for nigh six hundred years after his death bear witness to the strength of his personality (Fig. 3). He reigned twenty-one years, and died when fifty-six years old.[1] His mummy in the Cairo Museum, not yet unrolled, is that of a short man, measuring 1.65 m. in length.

Of his sister and wife, Aahotep II, little is known. The union brought forth four children—two sons, Amenmes and Uazmes,[2] and

[1] Petrie, *A History of Egypt*, I, 54. [2] Buttles, *The Queens of Egypt*, p. 71.

two daughters, Aahmes and Nebta. One of the sons was associated for a time with his father in governing the country. One daughter, Aahmes, married her half-brother, Thutmose I, the son of her father by Senseneb, probably a slave. Her portrait adorns the walls of the temple of Deir el Bahri (Fig. 5), and without doubt her expression is fascinating; the features are refined and it would be difficult to find a nobler countenance than that of this queen, the descendant of incestuous marriages of great-grandparents, grandparents, and parents. The length of her life is unknown.

Her husband and half-brother, Thutmose I, ascended the throne about 1535 B.C., led an expedition into Nubia, forced his way through the Cataract, and seized and strongly fortified the country. He then invaded Syria and reached Naharin, that is, the country from the Orontes to the Euphrates and beyond, where he slew or made prisoners many of his foes. At home he was a passionate and successful builder. He built the temple of Set at Nubt, near Negadah, the great temple of Medinet Abou, probably designed the temple of Deir el Bahri, added pylons and an obelisk to the temple of Karnak, and protected his country by rebuilding the frontier defenses. He died at the age of forty-eight, after celebrating the thirtieth anniversary of his coronation.

The authenticity of the mummy (Fig. 4) supposed to be that of Thutmose I is not quite certain, though the likeness to Thutmose II leaves little doubt that this mummy is that of Thutmose I or some near relative. It is 1.54 m. long. The cranium measures 0.18 by 0.133 m., and the narrow, long, refined face is that of a clever and cunning person.

The marriage of Aahmes with her half-brother, Thutmose I, had issue, two sons and two daughters, of whom both boys and one daughter died young. The second daughter, Queen Hatshepsut I, in spite of opposition, was associated with her father in the government of the kingdom. Thutmose I had married, beside Queen Aahmes, a woman of only half-royal lineage, Mut-nefert; and Hatshepsut, following the royal tradition, married her half-brother, Thutmose II, born from the latter marriage.

Thutmose II added a pylon to Karnak, decorated the temple with statues, and inscriptions relating to his work are met with as far as Barkal in the Sudan and the Oasis of Farafra. The mask, statues, and mummy of Thutmose II (Fig. 6) represent a smiling and amiable countenance, with features somewhat weaker than those of Thutmose I, whom he otherwise resembles. The body is thin, somewhat shrunken, and not very muscular, and measures 1.684 m., the bald head being 0.191 m. long by 0.149 m. broad, and the face wrinkled.

Thutmose's half-sister and queen, Hatshepsut, proved an exception to the rule that the female members of the family inherited the Egyptian crown but exerted no authority, for she overshadowed her husband and was the actual sovereign, and he merely the king-consort. She "acted as master of the country. The kingdom was subjected to her will. Egypt bowed its head."[1]

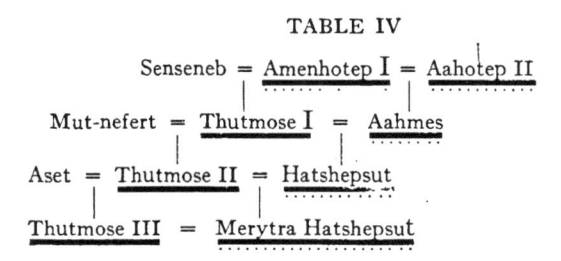

TABLE IV

```
       Senseneb = Amenhotep I = Aahotep II
                       |
  Mut-nefert = Thutmose I = Aahmes
                    |
   Aset = Thutmose II = Hatshepsut
                    |
   Thutmose III = Merytra Hatshepsut
```

After the death of Thutmose II, the queen, according to the custom of the country, shared the kingdom with her nearest male relative, Thutmose III, the son of her former husband by Asat, who apparently was not of royal birth.

To strengthen her position, the queen claimed direct descent from the god Amon, and her miraculous conception, birth, and education are recorded on the walls of the Luxor temple. With remarkable energy she restored many buildings, built the temple of Deir el Bahri, began the façade at Speos Artemides, brought an obelisk from Nubia to Luxor, and fitted out an expedition to the land of Punt, which returned with great treasure, quaint animals, and plants. Her reign was perhaps too peaceful, as it was probably during this period that some of the Asiatic provinces were lost to Egypt. A wise ruler, she exercised her power with justice and

[1] Maspero, *The Struggle of the Nations*, p. 42.

moderation during her long reign, and throughout the Nile Valley, from Buto in the Delta, by way of Beni-Hassan, Karnak and Thebes, El Kab, and Kom Ombo, to Assouan at the First Cataract of the Nile, and from the far rock cliffs of Sinai, sculptured stone and inscribed stele record the reign of Hatshepsut, fulfilling the wish voiced in her temple that her name may remain and live on in temple and land for "ever and ever." Nothing, unfortunately, is known about her personal appearance, as the Luxor and Deir el Bahri portraits are conventional and for the most part obliterated by her successors.

No less remarkable than Hatshepsut was her nephew and stepson, Thutmose III,[1] the son of a father descended from a series of incestuous marriages, and of a mother who was not of royal blood. After Hatshepsut's death he became one of the strongest rulers in Egyptian history; during her lifetime his influence had not been felt. His Majesty was somewhat short, measuring 1.615 m., his cranium was 0.196 m. long and 0.150 m. broad, and though he died at an advanced age his mummy with its distinguished features gives, in spite of the bald head, the impression of a youngish person. The upper teeth project greatly (Fig. 7).

His character stands forth with more of colour and individuality than that of any king of early Egypt, except Akhnaton. We see the man of a tireless energy unknown in any Pharaoh before or since, the man of versatility, designing exquisite vases in a moment of leisure; the lynx-eyed administrator, who launched his armies upon Asia with one hand and with the other crushed the extortionate tax-gatherer.[2]

Thutmose III left his mark on Heliopolis, where he erected the two famous obelisks, on Abu Sir, Memphis, Gurob, etc. Koptos was entirely rebuilt, Karnak was extended, Medinet Abou and Deir el Bahri were completed, more than thirty different sites in Egypt and Nubia were built over, and innumerable fragments of statues, sphinxes, etc., testify to the building activity of this great warrior.

His reign marks an epoch not only in Egypt, but in the whole East as we know it in his age. Never before in history had a single brain wielded the

---

[1] Thutmose III is held by some to have been the son of Thutmose I and not of Thutmose II. If that be true, he married not his sister but his niece. See Petrie, *A History of Egypt*, II, 78.

[2] Breasted, *A History of Egypt*.

resources of so great a nation and wrought them into such centralized, permanent, and at the same time, mobile efficiency, that for years they could be brought to bear with incessant impact upon another continent as a skilled artizan manipulates a hundred-ton forge hammer; although that figure is inadequate unless we remember that Thutmose forged his own hammer. The genius which rose from an obscure priestly office to accomplish this for the first time in history reminds us of an Alexander or of a Napoleon. He built the first real empire, and is thus the first character possessed of universal aspects, the first world hero. He made not only a world-wide impression upon his age, but an impression of a new order. His commanding figure, towering like an embodiment of righteous penalty among the trivial plots and treacherous schemes of the petty Syrian dynasts, must have clarified the atmosphere of Oriental politics as a strong wind drives away miasmic vapours. The inevitable chastisement of his strong arm was held in awed remembrance by the men of Naharin for three generations. His name was one to conjure with, and centuries after his empire had crumbled to pieces, it was placed on amulets as a word of power.[1]

He died at the age of sixty-three.

Thutmose III married his half-sister, Merytra Hatshepsut, Queen Hatshepsut's daughter, and also another woman, Sat-Aah. The number of his children is unknown, but he is said to have had eight daughters.

Amenhotep II, the son of Thutmose III and Merytra Hatshepsut, was 1.63 m. in height. He was associated with his father in government for some time, and ascended the throne when about eighteen to twenty years old, reigned for twenty-five years, and died at the age of forty-six. His physical strength was extraordinary, and he claimed that no one could bend his bow. (Fig. 8).

On the death of Thutmose III, the Syrian tribes almost simultaneously rose in revolt, but they had not reckoned with the boundless energy of the new king. Amenhotep II left Egypt with his army in April and already in May defeated the Syrians in a battle in which he with his own hand took eighteen prisoners and fifteen horses. He advanced with irresistible power, crossed the Euphrates triumphantly, returned to Egypt, and, equally successful in the South, conquered part of the Sudan.

Amenhotep II married Tiaa,[2] who may have been his half-sister by a mother not of royal birth. Their son, Thutmose IV (Fig. 9),

[1] Breasted, *op. cit.* [2] Buttles, *op. cit.*, p. 101.

an energetic lion-hunter in his youth, came to the throne at the age of twenty-four, and showed his energy by leading an expedition to Syria, from which he returned with a cargo of cedar and many prisoners. He contracted an alliance with Babylonia and with the Mitannian king, whose daughter, Mutemuya,[1] he married. He died at the age of thirty-three.

Thutmose IV was followed by his sixteen-year-old son, Amenhotep III, who married the celebrated Tiy (Fig. 11), a woman of uncertain origin, perhaps a Syrian princess of partly Egyptian descent, and also another Syrian princess, Kirgipa or Gilukhipa. The reign of this king was marked by great expansion of art and commerce due to peaceful development at home rather than by great conquests. He reigned for thirty-six years and died when about fifty-two years old (Fig. 10). Owing to their shorter reigns, Amenhotep II, Thutmose IV, and Amenhotep III built far less than their predecessors.

Amenhotep IV (Figs. 12 and 13), or Akhnaton, the last king of this dynasty to play a leading part in history, was the grandson of Mutemuya, a Syrian woman, and the son of Tiy, whose nationality, as just said, is uncertain, and his peculiar genius, therefore, may have been due to the foreign blood in his veins or to the powerful influence exerted on him by his mother.

The characteristic traits of Akhnaton were religious enthusiasm and a high moral standard. As Weigall has pointed out, he was the first Egyptian monotheist[2] and monogamist at a time when polytheism and polygamy were the fashion, and a pacifist when Egyptians were enjoying the fruits of their conquests. He erected an entirely new town, Akhetaton, now Tell el Amarna, which he adorned with the temples of Queen Tiy, of Baketaton, the king's sister, of Queen Nefertiti, and last, but most important of all, with the great temple of Aton. An *intellectuel* of the first order, he patronized a new and realistic form of art, but his fanatical hatred of the ancient religion led to the destruction or mutilation of countless ancient artistic treasures, and his neglect of the royal duties, his inertia and physical laziness brought about the loss of the Syrian kingdom. In truth, he showed in some of his actions as little common sense as some other religious reformers have done. Never-

[1] Breasted, *op. cit.*, p. 328.   [2] Weigall, *Akhnaton*.

theless, a monarch who founds a monotheistic religion in the teeth of the opposition of a most powerful priesthood, who builds a new town where he worships his god away from old associations and among congenial surroundings, who endows that new town with beautiful temples, who patronizes a new form of art, and who perhaps composed the magnificent hymn to Aton, cannot be considered as lacking in energy, or as a degenerate, or an effeminate person (Fig. 14).

The characteristics of the Eighteenth Dynasty were thus tireless energy, which enabled Egypt to resist its foreign foes, to carry the Egyptian flag abroad, and to establish wise government at home, and an enlightened taste for the fine arts most forcibly shown in the

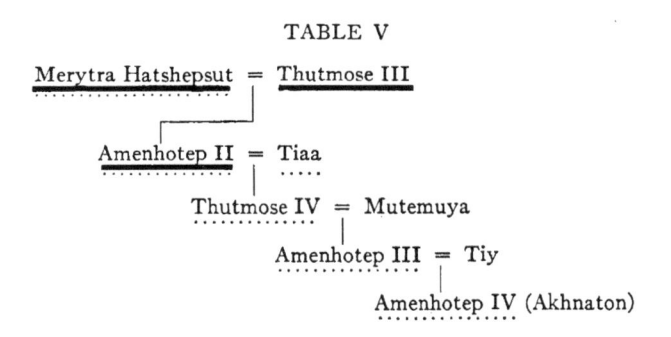

TABLE V

Merytra Hatshepsut = Thutmose III
        Amenhotep II = Tiaa
                Thutmose IV = Mutemuya
                        Amenhotep III = Tiy
                              Amenhotep IV (Akhnaton)

artistic reforms of Akhnaton. In these nine generations, issued from consanguineous marriages, there is no diminution of mental force. The energy characteristic of Ahmose I is found two hundred years afterwards in Akhnaton, used, it is true, for different objects and higher ideals, but as intense in 1375–1358 as it was in 1580–1557. Akhnaton's ideal may have been suggested by his mother, the clever queen Tiy; his energy and keen intellect he inherited, in part, at least, from his father.

In the absence of any data regarding the average number of children in Egyptian families, it is not possible to compare accurately the fertility of the consanguineous unions of the Eighteenth Dynasty with that of unrelated people from the same period; all that can be said is that without doubt these incestuous unions were blessed with many children. Moreover, the sexual power of the male members of the family is proved by the fact that they had families by their sisters, wives, and by other women as well. Table VI, giving the children known to have been born to the kings and queens of this dynasty, is necessarily incomplete, as the number of children born in and out of wedlock cannot even be guessed at, and indeed many of those mentioned in the table would have been entirely forgotten

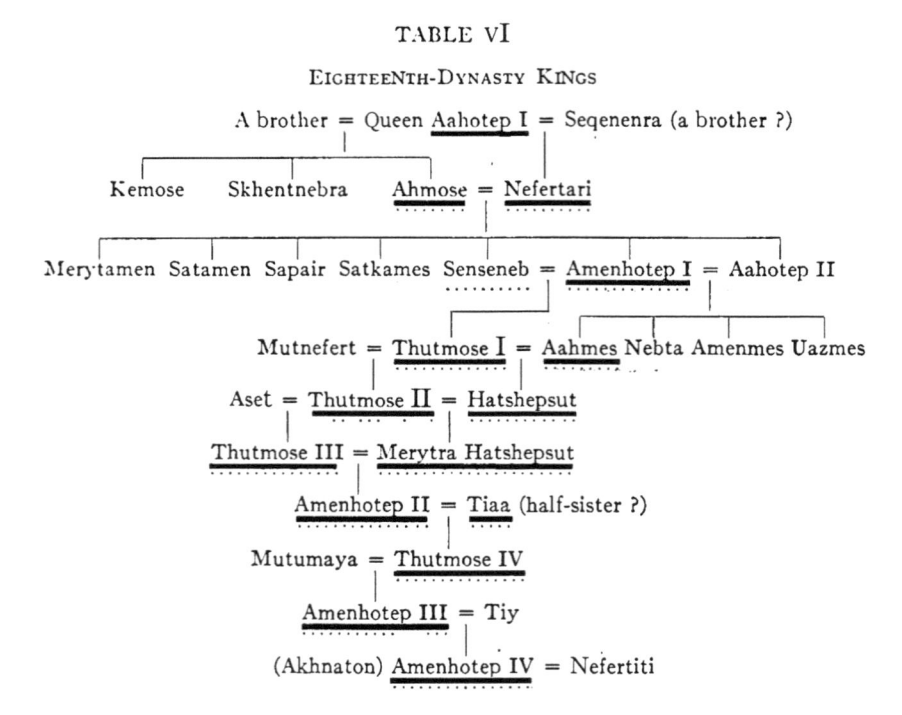

TABLE VI

EIGHTEENTH-DYNASTY KINGS

```
              A brother  =  Queen Aahotep I  =  Seqenenra (a brother ?)
                                  |
      ┌───────────┬──────────────┬─────────────┐
   Kemose    Skhentnebra      Ahmose   =   Nefertari
                                          |
   ┌──────────┬────────┬────────┬─────────┬───────────┐
Merytamen Satamen Sapair Satkames Senseneb = Amenhotep I = Aahotep II
                                                   |
                          ┌────────────────────────┼──────────────────┐
                     Mutnefert = Thutmose I = Aahmes Nebta Amenmes Uazmes
                                     |
                           Aset = Thutmose II = Hatshepsut
                                         |
                            Thutmose III = Merytra Hatshepsut
                                         |
                              Amenhotep II = Tiaa (half-sister ?)
                                         |
                                Mutumaya = Thutmose IV
                                         |
                                Amenhotep III = Tiy
                                         |
                        (Akhnaton) Amenhotep IV = Nefertiti
```

had it not been for the accidental discovery of some document or object inscribed with their names. The infants who died, the miscarriages, and the illegitimate children, etc., must remain an unknown quantity, though it can be asserted that the number of children born was certainly larger than that given in this table. In the case of the Eighteenth Dynasty, therefore, loss of prolificity did not follow consanguineous marriages.

The second evil usually attributed to consanguineous marriages is diminished duration of life in the offspring. The figures referring to this point given in Table VII are approximate only, for some monarchs may have lived a few years more or less; and further, as the mean duration of life in ancient Egypt is unknown, the value of the table is diminished; but in any case, an average duration of life of forty-four years cannot be considered as short.

TABLE VII

	Reign	Years	Age at Death
Ahmose I	1580–1557	22	55
Amenhotep I	} 1557–1501	56	56
Thutmose I			48
Thutmose III	1501–1447	54	63
Amenhotep II	1448–1420	26	46
Thutmose IV	1420–1411	8	33
Amenhotep III	1411–1375	36	45
Amenhotep IV	1375–1358	17	27

TABLE VIII

	Height	Cranial Measurements Length	Cranial Measurements Breadth
Ahmose	1.63	0.207	0.156
Amenhotep I	1.65	....	....
Thutmose I	1.54	0.180	0.133
Thutmose II	1.685	0.191	0.149
Thutmose III	1.61	0.196	0.150
Amenhotep II	1.67	0.191	0.144
Thutmose IV	1.65	0.184	0.143
Amenhotep III	1.56	0.194	0.148
Amenhotep IV	mummy incomplete	0.189	0.154

There is no evidence to show that idiocy, deaf-mutism, or other diseases generally attributed to consanguineous marriage ever occurred among the members of this dynasty, and as far as can be ascertained from mummified bodies, masks, and statues, the features of both men and women were fine, distinguished, and handsome.

The heights and cranial circumferences are shown in Table VIII. The kings, though not tall men, were by no means undersized, and their height is well maintained during nine successive generations.

The cranial measurements of 413 living modern Egyptians[1] give an average of 0.184 by 0.133 m., which almost exactly corresponds with the cranial measurements of Thutmose I.

The portraits and mummies are those of stout, well-nourished persons. Although the mummified body of Thutmose II, for instance, is now reduced to little more than skin and bone, the redundancy of the skin of the abdomen, thighs, and cheeks is a proof of the obesity of the king. Perhaps the most typical instance of pathological obesity in the family is seen in the portraits of the heretic king Akhnaton (1374-1356 B.C.) who is represented as a man with a thin face, neck, and legs, but with a very protuberant abdomen. There is no reason to doubt that the portraits of the monarch are faithful likenesses. True, the abdomen is rather prominent in other people represented at Tell el Amarna, owing chiefly to the cut of the dress, which, firmly tied below the umbilicus, caused the lower part of the abdomen to protrude; but in persons not wearing this dress the abdomen is flat, and even in men attired in the garment just described it is never as protuberant as in King Akhnaton. Where the king is represented distributing collars of gold, his abdomen actually hangs over the edge of the balcony, a most realistic piece of portraiture. The very thin calves of Akhnaton show that the artist faithfully copied nature. The king's obesity may have been partially responsible for his politics. Corpulent subjects generally dislike physical exertion, and his stoutness may have been the reason why, when the outlying provinces of his kingdom were threatened, he left unanswered the appeals for help and thus became responsible for the loss of some of the foreign possessions of Egypt. Another picture from Tell el Amarna may be referred to here.[2] It is divided into two halves, the left representing the household of Akhnaton, the right the household of his father, Amenhotep III. It shows that Akhnaton's obesity was inherited, for father and son show the same abdominal deformity. Indeed, the whole royal family is distinctly stout, in contrast with th three lean female servants on the extreme right. The mummy of Amenhotep III (1411-1375 B.C.) is in the Cairo Museum, and it

[1] *Archaeological Survey*, p. 25.
[2] *El Amarna*, i, ii, xviii.

is unfortunate that the body is in such a wretched state that its examination gives little information as to his corpulency.

The skull attributed to Akhnaton, according to Elliot Smith, presents a number of interesting and significant features. The cranium is broad and relatively flattened, its measurements being 0.189 m. in length and 0.154 m. in breadth, 0.136 m. in height, 0.099 m. minimal frontal breadth, with a circumference of 0.545 m. The form of the cranium, and the fact that it is exceptionally thin in some places and relatively thick in others, indicate, in Elliot Smith's opinion, that a condition of hydrocephalus was present during life; and Professor A. R. Ferguson is of the opinion that the signs of this disease are unquestionable. Whether the skull is Akhnaton's or not, it is interesting to find that hydrocephalus existed about thirty-five hundred years ago.

The result of this inquiry is that a royal family, in which consanguineous marriage was the rule, produced nine distinguished rulers, among whom were Ahmose, the liberator of his country; Thutmose III, one of the greatest conquerors and administrators that the world has ever seen; Amenhotep IV, the fearless religious reformer; the beloved queen Nefertari who was placed among the gods after her death; Aahmes, the beautiful queen, and Hatshepsut, the greatest queen of Egypt. There is no evidence that the physical characteristics or mental power of the family were unfavourably influenced by the repeated consanguineous marriages.

NINETEENTH-DYNASTY KINGS

The kings and queens of the Nineteenth Dynasty, a remarkably handsome set of people, were probably lineal descendants of those of the Eighteenth Dynasty.

Seti I (Figs. 15 and 16), in spite of his big and heavy jaw, presents a most noble and dignified appearance; he measures 1.665 m. in height, and his cranium 0.196 by 0.143 m. Ramses II (Fig. 17), the great historical figure of this dynasty, married two of his sisters, and had four children by the first, and three, or possibly four, by the second sister. He is said to have married two of his daughters, but the evidence on this point is not conclusive. By other wives and concubines the king is said to have had one hundred six other sons and forty-seven daughters, therefore this descendant of a long line of consanguineous marriages cannot be said to have been infertile. His features are strong and refined, the teeth excellent, and the only blemish is the complete baldness. The body measures 1.733 m., and his cranium 0.195 by 0.136 m. (Fig. 18).

Little is known about Ramses II's children (Fig. 20). One son, Khemwese, became high priest of Ptah, organized the thirtieth anniversary of his father's reign, was associated with the king in the

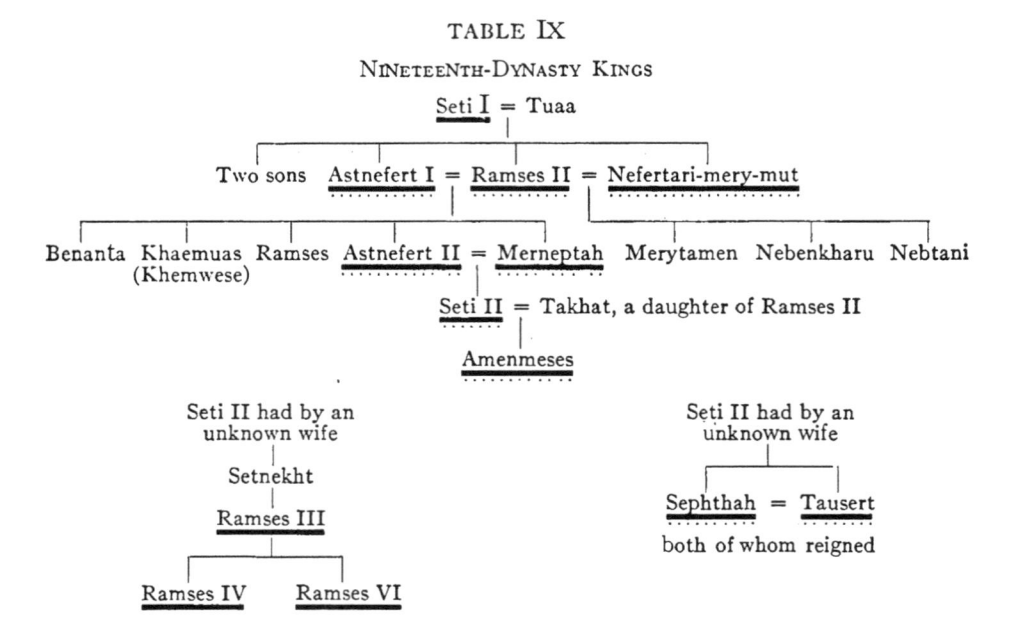

TABLE IX

NINETEENTH-DYNASTY KINGS

Seti I = Tuaa

Two sons   Astnefert I = Ramses II = Nefertari-mery-mut

Benanta Khaemuas Ramses   Astnefert II = Merneptah   Merytamen Nebenkharu Nebtani
         (Khemwese)

Seti II = Takhat, a daughter of Ramses II

Amenmeses

Seti II had by an unknown wife

Setnekht

Ramses III

Ramses IV   Ramses VI

Seti II had by an unknown wife

Sephthah = Tausert
both of whom reigned

administration of Egypt, and predeceased his father. The other children formed the powerful tribe of the Ramessides, which exerted considerable influence for many generations; one daughter, Benanta, was charmingly pretty.

Merneptah (Fig. 19), the son of Ramses II by his first sister, was more than middle-aged when he succeeded his father, and he, in spite of his years, dealt energetically with the foes of Egypt. When the Libyans threatened the very existence of Egypt, he assembled his nobles, stirred up their enthusiasm by an eloquent speech, and with their help inflicted a crushing defeat on the

EFFECTS OF CONSANGUINEOUS MARRIAGES 339

Libyans and their European mercenaries. Turning then to Palestine, he subdued the country and levied tribute on the land. "All lands are united, they are pacified. Every one that is turbulent is bound by King Merneptah."

TABLE X

	Height	Cranial Measurements
Seti I	1.665 m.	0.196 m. by 0.143 m.
Ramses II	1.733 m.	0.195 m. by 0.136 m.
Merneptah	1.714 m.	0.185 m. by 0.160 m.
Seti II	1.640 m.	0.187 m. by 0.141 m.
Sephtah*	1.638 m.	0.189 m. by 0.147 m.

* King Sephtah suffered from left talipes equino-varus.

Merneptah's building activities were not great, and his method of obtaining stone by breaking up ancient monuments, though closely imitated afterwards by Mehemet Aly and in still more recent

TABLE XI
TWENTY-FIRST DYNASTY, RAMESSIDE LINE

Of Thebes   Of Tanis

Herhor = Nezemt (?)   Nebseni = Thentamen = Nesibanebdadu

18 princes   19 princesses   Piankhi = Hent-taui I   Pasebkhanu I (?)

                                    Pinezem I = Maatkara
                                              Masaherta

                                    Menkheperia = Astemkheb I

Hent-taui II (2) = Tahenthuti (1) = Nasibadadu

                    Nesikhonsu = Pinezem II = Astemkheb II

                    Nesitanebasheru

times by British administrators, is not to be commended. He died after a reign of ten years, when approximately seventy years old, and is probably the Pharaoh of the Exodus, commonly believed to have been drowned in the Red Sea. His mummy measures 1.714 m., his cranium 0.185 by 0.160 m. The aorta was calcareous.

Merneptah married Astnefert II, most probably his sister. Their son and successor, Seti II (Fig. 21) died (murdered?) after a very short reign, during which he carried out many important public works. He was probably fairly advanced in years at the time of his death.

The heights and cranial measurements of the Ramessides are shown in Table X.

Table XI gives a résumé of the chief marriages of the Twenty-first Dynasty, and shows that consanguineous marriages were common, and marriages between brother and sister very few.

King Herhor married Nezemt, who was probably a near relative and possibly his sister, and at Karnak she is represented at the head of a long list of her children, eighteen princes and nineteen princesses. The grandson Pinezem I reigned over forty years, but very little is known about the rest of the family.

ETHIOPIAN KINGS

The Ethiopian Dynasty also followed the custom of close intermarriage. Queen Amenertas married her brother Piankhi II, and their daughter Shepenapt III married her half-brother Taharka, the

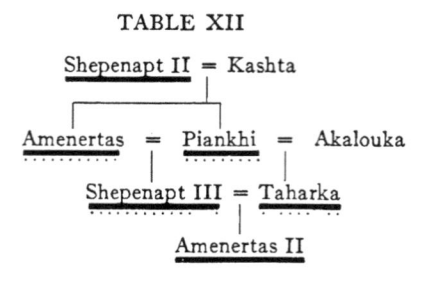

TABLE XII

Shepenapt II = Kashta
└─────┬─────┘
Amenertas = Piankhi = Akalouka
         │   │
    Shepenapt III = Taharka
              │
         Amenertas II

son of Akalouka, and a child, Amenertas II (and possibly others) was born from this consanguineous marriage. Taharka was a man of foresight, power, and courage, but unfortunately we know practically nothing of Amenertas II.

PTOLEMAIC KINGS

I. DIRECT LINE

The history of the Ptolemies is of special interest to the student of heredity, because the first four kings of the family not sprung from consanguineous unions, can be compared with the later kings who were born when such marriages had become the rule.

The founder of the dynasty, Ptolemy I Soter I (Fig. 27, 1), a favourite general and companion of Alexander the Great, enjoyed so great a popularity and influence that at the death of Alexander the satrapy of Egypt fell to him without any opposition, and he lost no time in establishing himself firmly in his new government. He first guarded himself against an attack from the west by occupying Cyrene, which became a province of Egypt, murdered Cleomenes, the financial controller who had been appointed by Alexander the Great, defeated the regent, Perdiccas, who had marched against Egypt, and put him to death.

At the second settlement of the empire (321 B.C.), Ptolemy was again awarded Egypt, with whatever lands he could conquer to the west. He seized both Cyprus and Syria, but he evacuated the last province temporarily, as his large army and the powerful fleet he had equipped were only just strong enough to rule and defend Egypt, Cyrene, and Cyprus. Indeed, Ptolemy was averse to any increased responsibility unless quite sure of his ground, and hence he prudently declined the royal dignity which some of his followers endeavoured to thrust upon him until the death of the sons of Alexander the Great had removed the only legitimate claimants to the throne.

The fleet and fortifications secured Egypt against every attempt at invasion from the eastern frontier. The strength of the Egyptian preparations was demonstrated when the attack of Antigonus by land and by sea failed to reach Alexandria, and the would-be invader finally asked for peace. Later on, Antigonus and Demetrius were defeated by the great coalition, and then Ptolemy who, it must be confessed, had been but a lukewarm supporter of the allies, secured lower Syria and Phoenicia as his share of the plunder. Shortly afterwards, the reoccupation of Cyprus, which he had given up temporarily, his appointment as protector of the league of free cities on the coast and islands of Asia Minor, and his settlements on the coasts of the Red Sea gave him, backed by his fleets, the command of the sea.

At home, the relations between the king and the native Egyptian population were so friendly that the latter gladly enlisted under Ptolemy's banner, and the large turbulent population of natives, Greeks, Persians, Syrians, etc., was kept well in hand. Ptolemy succeeded—and that was perhaps his most wonderful achievement—in founding in Egypt the cult of Serapis, a divinity adored by both Greeks and natives. Science and art were encouraged, the celebrated Museum was founded, Alexandria became the great scientific centre of the world, trade was encouraged, agriculture developed, exchange made easier by the new coinage, and every department of state was improved by the new ruler.

Ptolemy abdicated in 285 B.C. and died two years afterwards at the age of eighty-four. He had married, probably at Alexander's instigation, a Persian princess, Artakama, about whom nothing is known. Far more celebrated than this first wife was his mistress, Thais, the courtesan, who had at least two children by him. His second legimate wife was Euridike, the daughter of Antipater, and by her he also had several children. His third wife, Berenike I, a grandniece of Antipater, supposed without any reason to have been Ptolemy's step-sister, was the mother of several children by another husband at the time of her marriage with the king. Her influence over him was so great that she persuaded him to put aside Euridike's son and to adopt her own son as his heir. Several other children were born, and the king added to his family, already very large, by adopting all his step-children. Divorce from his second wife is nowhere mentioned, and Ptolemy was doubtless living with both his second and third wife at the same time.

The bold and patient father of the Ptolemaic dynasty was a political genius of the first order, a great soldier, a cunning diplomat, an able financier, a promoter of exploration, a master of foreign and home affairs, a religious reformer, and a protector of art, science, commerce, and agriculture. His private life, on the other hand, judged by our present standard, was far from edifying.

Ptolemy II Philadelphus (born 309, died 246) (Fig. 24), son of the first king, married Arsinoë I (Fig. 25), the daughter of the king of Thrace, and later on his own sister, older than himself, by whom he had no issue. His character, like his father's, was bold and cunning, and again like his father, he had, in spite of his devotion to his sister, many mistresses:[1] Didgona, a native of Egypt, Bilisticha, Agathoclea, Stratonike, Clio, his cup-bearer, who clothed in a tunic only and holding a cornucopia in her hand, was represented in many statues, to the scandal even of Alexandria, Myrtium, a most notorious and common prostitute who owned the finest houses in Alexandria, Mnesis and Pothina the flute-player, and many others. His effigies on the coins of the period show a stout, plethoric man (Fig. 27, 7) with rather fine classical features, and his sister, Arsinoë Philadelphus (Fig. 27, 8), looks a buxom, handsome woman with regular features. The king died at the age of sixty-three, after having been a martyr to gout.

To look upon Ptolemy II as a common debauchee is doing him a great injustice. He patronised science and art, subsidised the Museum and added considerably to the library, which owned the unprecedented number of 400,000 volumes. The famous Septuagint version of the Bible possibly dates from this time. His foreign politics were successful, and at home his reign appears to have been peaceful.

Allowing for all exaggeration, the "Praise of Ptolemy" by Theocritus shows in what esteem he was held by his contemporaries:

> That king surpassingly is excellent
> For wealth, wide rule by sea and o'er much continent.
>
> In many a region many a tribe doth till
> The fields, made fruitful by the shower of Zeus;
> None like low-lying Egypt doth fulfil
> Hope of increase, when Nile the clod doth loose,
> O'er-bubbling the wet soil: no land doth use
> So many workmen of all sorts, enrolled
> In cities of such multitude profuse,
> More than three myriads, as a single fold
> Under the watchful sway of Ptolemy the bold.

---

[1] Athenaeus *Deipnosophists* xiii. 40.

>Part of Phoenicia, some Arabian lands,
>Some Syrian, tribes of swart Aethiopes,
>All the Pamphylians, Lycians he commands,
>And warlike Carians; o'er the Cyclades
>His empire spreads; his navies sweep the seas;
>Ocean and rivers, earth within her bounds
>Obeys him: and a host of chivalries,
>And shielded infantry, with martial sounds
>Of their far-glittering brass, the warrior-king surrounds.
>
>For o'er the broad lands of that happy sept
>The bright-haired Ptolemy strict ward hath kept.
>
>His whole inheritance he cares to keep,
>As a good king. Himself hath garnered more:
>Nor useless in his house the golden heap,
>Increased like that of ants.
>
>   [Theocritus *Idylls*. xvii]

The third Ptolemy, Euergetes I (Fig. 27, 2), married Berenike of Cyrene (Fig. 27, 3). He was a successful warrior and diplomatist, and a patron of science and religion. The Museum and Library continued to flourish under his reign; he invited great savants, including Eratosthenes, to settle in Egypt, reformed the calendar, and built the temple of Edfou. Of all the Ptolemies, he was the only one whose private life was exemplary. He died when about sixty-three years old. Physically, there was a great resemblance between him and his father.

Ptolemy IV Philopator (Fig. 27, 4), the son of Ptolemy III by a princess of Cyrene, succeeded his father, and his life is of great interest, for had he been the child of a consanguineous marriage, his shameful characteristics would doubtless have been attributed to the close relationship between the parents.

The king succeeded,

in the heyday of youth, with his education completed by the greatest masters, to a great empire, a full treasury, and peace at home and abroad. Yet, in the opinion of our Greek authorities, Polybius and Strabo, no member of the dynasty was more criminally worthless, nor so fatal to the greatness and prosperity of Egypt.[1]

[1] Mahaffy, *A History of Egypt: Ptolemaic Dynasty*, p. 127.

EFFECTS OF CONSANGUINEOUS MARRIAGES

Shortly after his ascent to the throne, the queen-mother Berenike and his brother Magas were murdered. Whether Ptolemy IV had a share in planning these murders is uncertain, but undoubtedly the fact that Sosibius, the chief actor, had considerable influence on the king threw some suspicion on the latter. His debauchery shocked his contemporaries. He loved to surround himself with low courtesans who treated him with scant respect, and his Greek mistress, Agathoclea, and her brother Agathocles, at one time the real rulers of the country, prevented him from taking a legitimate wife until the mistress had given up all hopes of having a child. So great was this woman's influence over him that Strabo simply calls him "Philopator, he of Agathoclea." Finally he married his sister, Arsinoë III (Fig. 27, 5), who was afterwards murdered by Agathocles.

The disreputable private life of Ptolemy IV did not interfere with his considerable diplomatic ingenuity, administrative skill, and military efficiency. On Antiochus attacking Egypt, an army was quickly raised, and the king, accompanied by his sister Arsinoë, defeated his foe at Rapha, and this victory and his strong government so impressed his neighbours that, during his lifetime, Egypt was not attacked again. In spite of his debauchery, he interested himself in intellectual pursuits, wrote tragedies, added to Philae, to Ar-hes-Nefer,[1] and built temples at Edfou, Alexandria, and probably at Naucratis also. His handling of home affairs, on the other hand, was not altogether successful; rebellion in Lower Egypt had to be quelled, and at the time of his death Egypt and Nubia were in a state of anarchy. The employment of native officers and soldiers ultimately led to a revolution, for he realized as little as some administrators do now that one cannot give away power and at the same time retain it.

Allowing, then, for the exaggerations of Polybius, of Strabo, and of the Jews, whom he had offended, the king may be described as a man whose life was soiled by culpable weakness and debauchery, but to some extent redeemed by a love of art and letters, and who, in his political actions, showed considerable ability and originality. The only known child of Ptolemy IV and his sister was

[1] Mahaffy, *op. cit.*, p. 138.

Ptolemy V Epiphanes (born 209), and as both king and queen died in 204, their other progeny, if any, cannot have been numerous.

Ptolemy V was only five years old when he came to the throne. He was betrothed to Cleopatra, a Syrian princess, when eleven years of age (198 B.C.) and married her five years afterwards.

On the coins of the period we see a stout, distinctly good-looking young man (Fig. 27, 6). He enjoyed a great reputation as an athlete and was fond of field sports, and like his forefathers, he was cruel, treacherous, and tyrannical whenever it suited his purpose to be so. His foreign policy certainly was not a success, but, as Mahaffy explains, he is hardly to be blamed for the sore diminution of the Egyptian empire during his reign; for the rise of the Romans, the astuteness of Antiochus, the invasion of his island empire by Philip, and his predecessor's mistaken policy of arming the natives were all factors which would have beaten the strongest man. He died at the age of twenty-nine, and it is not improbable that he was murdered.

The marriage of Ptolemy V Epiphanes with the Syrian princess was blessed with at least four children. One son, Ptolemy VI Eupator, died young. Another son, Ptolemy VII Philometor (Fig. 27, 9), the descendant of consanguineous grandparents, was seven years old when he ascended the throne (181 B.C.) and was killed at the age of forty-three (145 B.C.). When still a boy of fifteen he, with his sister-wife Cleopatra II, successfully organized the resistance to King Antiochus, quelled rebellions in Upper and Lower Egypt, reconquered and pacified Nubia. In Upper Egypt he did considerable building work. His quarrels with his brother, the clever and unscrupulous Ptolemy IX Euergetes II, would fill a volume. His treatment of his brother was magnanimous, for having taken him prisoner, he spared his life, and forgetting the past suggested they should form a new alliance by a marriage between his own daughter and Euergetes, to whom he left Cyrene. The fear of the Romans may possibly have made these arrangements advisable, but it is only fair to assume that his natural kindness and the ties of blood urged him to follow this course. King Philometor was the Ptolemy, "virtuous, pious, and kindest of men," to whom the companions in arms in Cyprus dedicated a crown of gold in the temple

EFFECTS OF CONSANGUINEOUS MARRIAGES 347

of Delos. They thank him for his benefactions to them and their homes, but they especially admire the kindness and magnanimity with which he made friendship and peace.

Cleopatra Thea, one of the children born of the incestuous marriage between Philomator and his sister, was married to Alexander Bela, king of Syria, and when her father and husband quarrelled,

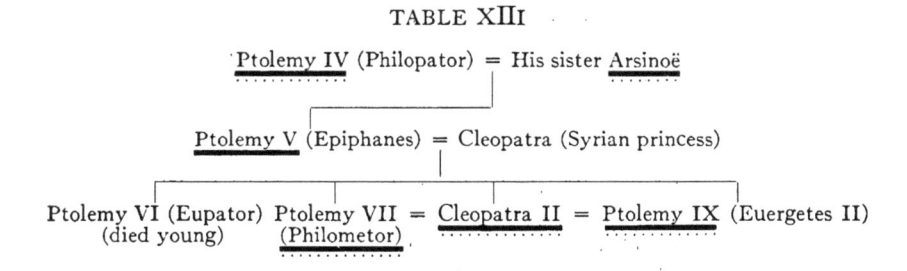

TABLE XIII

Ptolemy IV (Philopator) = His sister Arsinoë
|
Ptolemy V (Epiphanes) = Cleopatra (Syrian princess)
|
Ptolemy VI (Eupator)   Ptolemy VII = Cleopatra II = Ptolemy IX (Euergetes II)
(died young)   (Philometor)

she left the latter and married her husband's rival, Demetrius II. The fortunes of war having compelled her second husband to fly the country and to marry the daughter of his captor, Cleopatra Thea at once retaliated by marrying Demetrius' brother, Antiochus VII Sidetes. The queen had children by all these husbands. She was not, as has been suggested, a weak simpleton, but a wicked, energetic woman, who shed blood whenever the success of her plans required

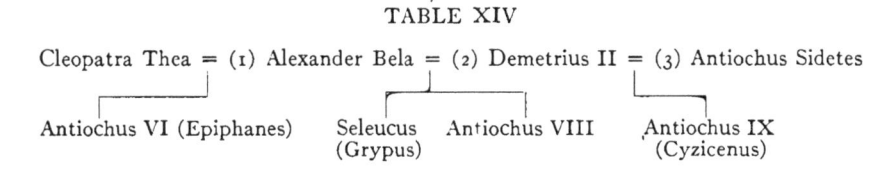

TABLE XIV

Cleopatra Thea = (1) Alexander Bela = (2) Demetrius II = (3) Antiochus Sidetes
| | |
Antiochus VI (Epiphanes)   Seleucus   Antiochus VIII   Antiochus IX
                           (Grypus)   (Cyzicenus)

it. She betrayed her husband, Demetrius II, who was assassinated with her knowledge, murdered her son Seleucus, and another son, Antiochus VIII, escaped the same fate only by compelling his mother to drink the poison she had prepared for him. There was no lack of energy, though for evil, in this queen, the offspring of an incestuous union.

After her brother-husband's death, Cleopatra II married her other brother, Ptolemy IX Euergetes II (Fig. 27, 10), by whom she is supposed to have had one son, Memphites, who was assassinated by his own father. The story, however, is so obscure and improbable that its truth may well be doubted. Ptolemy Euergetes II, nicknamed Physkon (Sausage), also married his wife's daughter, Cleopatra III (Fig. 27, 11), at once his niece and step-daughter, after, it is said, outraging her.

It is difficult to estimate justly the character of this king, the greatest historians differing in their opinion of him; but the appreciation given by Mahaffy appears so equitable and temperate that I cannot do better than reproduce it here:

> Our Greek authorities tell us of nothing but the crimes and follies of Physkon, tempered by Greek distractions of writing memoirs, and of discussions with the learned Greeks of the Museum. All the world, not to say his own nation, are described as filled with horror at his enormities. If we turn to inscriptions and to papyri we find the king and his queens commemorated in friendly dedications to and by his officers in Delos, in Cyprus and in Egypt. He extends the commercial bounds of Egypt to the south and east; he keeps Cyrene perfectly still and undisturbed, probably under the viceroyalty of his son Apion. He so far manages to control two ambitious queens, probably at deadly enmity, that at the very close of his life they both appear associated with him in the royalty as if nothing had happened to disturb the peace of the palace. Throughout the country the legal and fiscal documents still extant show the prevalence of law and order.
>
> Modern criticism, suspicious of the exaggerations familiar to ancient rhetoricians, may lighten the burden of crimes and maledictions with which he is charged, but it is not possible to wipe out all the lines of this repugnant caricature. He was, in any case, an energetic figure, a despot without scruples, but not without intellect, who seems to have summed up in himself and carried away all the virility of his race.[1]

His wife and niece, Cleopatra III, a masterful woman, had an almost pathological hatred for her first son. Again and again did she endeavour to remove him from the throne and to place the crown of Egypt on the head of her second son, Ptolemy XI Alexander. "Never, that we know of," wrote Pausanias, "was there a king so hated by his mother." For many years the history of Egypt is that of the quarrel and intrigues of this strong-minded woman and her two sons. The first son, Ptolemy X, nicknamed Lathyrus, married his sister, Cleopatra IV, during his father's reign, and a son had

[1] Mahaffy, *op. cit.*, p. 202a.

been born when his mother, Cleopatra III, compelled the young king to repudiate his wife and to marry his other sister, Cleopatra Selene, who had two sons by him. When Lathyrus had to fly from Egypt, Selene retired to Syria, where she married three husbands in succession and was finally put to death by Tigranes, king of Armenia, after having had four, probably five, and perhaps more sons, by her four husbands; of these the first was her brother, the second and the third her cousins (the second being himself a descendant of an incestuous marriage), and the fourth her step-son and second cousin. She is the only Cleopatra who is not guilty of one or more murders during her adventurous career.

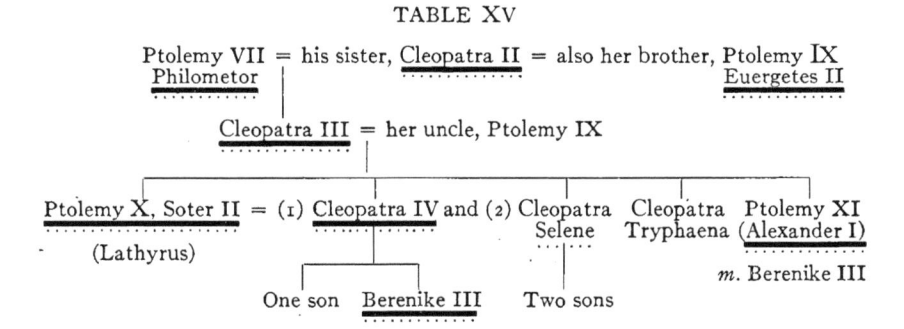

TABLE XV

Ptolemy VII = his sister, Cleopatra II = also her brother, Ptolemy IX
Philometor   Euergetes II

Cleopatra III = her uncle, Ptolemy IX

Ptolemy X, Soter II = (1) Cleopatra IV and (2) Cleopatra   Cleopatra   Ptolemy XI
(Lathyrus)   Selene   Tryphaena   (Alexander I)
                                                                       m. Berenike III
            One son   Berenike III   Two sons

Meanwhile, Cleopatra IV, the first wife of Ptolemy X Lathyros, had gone to Cyprus, enlisted a number of mercenaries, proceeded to Syria, married Antiochus IX, and attacked Antiochus VIII, the husband of her sister Tryphaena. The sister, getting the upper hand, had her put to death.

Cleopatra III's last daughter, Tryphaena, married Antiochus VIII Grypos, and after perpetrating the crimes mentioned above was herself murdered by Antiochus XI.

The history of the four Cleopatras, the daughters and granddaughters of incestuous marriages, is a long relation of intrigues and appalling crimes. All had sons and grandsons of whom some are known by name. Very probably many more have been entirely forgotten.

Ptolemy X Lathyrus died in 80 B.C. at the age of sixty-two. His brother and rival Ptolemy Alexander I had been killed in 88 B.C.

He was probably about forty years old at the time, and was said to have repaid his mother's kindness to him by murdering her. He resembled her physically, for she was nicknamed κόκκη and he κόκκης, "the red one." It is difficult to form an estimate of these two brothers' characters, so completely overshadowed are they by the striking personality of the queen-mother. She it is who occupies the stage; a clever, daring, ruthless, intriguing woman, who for thirty years was the all-powerful ruler of Egypt, and certainly her incestuous origin did not prevent her from displaying remarkable energy.

Lathyrus, by his marriage with his sister Cleopatra IV, had a daughter, Berenike III, who married her uncle Ptolemy XI Alexander I, and one son, who was murdered. Posidonius of Rhodes, a contemporary, draws a portrait of this sovereign which is not without humour:

> The dynast of Egypt, hated by the people, but flattered by those round him, lived in great luxury, and could not walk otherwise than supported by two acolytes; but in banquets, when he became excited, he jumped from the couch, and executed, barefoot, dances with greater agility than professional dancers.

When Ptolemy XI Alexander I died, his son, Ptolemy XII Alexander II, by a second wife, following the advice of Sylla, married his step-mother, and was murdered shortly afterwards, after putting his wife to death.

The direct line of the Ptolemies now comes to an end, not because the women had become barren, or the men unable to beget children, but because all the male descendants born in legitimate wedlock had been killed or exiled.

II. INDIRECT LINES

Ptolemy X Lathyrus (Fig. 27, 12) had left two illegitimate sons, and one of them, nicknamed Auletes, the flute-player, now laid claim to and ascended the throne, the other son being made king of Cyprus. The latter retained his throne until the Romans occupied the island, when rather than submit to this indignity he poisoned himself.

Auletes married Cleopatra V Tryphaena II, who was called his sister in official records, though there is no proof that she stood in such relationship to him. His daughter, Berenike IV, was probably by this wife, and by a second wife the king had another family, the most prominent member of which was Cleopatra VII, the great Cleopatra.

Auletes is stated to have been an idle, drunken, and wicked man, the whole of these accusations resting on about half a dozen anecdotes, which have as little value as have nowadays the countless stories about royalty. A curious passage of Strabo[1] shows that a good deal of the indignation of ancient Greek authors was due to the king's passion for what would be now considered an artistic occupation. Strabo says:

> Besides other deeds of shamelessness, he acted the piper; indeed, he gloried so much in the practice that he scrupled not to appoint trials of skill in his palace: on which occasions he presented himself as a competitor among other rivals.

What would Strabo have said of Frederick the Great, or of Ludwig of Bavaria, or of the Royal Duke who played the violin obbligato for a distinguished singer at a public concert?

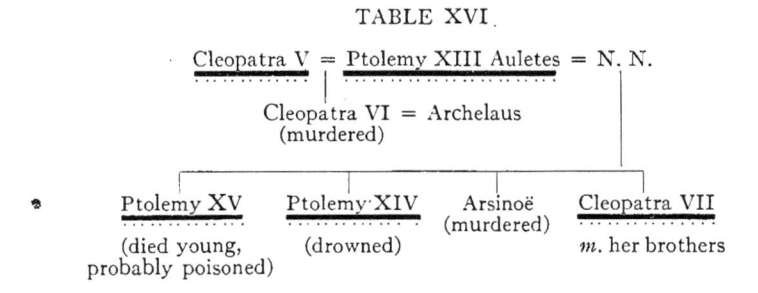

TABLE XVI.

Cleopatra V = Ptolemy XIII Auletes = N. N.
|
Cleopatra VI = Archelaus
(murdered)

Ptolemy XV   Ptolemy XIV   Arsinoë   Cleopatra VII
(died young, (drowned)   (murdered)   m. her brothers
probably poisoned)

The king had no easy task. He, a bastard, had to defend his throne against those who had perhaps a more legitimate claim to the throne. No doubt he fleeced his country, but let it be remembered in his favour that his only chance of keeping the throne was by bribing *the whole of the Roman senate*, and by becoming the prey of Roman money-lenders. His financial struggles, and indeed his whole history, curiously resemble the history of some very modern rulers. To keep himself on the throne at all was a truly marvellous

[1] Strabo xvii. 1, 11.

feat, and however disgraceful his private life may have been, his cleverness and genius for intrigue were remarkable.

His son, generally described as a puppet in the hands of his attendants, clearly was not responsible for the murder of Pompey. He fought a gallant fight against Julius Caesar, and though but a boy without experience, behaved with decision and bravery and perished in battle.

A just estimate of the great Cleopatra (Fig. 26) is an almost hopeless task, for the accounts of her life, as Weigall has pointed out, are written by her enemies. Her amours with Caesar and with Antony must not be judged according to our standard, and though it would probably be going too far to maintain that her intrigues with these two men were for political reasons only, there can be no doubt that, had she resisted either of them, Egypt would have been lost to her and to her dynasty. It is sheer nonsense to look upon Caesar or Antony as the unfortunate victim of a designing woman. By the time Caesar met Cleopatra he was an elderly man, who had ruined the wives and daughters of an astonishing number of his friends, and whose reputation for such seductions was of a character almost past belief. Antony also was not a boy but a man of the world, *une homme à femmes*, who had seduced many women. Cleopatra at that time was a girl twenty-one years old, against whose character not one shred of trustworthy evidence has been advanced. The prodigality, the luxury and licence of her court were those of every eastern court of her time, and no great blame can be attached to her endeavouring to please Caesar and Antony by sumptuous entertainments. The responsibility for such waste of money should be put with much greater justice at the door of those who allowed her to squander fortunes on their amusement.

Certainly, the audacity, cleverness, and resources of this Egyptian queen, the last offspring of many incestuous marriages, compel our admiration, and had not Caesar's murder put an end to her ambitions, she might have become the empress of the world! She was musical, artistic, and encouraged science; her good spirits were proverbial, and induced her to play harmless and rather pointless practical jokes. She was considered a very fine linguist, perhaps not a great achievement in a town where, to this day, every

TABLE XVII
Ptolemaic Dynasty

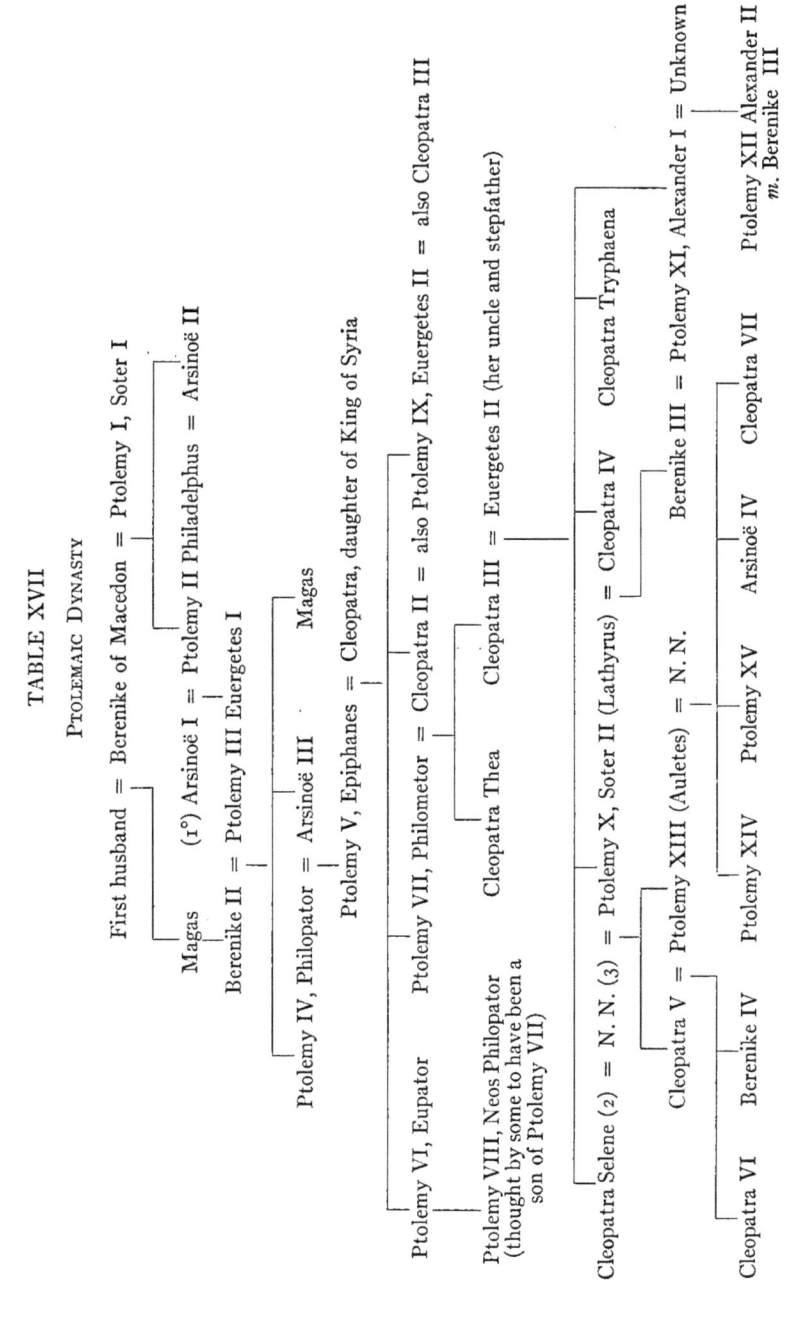

First husband = Berenike of Macedon = Ptolemy I, Soter I

(1°) Arsinoë I = Ptolemy II Philadelphus = Arsinoë II

Magas

Berenike II = Ptolemy III Euergetes I

Ptolemy IV, Philopator = Arsinoë III   Magas

Ptolemy V, Epiphanes = Cleopatra, daughter of King of Syria

Ptolemy VI, Eupator   Ptolemy VII, Philometor = Cleopatra II = also Ptolemy IX, Euergetes II = also Cleopatra III

Ptolemy VIII, Neos Philopator (thought by some to have been a son of Ptolemy VII)

Cleopatra Thea   Cleopatra III = Euergetes II (her uncle and stepfather)

Cleopatra Selene (2) = N. N. (3) = Ptolemy X, Soter II (Lathyrus) = Cleopatra IV   Cleopatra Tryphaena

Cleopatra V = Ptolemy XIII (Auletes) = N. N.   Berenike III = Ptolemy XI, Alexander I = Unknown   Ptolemy XII Alexander II *m.* Berenike III

Cleopatra VI   Berenike IV   Ptolemy XIV   Ptolemy XV   Arsinoë IV   Cleopatra VII

inhabitant speaks three languages as a rule, where many can converse in five, six, or seven tongues, and official correspondence is carried on in three languages.

Of her physical appearance we know but little. Her portraits, if authentic, do not give one the idea of a very beautiful woman, and her charm was probably one of manner. Dion Cassius says:

> She was splendid to hear and to see, and was capable of conquering the hearts which had resisted most obstinately the influence of love and those which had been frozen by age.

Another author[1] expresses himself as follows:

> Now her beauty, as they say, was not in itself altogether incomparable nor such as to strike those who saw her: but familiarity with her had an irresistible charm, and her form, combined with her persuasive speech and the peculiar character which in a manner was diffused about her behaviour, produced a certain piquancy. There was a sweetness in the sound of her voice when she spoke.

The two charges of cruelty always brought against her are that she murdered her sister, Arsinoë IV, and her brother, Ptolemy XV. The blame for the murder of her sister is minimized by the fact that Arsinoë, who had declared war against her, would have shown no mercy had she won the day; and with regard to Ptolemy XV, there is no proof that he was murdered, and if he was, the deed was done at Rome when Cleopatra was entirely under Caesar's influence, and in his power. Her end, when rather than grace her conqueror's triumph she committed suicide, was that of a plucky woman (Fig. 27, 13).

Cleopatra had one son by Julius Caesar and three children by Antony. The son was murdered and two children are known to have married and to have had children.

III. SUMMARY

The Ptolemies born from consanguineous unions were neither better nor worse than the first four kings of the same family issued from non-consanguineous marriages, and had the same general characteristics. Their conduct of foreign affairs and of internal administration was in every way remarkable and energetic. They

---

[1] Plutarch *Life of Antonius* 27.

were not unpopular in their capital, and the Alexandrians rallied round their rulers when the Romans entered Egypt, and resisted the foreigner.

Though much has been written about the awful sexual immorality of the Ptolemies, they must not be judged by comparison with the morals of this century, but an opinion must be based on the study of the literature and customs of the time. The chief characteristic of the Alexandrian literature is its eroticism, and the standard of morality was as low as it possibly could be. The spirit of disparagement which existed always led to a systematic slandering of the reigning king; and, later on, the Romans industriously blackened the character of their future opponents. Thus it is not unlikely that the Ptolemies were better than they have been painted. Their standard of morality was certainly not lower than that of their fellow-townsmen.

The children from these incestuous marriages displayed no lack of mental energy. Both men and women were equally strong, capable, intelligent; and wicked. Certain pathological characteristics doubtless ran through the family. Gout and obesity weighed heavily on the Ptolemies, but the tendency to obesity existed before consanguineous unions had taken place.

The male and female effigies on coins are those of very stout, well-nourished persons. The theory that the offspring of incestuous marriages is short-lived receives no confirmation from the history of the Ptolemies.

The length of life of the Ptolemaic kings was as follows:

	Age at Death
Ptolemy I Soter	84
Ptolemy II Philadelphus	62
Ptolemy III Energetes	63
Ptolemy IV Philopator	39 (murdered?)
Ptolemy V Epiphanes	28 (killed?)
Ptolemy VI Eupator	— (?)
Ptolemy VII Philometor	42 (killed?)
Ptolemy IX Euergetes II	60
Ptolemy X Soter II (Lathyros)	61
Ptolemy XI Alexander I	62
Ptolemy XII Alexander II	29 (killed?)
Ptolemy XIII Auletes	59
Ptolemy XIV and Ptolemy XV	— (both killed young)

Omitting those who died violent deaths, the average length of life of the Ptolemies was sixty-four years. Several women of the family reached an advanced age, amounting in three cases to over sixty years. Owing to the lack of statistics in ancient Alexandria, it is impossible to compare the length of life of Ptolemaic kings with that of other Alexandrian families. But when we consider the nature of these lives, diversified by intrigues, murders, wars, and debauchery, we may admit that the Ptolemies possessed remarkably strong constitutions.

Sterility was not a result of these consanguineous marriages. No case of idiocy, deaf-mutism, etc., in Ptolemaic families has been reported. With regard to the theory that hereditary pathological tendencies are "reinforced" by consanguineous marriages, cousins or near relatives who marry are not usually affected with, nor predisposed to, deaf-mutism, idiocy, epilepsy, nor to the other infirmities which are said to threaten the children of consanguineous parents. There can be no question of any reinforcement of a hereditary tendency which does not exist on either side. The history of the Ptolemies does not show that their predisposition to obesity or to gout was increased by their consanguineous marriages. Had the families of these monarchs suffered from some hereditary disease, the local satirists would have made capital of it, with due exaggeration, and the fact that they were silent is of the utmost importance.

DESCRIPTION OF PLATES LXIII–LXXI

(The following described figures are referred to in the text by number only.)

PLATE LXIII

FIG. 1.—Nefertari.

FIG. 2.—Queen Nefertari, wife of Ahmose I. From a wooden statue at Turin (Alinari).

FIG. 3.—Amenhotep I. (British Museum.) (W. A. Mansell.)

PLATE LXIV

FIG. 4.—Mummified head of Thutmose I. From G. Elliot Smith's *Catalogue général des antiquités égyptiennes du Musée du Caire*, Cairo, 1912.

FIG. 5.—Queen Aahmes. From E. Naville's *The Temple of Deir-el-Bahri*, London, 1898.

FIG. 6.—Mummified head of Thutmose II. (Bonfils.) (Cairo Museum.)

PLATE LXIII

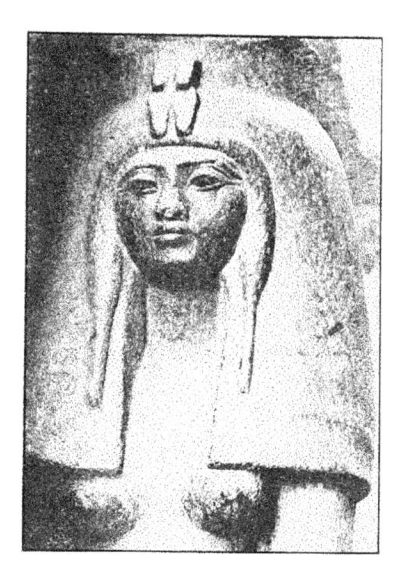

FIG. 1

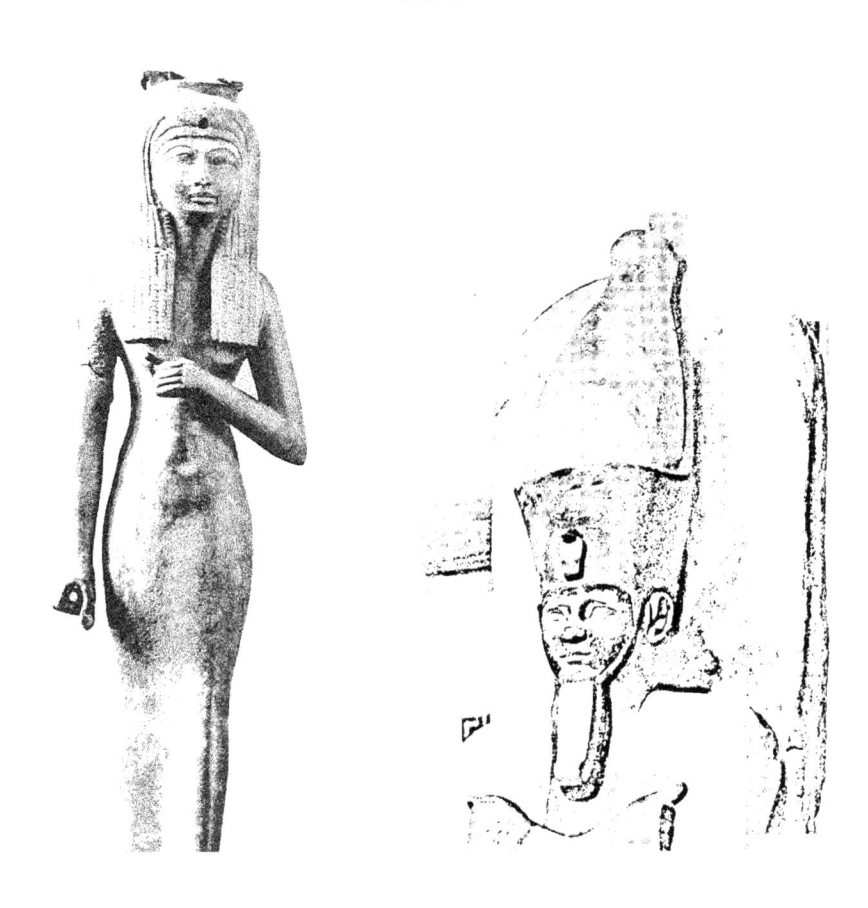

PLATE LXIV

Fig. 4

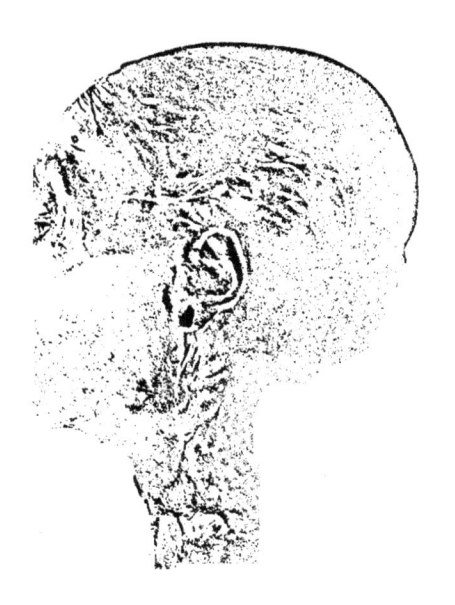

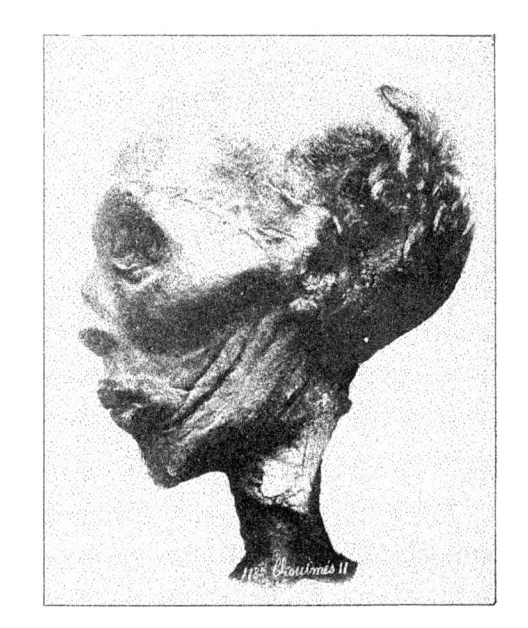

Fig. 6

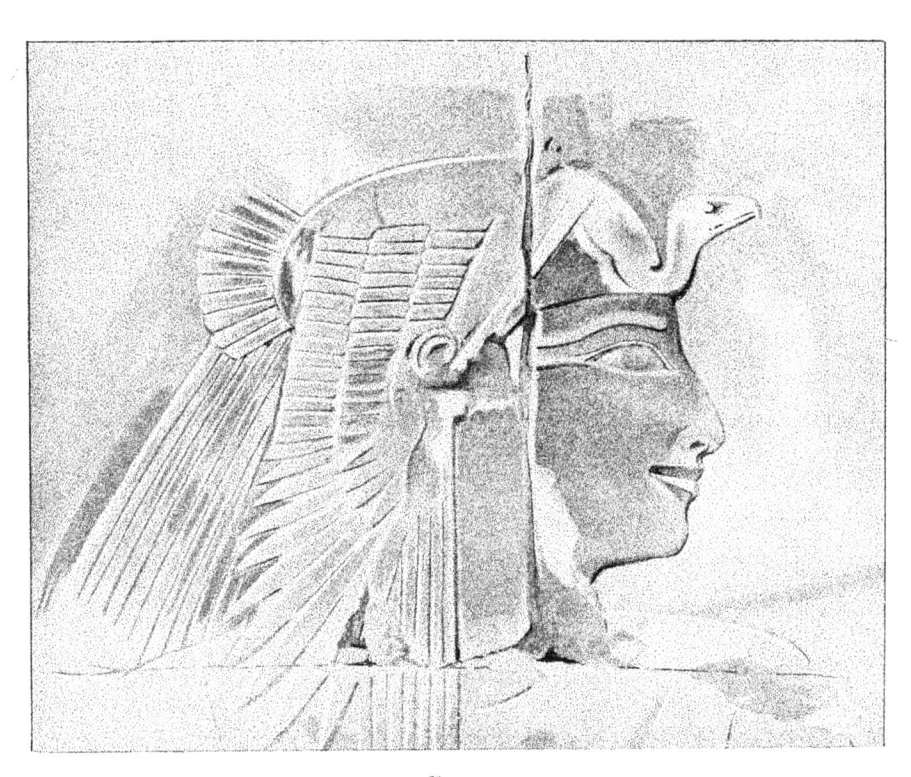

Fig. 5

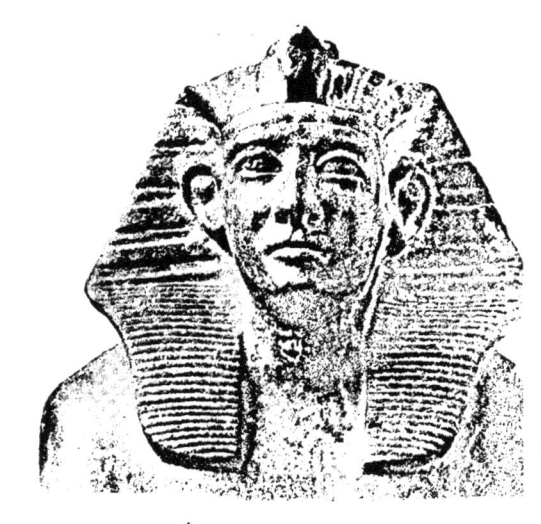

FIG. 10

FIG. 7

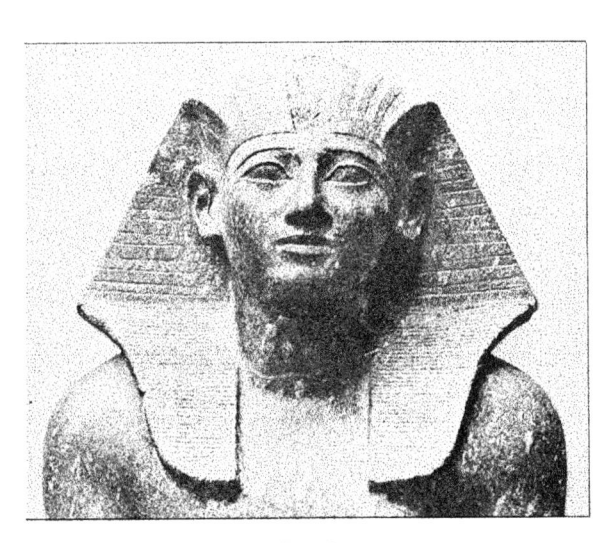

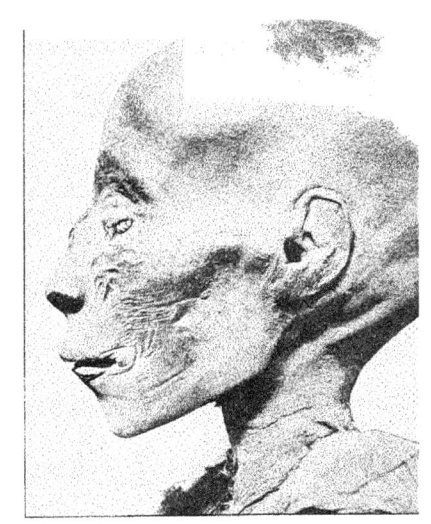

FIG. 8

FIG. 9

PLATE LXVI

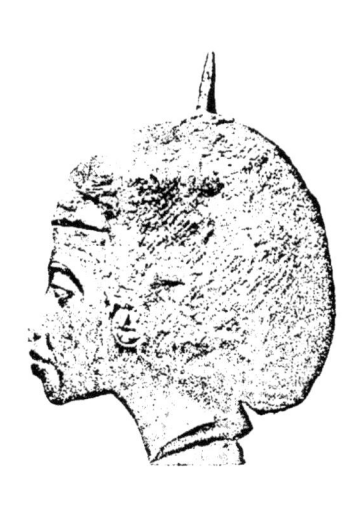

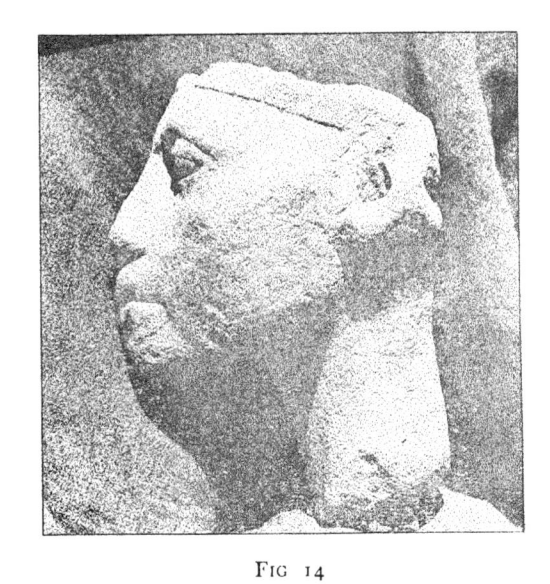

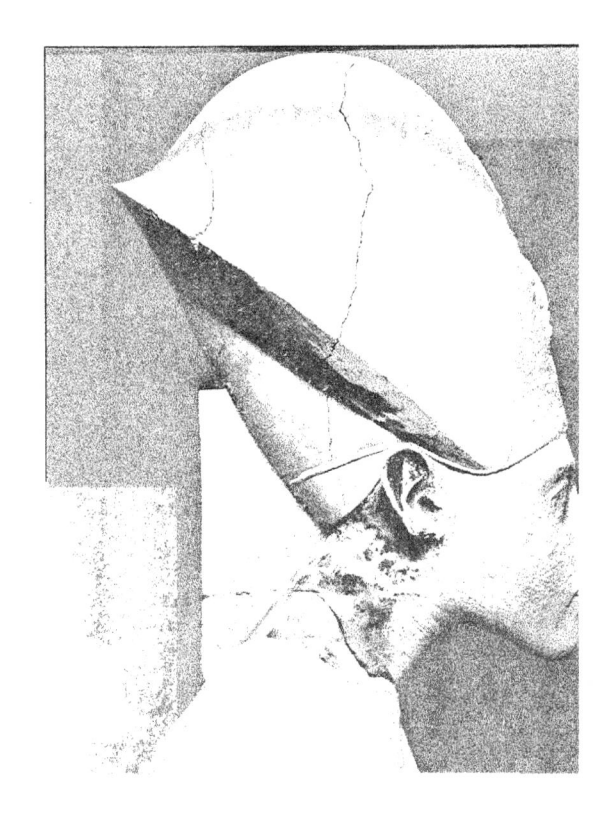

Fig 11

Fig 14

PLATE LXVII

Fig. 15

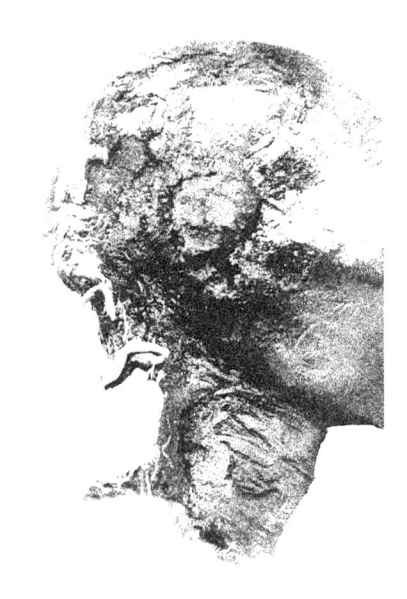

Fig. 16

Fig. 17

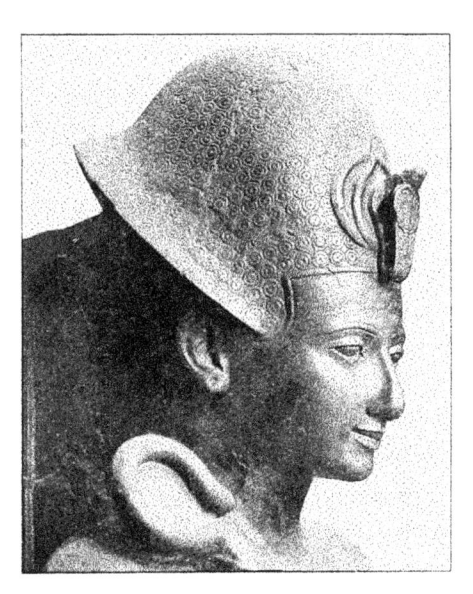

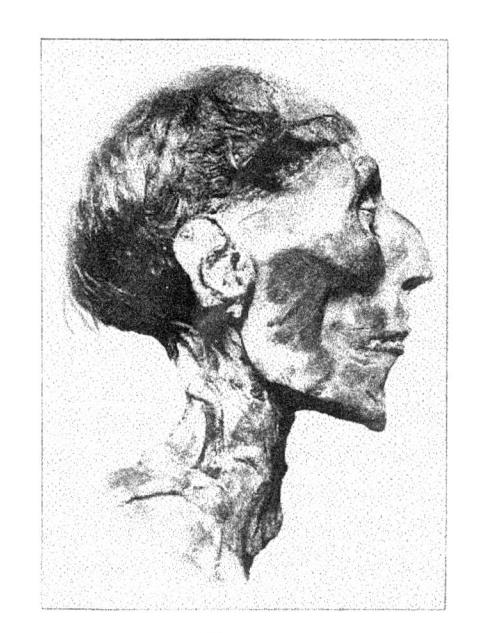

Fig. 18

PLATE LXVIII

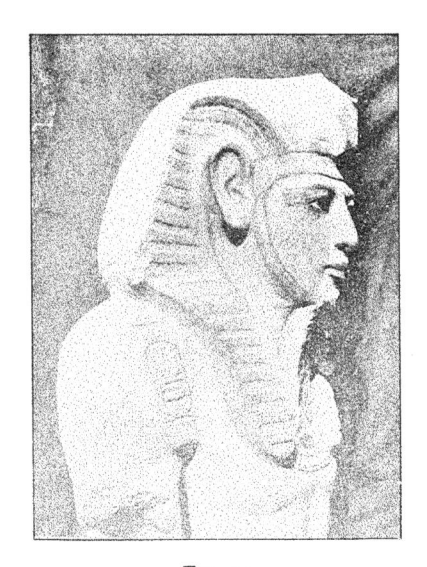

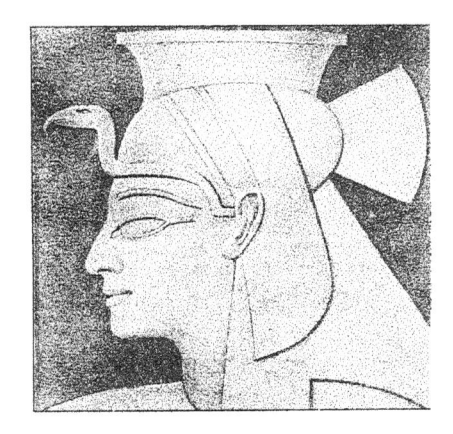

Fig. 19

Fig. 20

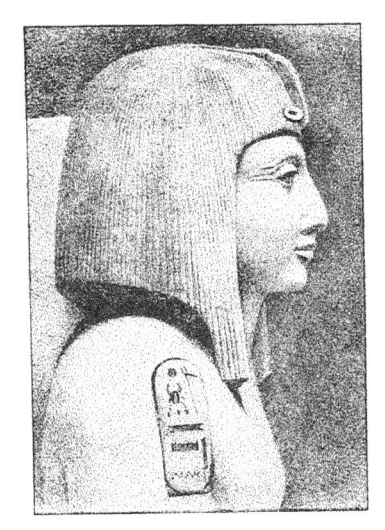

Fig. 21

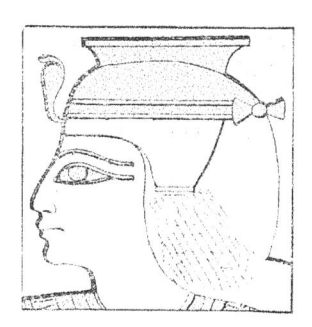

Fig. 22

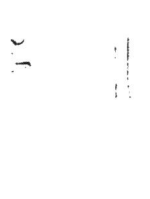

Fig. 23

PLATE LXIX

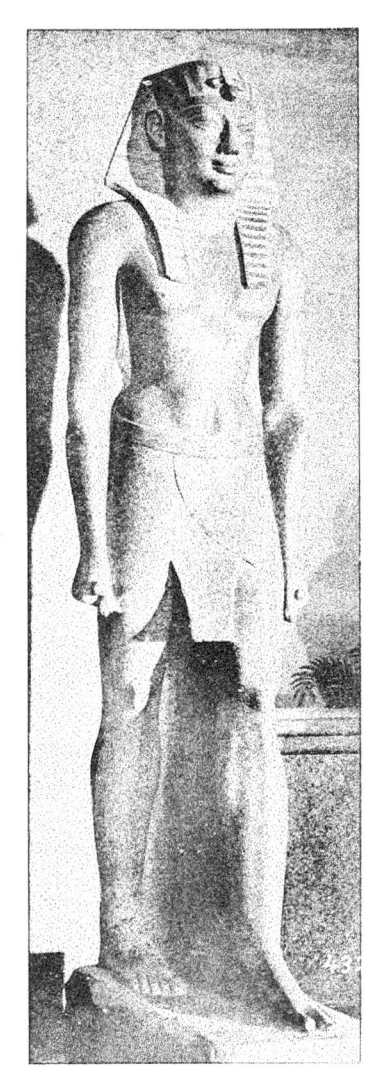

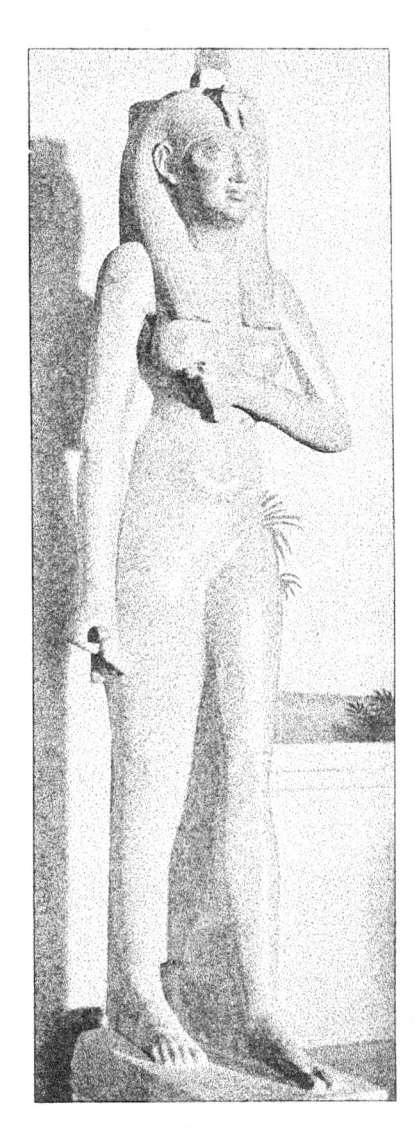

FIG. 24

FIG. 25

PLATE LXX

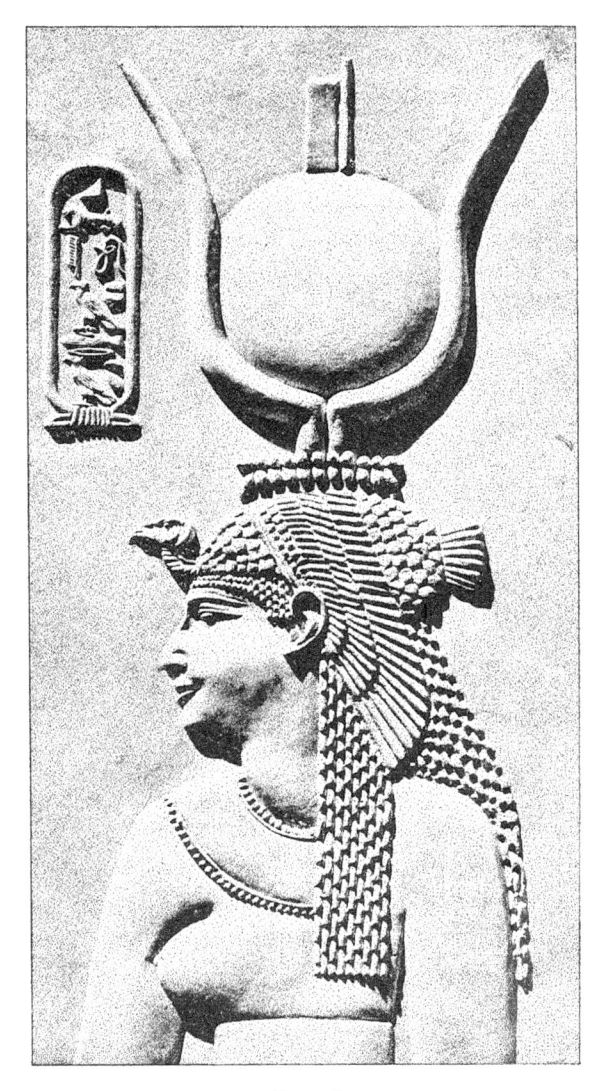

Fig. 26

PLATE LXXI

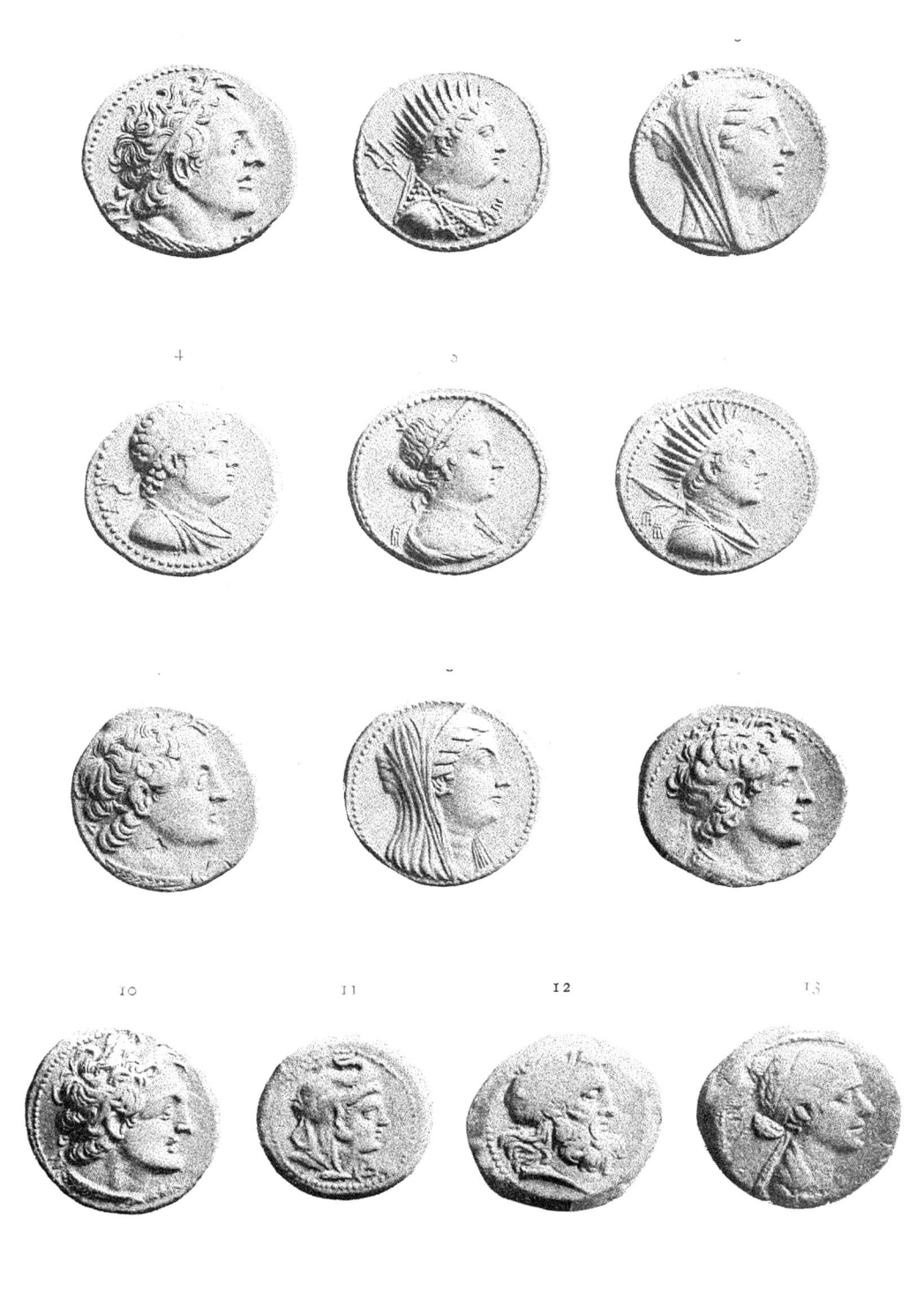

EFFECTS OF CONSANGUINEOUS MARRIAGES 357

PLATE LXV

Fig. 7.—Thutmose III. (British Museum.)
Fig. 8.—Amenhotep II. (Karnak.) From Legrain's *Catalogue général des antiquités égyptiennes du Musée du Caire*, Cairo, 1906.
Fig. 9.—Mummified head of Thutmose IV. From G. Elliot Smith's *Catalogue général des antiquités égyptiennes du Musée du Caire*, Cairo, 1912.
Fig. 10.—Amenhotep III. From Legrain's *Catalogue général des antiquités égyptiennes du Musée du Caire*, Cairo, 1906.

PLATE LXVI

Fig. 11.—Queen Tiy. (Berlin.)
Fig. 12.—Amenhotep IV. (Berlin.)
Fig. 13.—Amenhotep IV or Akhnaton. From a statue in the Louvre.
Fig. 14.—Death mask of Akhnaton.

PLATE LXVII

Fig. 15.—Seti I, offering. (Abydos.)
Fig. 16.—Seti I. (Bonfils.) (Cairo Museum.)
Fig. 17.—Ramses II.
Fig. 18.—Mummified head of Ramses II. (Bonfils.) (Cairo Museum.)

PLATE LXVIII

Fig. 19.—Merneptah. Gray granite figure from his temple at Thebes.
Fig. 20.—Merytamen, daughter of Ramses II.
Fig. 21.—Seti II. From his statue.
Fig. 22.—Takhat. From tomb of Amenmeses.
Fig. 23.—Amenmeses. From his tomb.

PLATE LXIX

Fig. 24.—Ptolemy II Philadelphus. (Vatican, Rome.)
Fig. 25.—Arsinoë II, ux. Philadelphus. (Vatican, Rome.)

PLATE LXX

Fig. 26—Cleopatra VII. (Bonfils.) (Dendera.)

PLATE LXXI

Fig. 27.—Images of royal Egyptians as portrayed on coins of the period. (1) Ptolemy I (Soter); (2) Ptolemy III (Euergetes); (3) Berenike II; (4) Ptolemy IV (Philopator I); (5) Arsinoë III (Philopator XV); (6) Ptolemy V (Epiphanes); (7) Ptolemy II (Philadelphus); (8) Arsinoë II; (9) Ptolemy VII (Philometor); (10) Ptolemy IX (Euergetes II); (11) Cleopatra III; (12) Ptolemy X (Lathyrus); (13) Cleopatra VII.

APPENDIX

CHRONOLOGICAL LIST OF EGYPTIAN KINGS AND DYNASTIES[1]

(N.B.—All dates with asterisks are astronomically fixed.)

	B.C.
Predynastic kingdoms already flourishing	4500
Introduction of calendar and earliest fixed date in history	*4241
Kingdoms of Upper and Lower Egypt probably flourishing by	4000
Accession of Menes and beginning of dynasties	3400
FIRST AND SECOND DYNASTIES	3400–2980

Eighteen kings, 420 years, ruling at Thinis. Tombs in Abydos and vicinity. Wars with Libyans, with Beduin of East, with Delta. Mining in Sinai. Stone masonry and arch introduced. (Recent investigations would indicate that we may possibly have to push back the beginning of the First Dynasty a number of centuries, possibly even before 4000 B.C.)

OLD KINGDOM—2980–2475 B.C.

THIRD DYNASTY	2980–2900

Zoser to Snefru, 80 years, ruling at Memphis. Zoser builds terraced pyramid of Sakkara, the oldest existing large stone building; continues mining in Sinai; wise man Imhotep. Snefru builds first real pyramids: one at Medûm, another at Dahshur; sends fleet to Lebanon (earliest known sea voyage and expedition into Syria in history); continues mining in Sinai.

FOURTH DYNASTY (Memphis), 150 years	2900–2750

Pyramids at Gizeh and Abu Roash.

1. Khufu, 23 years	2900–2877

Great Pyramid of Gizeh. Highest prosperity of Old Kingdom.

2. Dedefre, 8 years	2877–2869
3. Khafre, x years. Second Pyramid of Gizeh 4. Menkure, x years. Third Pyramid of Gizeh	2869–2774
5. ......, x years.	
6. ......, 18 years	2774–2756

[1] From J. H. Breasted's *A History of the Ancient Egyptians* (1920).

APPENDIX

	B.C.
7. Shepseskaf, 4 years	2756–2752
8. ......, 2 years	2752–2750

Triumph of Heliopolis and solar theology (2750).

FIFTH DYNASTY, Memphis, 125 years 2750–2625
Offices become hereditary. Pyramids at Abu Sir and Sakkara.
1. Userkaf, 7 years .... about 2750–2743
   First Pharaoh recorded at First Cataract.
2. Sahure, 12 years .... about 2743–2731
   Mining in Sinai. First expedition to Punt (Ophir). Naval expedition to Phoenicia. Earliest colonnades.
3. Neferirkere, x years ⎫
4. Shepseskere, 7 years ⎬ 2731–2721
5. Khaneferre, x years ⎭
6. Nuserve, 30 years 2721–2691
7. Menkuhor, 8 years 2691–2683
8. Dedkere-Isesi, 28 years 2683–2655
   First Pharaoh recorded at Hammamât. Second expedition to Punt.
9. Unis, 30 (+x) years 2655–2625
   Earliest Pyramid Texts.

SIXTH DYNASTY, Memphis, 150 years 2625–2475
Pyramids at Sakkara. Appearance of landed nobles detached from court.
1. Teti II, x years ⎫ 2625–2590
2. Userker, x years ⎭
3. Pepi I, 20 years 2590–2570
   Residence now first called Memphis. Five primitive expeditions into Sinai. Earliest expedition into Palestine in history. Control of Northern Nubia. Nubian mercenaries common in Egyptian army.
4. Mernere I, 4 years 2570–2566
   Canal in First Cataract. Pharaoh receives homage of Nubian chiefs at First Cataract. Harkhuf's trading expeditions to far south, Yam, and the Sudan—earliest expeditions into inner Africa.
5. Pepi II, 90 (+x) years (longest reign in history) 2566–2476
   Harkuf's trading expeditions in Sudan continue. Mekhu and Sebui's expeditions in Sudan. Campaigns in Northern Nubia. Loose sovereignty in Northern Nubia. Expeditions to Punt (Ophir) common. Commerce with Lebanon and Aegean. Decline of Memphis.
6. Mernere II, 1 year 2476–2475
   Fall of Old Kingdom.

                                                                    B.C.
SEVENTH AND EIGHTH DYNASTIES. Known total 30 years...... 2475-2445
    Collapse of Memphis.

NINTH AND TENTH DYNASTIES, Heracleopolis, estimated 285 years. 2445-2160
    Eighteen feeble kings residing at Heracleopolis. Rise of Thebes
    under Intefs. Struggle with Thebes; tombs at Siut; fall of
    Heracleopolis; triumph of Thebes.

MIDDLE KINGDOM, 2160-1788 B.C.

ELEVENTH DYNASTY, Thebes, 160 years...................... 2160-*2000
    Pyramids at Thebes.
  1. Horus Wahenekh-Intef, 50 (+x) years.
      Tomb at Thebes.
  2. Horus Nakhtneb-Tepnefer-Intef, x years.
  3. Horus Senekhibtowe-Mentuhotep, x years.
  4. Nibhapetre-Mentuhotep, x years.
      Tomb at Thebes.
  5. Nibtowere-Mentuhotep, 2 (+x) years.
      Expedition to Hammamât.
  6. Nibhepetre-Mentuhotep, 46 (+x) years.
      Expedition against Nubia. Earliest temple at Thebes.
  7. Senekhkere-Mentuhotep, 8 (+x) years.
      Expedition to Hammamât and Punt.

TWELFTH DYNASTY, Thebans, 213 years..................... *2000-*1788
    Residence at Lisht and in Fayum.
  1. Amenemhet I, 30 years................................. *2000-*1970
      Feudal organization perfected; great prosperity. Sesostris I,
      10 years coregent (1980-1970). Expedition into Wawat
      (1971). Canal connecting Nile and Red Sea; frequent
      intercourse with Syria; Egyptians in Syria. Pyramid at
      Lisht.
  2. Sesostris I, 45 years.................................. *1980-*1935
      Ten years coregent with Amenemhet I. Nubian conquest
      carried into Kush—first foreign campaign led by a Pharaoh
      personally. Amenemhet II, 3 years coregent. Pyramid
      at Lisht.
  3. Amenemhet II, 35 years................................ *1938-*1903
      Three years coregent with Sesostris I; expeditions to Sinai,
      Nubian mines, Punt. Three years coregent with Sesostris
      II. Pyramid at Dahshur.
  4. Sesostris II, 19 years.................................. *1906-*1887
      Three years coregent with Amenemhet II. Traffic with
      Punt. Pyramid at Illahun.

APPENDIX

B.C.

5. Sesostris III, 38 years..................................*1887-*1849
    New canal through First Cataract. Subjugation of Lower Nubia to Second Cataract complete. Expeditions thither in years 8, 12, 16, 19. Southern frontier established at Semneh in year 8 (1879). First campaign of Middle Kingdom in Syria. Semitic traders in Egypt. Monuments of Egyptian officials in Gezer (Palestine). Commerce with Aegean. Nomarchs decline. Oldest known drama; strophic poetry; tales. "Messianic" prophecy, earliest Book of the Dead. Coregency with son. Pyramid at Dahshur.
6. Amenemhet III, 48 years..............................*1849-*1801
    Coregency with father. Great development of resources; nomarchs suppressed; activity in Sinai; regulation of Nile and irrigation; Lake Moeris; Fayum exploited; Labyrinth. Pyramid at Dahshur, possibly also at Hawara.
7. Amenemhet IV, 9 years................................*1801-*1792
    Decline of Middle Kingdom.
8. Sebeknefrure (queen), 4 years.........................*1792-*1788
    Fall of Middle Kingdom.

THIRTEENTH TO SEVENTEENTH DYNASTIES, 208 years........... *1788-1580
    Great confusion, usurpation, civil war. Hyksos rule about 100 years (1675-1575?). Horse introduced. Sekenenre king at Thebes, mummy in Cairo.

EMPIRE, FIRST PERIOD, 1580-1350 B.C.

EIGHTEENTH DYNASTY, Thebes, 230 years.................... 1580-1350
1. Ahmose I, 22 (+x) years.............................. 1580-*1557
    Expulsion of Hyksos by 1580. Extermination of landed nobles; lands revert to crown. First standing army; military state organized. Campaign in Syria. Tomb at Thebes; mummy at Cairo.
2. Amenhotep I, 10 (+x) years.
    Campaign in Syria; against Libyans. Tomb at Thebes; mummy at Cairo.
3. Thutmose I, 30 (+x) years. }*1557-*1501
    Conquest of Kush to above Third Cataract. Conquest of Syria, tablet of victory on Upper Euphrates.
4-5. Thutmose III, including Thutmose II and Hatshepsut, 54 years..*1501-*1447
    Accession of Thutmose III and Hatshepsut, May 3, 1501. Feuds in royal family. Coregents supplanted about 1496 by

B.C.

6. Thutmose II, about 3 years......................about 1496–1493
   Expedition against Nubia. Accepts coregency of Thutmose III. Mummy at Cairo. Succeeded by

4–5. Thutmose III and Hatshepsut.......................... 1493–1480
   Splendid buildings and expedition to Punt by queen. She dies 1481 (1470). Tomb at Thebes.

4. Thutmose III alone, 33 years........................... *1479–*1447
   Seventeen campaigns in Asia (1479–1459). Asiatic empire consolidated; frontier established on Upper Euphrates. Egyptian fleet developed. Empire organized from Euphrates to Fourth Cataract. First great empire in history. Great buildings; vast wealth. Son made coregent (1448). King dies, March 17, 1447. Tomb at Thebes; mummy at Cairo.

7. Amenhotep II, 26 (+x) years........................... *1448–1420
   Coregent with father. Campaign to Euphrates; to Napata. Empire maintained. Mummy still in tomb at Thebes.

8. Thutmose IV, 8 (+x) years............................. 1420–1411
   Campaign in Asia; in Nubia. Asks and secures Mitannian princess in marriage. Tomb at Thebes; mummy at Cairo.

9. Amenhotep III, 36 years............................... 1411–1375
   Greatest splendor of the empire. Imperial Thebes; vast temples; clear-story architecture evolved. Campaign in Nubia. Amarna Letters. Pharaoh marries Mitannian princess Gilukhipa. Cyprus vassal kingdom. Hittites seize Pharaoh's north Syrian dependencies; Khabiri Semites begin migration into Syria and Palestine. Decline of empire. Commerce with Babylonia, Syria, Aegean; Egyptian monuments in Crete and Mycenae. Tomb at Thebes; mummy at Cairo.

10. Ikhnaton (Amenhotep IV), 17 (+x) years................ 1375–1358
    Introduction of earliest monotheism. Religious revolution. Thebes forsaken, Amarna, and Amarna Letters. Hittites seize Syria to Amor. Khabiri Semites invade Palestine, Hebrews with them. Complete dissolution of Egyptian Empire in Asia. Tomb at Amarna. Fall of Eighteenth Dynasty. Disorganization.

11. Sakere, x years.
12. Tutenkhamon, x years.
    Return to Thebes, Amon partially restored. }........... 1358–1350
13. Eye, 3+x years.
    End of empire, first period (1350).

APPENDIX 363

B.C.
EMPIRE, SECOND PERIOD, 1350 TO ABOUT 1150 B.C.

NINETEENTH DYNASTY, City of Ramses, 145 years.............. 1350–1205
1. Harmhab, 34 (+x) years...........................about 1350–1315
   Restoration of traditional religion; triumph of Amon. Reorganization of government; Thebes restored. Campaign in Nubia.
2. Ramses I, 2 years................................about 1315–1314
   Great Hall of Karnak begun.
3. Seti I, 21 (+x) years............................about 1313–1292
   Palestine recovered; first conflict with Hittites. Campaign against Libyans. Great Karnak Hall continued. Nubian gold mines exploited. Tomb at Thebes; mummy at Cairo.
4. Ramses II, 67 years..............................about 1292–1225
   Nubian gold mines exploited. Asiatic war, chiefly with Hittites (1288–1271). Penetrates to North Syria, but Syria not recovered. Treaty with Hittites (1271). Great Karnak Hall completed; immense buildings everywhere. Decay of art and architecture begin. Hebrew oppression (?). Semitic influences. Libyan aggression. Tomb at Thebes; mummy at Cairo.
5. Merneptah, 10 (+x) years.........................about 1225–1215
   Asiatic campaign, "Israel" among defeated, year 3. Libyans and northern allies defeated in Delta, year 5. Tomb at Thebes; mummy at Cairo.
6. Amenmeses, x years...............................about 1215
   Tomb at Thebes.
7. Siptah, 6 (+x) years.............................about 1215–1209
   Tomb at Thebes.
8. Seti II, 2 (+x) years............................about 1209–1205
   Exodus of Jacob tribesmen (?). Tomb at Thebes; mummy at Cairo.

Complete anarchy and Syrian usurper..................about 1205–1200

TWENTIETH DYNASTY, City of Ramses, 110 years.............. 1200–1190
1. Setnakht, 1 (+x) years..........................about 1200–1198
   Order restored. Tomb at Thebes; mummy at Cairo.
2. Ramses III, 31 years............................about 1198–1167
   First War: Defeat of Libyans and northern "sea peoples" in western Delta, year 5 (about 1193). Second War: Defeat of northern "sea peoples" in Syria, year 8 (about 1190). Third War: Second defeat of Libyans and "sea peoples" in western Delta, year 11 (about 1187). Fourth

War: Campaign in Amor (about 1185). Increase of mercenaries in army. Increasing power of Amon. General decline. Tomb at Thebes; mummy at Cairo.

		B.C.
3. Ramses IV, 6 years................................about		1167–1161

Tomb at Thebes; mummy at Cairo.

4. Ramses V, 4 (+x) years...........................about   1161–1157
Tomb at Thebes; mummy at Cairo.
5. Ramses VI, x years................................about   1157–1150
Tomb at Thebes; mummy at Cairo.

DECADENCE 1150–663 B.C.

6–7. Ramses VII and VIII, x years ....about   1150–1142
8. Ramses IX, 19 years...............................about   1142–1123
Decay of Thebes begins. Royal tombs robbed. Tomb at Thebes. Power of high priest of Amon rapidly increasing.
9. Ramses X, 1 (+x) years...........................about   1123–1121
Tomb at Thebes.
10. Ramses XI, x years................................about   1121–1118
Tomb at Thebes.
11. Ramses XII, 27 (+x) years.........................about   1118–1090
Pharaoh reduced to a mere puppet. Delta kingdom founded at Tanis by Nesubenebded (Smendes). Sends gift to Tiglath-pileser I (?). High priest of Amon, Hrihor, seizes throne at Thebes. Pharaoh's tomb at Thebes.

TANITE-AMONITE PERIOD, 1090–945 B.C.

Twenty-first Dynasty, Tanis, 145 years ....about   1090–945
Libyans migrate steadily into Delta and fill army as mercenaries.
1. Nesubenebded, Tanite } x years...............about   1090–1085
2. Hrihor, high priest at Thebes
Egyptian power in Asia gone.
3. Pesibkhenno I, 17 (+x) years......................about   1085–1067
4. Paynozem I, 40 (+x) years.........................about   1067–1026
5. Amenemopet, 49 (+x) years........................about   1026–976
6. Siamon, 16 (+x) years.............................about   976–958
7. Pesibkhenno II (Psusennes), 12 (+x) years...........about   958–945
Libyans seize throne. End of Tanite-Amonite period.

LIBYAN PERIOD, 945–712, B.C.

Twenty-second Dynasty, Bubastis, 200 years..........about   945–745
1. Sheshonk I, 21 (+x) years.........................about   945–924
Campaign in Palestine; Jerusalem captured. Gezer presented to Solomon. Campaign in Nubia.

APPENDIX

	B.C.
2. Osorkon I, 36 (+x) years............about	924–895
3. Takelot I, 23 (+x) years............about	895–874
4. Osorkon II, 30 (+x) years............about	874–853
5. Sheshonk II, oo years.	

Died about 877 B.C. during coregency with Osorkon II.

6. Takelot II, 25 (+x) years............about	860–834

Probably contributed 1,000 men against Shalmaneser II at Qarqar (854). Seven years coregent with Osorkon II.

7. Sheshonk III, 52 years............about	834–784
8. Pemou, 6 (+x) years............about	784–782
9. Sheshonk IV, 37 (+x) years............about	782–745

Rise of independent kingdom in Nubia.

TWENTY-THIRD DYNASTY, Bubastis, 27 years............about	745–718
1. Pedibast, 23 (+x) years............about	745–721

NUBIAN PERIOD, 722–661 B.C.

2. Osorkon III, 14 (+x) years............about	720–718

Conquest of Piankhi. Tefnakhte of Sais.

3. Takelot III, x years.

TWENTY-FOURTH DYNASTY, Sais, 6 years............about	718–712

Bekneranef (Bocchoris), 6 (+x) years. Slain by Shabaka.

TWENTY-FIFTH DYNASTY, Napata, 50 years............	712–663
1. Shabaka, 12 years............	712–700

Gains all Egypt. Incites revolt in Syria and Palestine against Sargon. Aegypto-Nubians under Taharka defeated by Sennacherib at Altaqu (701).

2. Shabataka, 12 years............	700–688
3. Tabarka (Tirhaka), 26 years............	688–663

Defeats Esarhaddon (673).

Assyrian Supremacy............	670–660

Taharka defeated by Esarhaddon; Memphis taken by Assyrians; Delta becomes Assyrian province (670). Delta rebels; Ashurbanipal retakes Memphis (668–666). Taharka retires to Napata.

4. Tanutamon............	663–655

Nubians resume control of Delta (663). Rise of Psamtik of Sais. Beginning of Twenty-sixth Dynasty (663). Nubians expelled by Ashurbanipal; Thebes plundered (661). Nubians return to Thebes and hold Upper Egypt (661–655); Nubian rule at Thebes ended by 654.

	B.C.
TWENTY-SIXTH DYNASTY, Sais, 138 years	663–525
1. Psamtik I (Psammeticus), 54 years	663–609

Several years under Assyrians.

RESTORATION, 660–525 B.C.

Alliance with Gyges of Lydia. Thebes gained (by 654). Renaissance in art, religion, literature, and government. Archaizing, retrospective age. Great prosperity.

2. Necho, 16 years	609–593

Invades Palestine; defeats Josiah; advances to Euphrates. Defeated at Carchemish by Nebuchadrezzar (605). Egypt again loses Syria, Palestine. Circumnavigation of Africa.

3. Psamtik II, 5 years	593–588

Campaign in Nubia.

4. Apries (Hophra), 19 years	588–569

Egyptian fleet developed. Phoenician coast taken. Unsuccessful invasion of Palestine against Nebuchadrezzar (586).

5. Amasis (Ahmose II), 44 years	569–525

Nebuchadrezzar attempts invasion of Egypt (568). Death of Apries (567 or 566). Alliance with Polycrates of Samos. Greeks numerous in Egypt; Naucratis built. Great prosperity. Egyptian navy greatly increased; Cyprus tributary. Alliance with Babylonia, Lydia (Croesus), and Sparta against Cyrus (547).

6. Psamtik III, a few months	525

Conquest of Egypt by Cambyses, the Persian. Egypt becomes a Persian province.

INDEX

INDEX

Aahmes, Queen, 356
Aahotep I, Queen, 325
Abnormalities of teeth, 268-321
Abou Menas, 236
Abscesses, alveolar, in ancient Egyptians, 123, 146, 301
Acetabulum, 179
Achondroplasia, 37, 46
Adipocere, 62
Ahmose I, 325
Akhnaton, 330, 333, 336
Alcohol, 29
Alexander the Great, 94, 104, 341
Alexandria, 63, 94, 141, 276
Alexandria Museum, 94, 139
Alveolar abscesses, 146, 161
Amenhotep I, 327
Amenhotep II, 171, 172, 174
Amenhotep III, 168, 170, 177, 178
Amenhotep IV, 337
Amon, the god, 329
Amset, the human-headed, 58
Amulets, 195
Anhapon, Queen, 174
Anomalies of teeth, 273, 279
Anthracosis, 15
Antinoë, 139, 152, 240, 300
Aorta: calcified, 23; of King Merneptah, 20
Archaeological Survey of Nubia, 1, 93, 272
Arsinoë I, Queen, 343
Arteries: diseases of, 13, 20; histology of, 13, 74; lesions of, 13, 20; method of isolating, 22
Arteriosclerosis: 13; in the aorta of King Merneptah, 20
Arthritis: 96, 164, 184, 212; deformans, 100, 119, 212-67
Ashmolean Museum, 49
Assuan dam, 50, 93, 225
Atheroma, 27
Atrophy, 17, 219
Attrition of teeth, 159, 283
Auletes, 351

Bacteria, 6, 16, 33, 176
Baldness, 173
Bandages, 128, 177
Baudouin, Professor Marcel, 185, 194, 307
Beni-Hassan, tombs of, 47, 49, 210
Bes, the god, 47
Bilharzia hematobia, 17, 18
Biliary calculi, 50
Bitumen, 21, 54
Blackheads, 173
Bladder, 59
Blood, 56
Blood vessels, histological examination of, 24
Bos primigenius, 188
Bouchard's nodosities, 104, 132
Brain, 141
Breasted, Professor J. H., 37, 272
Breccia, Professor E., 3, 94, 139, 229, 270
Broca, Paul, 46, 199
Bronze period, 185, 198

Cairo Medical School, 56, 83
Cairo Museum, 32, 38, 44, 66, 166
Caithness, prehistoric remains at, showing pathology, 185
Calcification of arteries, 25
Calculi: biliary, 50; urinary, 11
Caries: 144, 161, 291; distribution of, in ancient times, 292
Cave bear, 187
Chatby, 94, 104, 270
Chnoum-hotep, the dwarf, 37, 38, 48
Chronological table of kings, 358
Chronology, 272
Cleopatra Thea, 347
Cleopatra III, 348
Cleopatra VII, the Great, 352
Clubfoot, 42, 49, 178
Cocheral, 195
Coptic bodies, lesions in, 96, 114, 139, 241
Copts, 21, 96, 300
Corpuscles, absence of blood, 28, 56
Coxa vara, 216, 257

369

INDEX

Crocodile, spondylitis in Miocene, 184
Cuvier, 196
Cynocephalus, 188

Darwin, Charles, 124
Darwin, George, 322
Dead, methods of preserving the, 56, 140
Decalcification, 22, 113
Deformed persons, 35, 42, 49
Delta of the Nile, 226
Dental: abscesses, 146; anomalies, 273; lesions, 268
Dentistry, absence of, in ancient Egypt, 123, 314
Desiccation, 88
Diastemae in ancient Nubians, 277
Diodorus Siculus, 52, 324
Dwarfs, 35–48

Embalming: 51–56, 127; incisions in, 56, 134; materials, 59–61, 127
Embolism, 27
Exostoses, 100

Faras, 156, 229, 308
Fayoum Pyramid, 98, 223
Ferguson, A. R., 32
Food of ancient Egyptians, 30, 124, 288
Fouquet, Dr., 3, 54, 55, 93, 224
Fractures, 96, 157, 162

Gavial, spondylitis deformans in Miocene, 184
Greek period, diseases of, 20, 55, 120, 228

Haemoglobin, 61
Hatshepsut I, Queen, 328
Hearst Expedition of the University of California, 66, 269
Heart, histological examination of the, 76, 141
Heliopolis, 303
Heredity, 322
Hernia, 172
Herodotus, 51
Histology, 1, 11, 32, 49
Hunchbacks, 35, 48, 49
Hydrocephalus, 170
Hyksos, 171, 326
Hypertrophy, 150

Idiocy, 322
Ikhnaton, 168
Insects, 99
Intestines: histological examination of, 83; methods of preservation of, 58

Jones, Dr. F. Wood, 3, 117, 216, 257

Kabyl tribes, 201
Kabylia, 201, 202
Kawamil, 224
Khebsennuf, 58
Kidneys: histological examination of, 17, 19, 81; method of preservation of, 57
Kjoekken-moeddings, 224
Kom el Shougafa, 179, 215, 232, 236, 372

Le Baron, J., 185
Lesions, osteo-arthritic, 185
Liver: histological examination of, 12, 77; method of preservation of, 58, 142
Looss, Professor, 50
Lordosis, 39, 45
Lortet, Professor, 3, 188
Lozère, 196
Lucas-Championnière, 199–206
Lumbago, 213
Lungs, histological examination of, 15, 79, 141

Malaria, 151
Malposition of teeth, 158
Mammary glands, 86
Mandible, 122
Marriages, consanguineous, physical effects of, 322
Maspero, Sir Gaston, 14, 46, 165
Merawi, 156, 229, 287
Meritamon, Princess, 177
Merneptah, King, 167, 172, 173, 338
Method, in technique, 1, 63
Methods of preservation, 59
Miocene, pathological vertebrae from the, 184
Monkeys, spondylitis deformans in ancient sacred, 188
Mummery, J. R., 268
Mummies: histology of, 1, 15, 49–92; microscopic examination of, 1, 11, 20; royal, 166

INDEX

Mummification, 20, 32
Muscles, histological examination of, 70
Myrrha, on marriage, 323

Nails, method of preservation of, 66, 70
Natron, 51, 60
Nefer, teeth of Queen, 276
Nefermaat, 96, 238
Nefertari, Queen, 326
Neolithic trephining, 195
Nerves, histological examination of, 72
New Caledonia, 209
Nibsoni, 172
Nodules of ancient teeth, 281
Nofritari, Queen, 173
Notmit, Queen, 173
Nubia, 118, 156, 245, 328

Obesity, 167, 170
Ossarium of Sedec, 198
Osseous lesions in ancient Egyptians, 93–126, 147–50
Osteo-arthritic lesions, 212–67
Osteomyelitis, 163
Osteophytes, 212–67
Osteosarcoma, 179
Ovary, 143
Overbites in ancient Egyptians, 279

Palaeopathology, definition of, 139
Papyrus, Berlin medical, 49
Papyrus, Ebers, 49
Paralysis, facial, 49
Pathological anatomy, 11, 166
Penis, 59
Periarthritis, 189
Periodontitis, 161, 304, 306, 312
Peroneal artery, atheroma in, 25
Persian occupation, 102, 127
Petrie, Professor Flinders, 11, 17, 40, 49, 54, 96, 223
Pettigrew, 53
Phtah, the god, 47
Poncet, Professor, 3
Pott's disease, 3, 42
Predynastic mummies, 12
Priest of Amon, 3, 54, 167
Prunière, 3, 196
Psoas abscess, 3

Ptolemaic kings, 341
Ptolemy I, 93, 341
Ptolemy II, 343
Ptolemy III, 344
Ptolemy IV, 345
Ptolemy V, 346
Ptolemy VI, 346
Ptolemy VII, 346
Ptolemy IX, 346
Punt, Queen of, 44, 48
Pyorrhoea alveolaris, 177, 214, 307
Pyorrhoea marginalis, 306

Ramses II, 172, 173, 337
Ramses III, 167
Ramses V, 172, 175
Ranefer, liver of, 12
Ras el Tin, 215, 233, 279
Raymonden, 184
Rhinoceros, pathology in Miocene, 189
Rickets, 43, 47, 49, 313
Rietti, Arnoldo, 93, 186
Roman cemetery, 179
Roman period, 113, 123
Rondelles, 195
Royal mummies, pathology of the, 166–76

Saknounrâ Tionâken, 171
Salt, 59, 60, 141
Sarcolemma, 71
Sawdust, 59
Schmidt, Professor, 56, 60, 61
Sciatica, 213
Scrotum, 59
Seti I, 172, 290, 337
Shattock, Mr., 20
Shellal, 225
Simpson, Hilton, 206–10
Sinai, Desert of, 88
Siptah, 178
Skin, 32, 66, 175
Skin, histological examination of, 66
Smallpox, 32, 175
Smith, Professor G. Elliot, 3, 11, 32, 50, 100, 165, 170, 172, 268
Solutrean period, 187
Spleen: 143; hypertrophy of, 150
Spondylitis deformans: 96, 163, 184, 188, 212–67; in sacred sheep, 188

INDEX

Steatopygia, 45, 49
Stomach, 85
Sudan, 156
Surgery, prehistoric, 195
Sweat glands, 68
Syphilis, 29, 94, 158, 313

Talipes equino-varus, 42, 48, 178
Teeth: condition of, 120, 131; diseases of, 120, 268; lesions of, 144, 177
Testicles, 85
Thutmose I, 328
Thutmose II, 167, 172, 174, 328
Thutmose III, 172, 174, 329, 330
Thutmose IV, 331
Tiaa, Queen, 331
Tiy, Queen, 332
Tobacco, 29
Tourah, 226, 303
Trepanations, multiple, 195, 197
Trepanning, 194

Trephining: 194; absence of, in Egypt, 200; prehistoric, 195
Tuamantef, the jackal-headed, 80
Tuberculosis of the spine, 3, 42
Tumor of the pelvis, 179

Ulcers, 174
Urinary calculi, 11
Ursus spelaeus, 187

Variola, 32, 175
Veddahs of Ceylon, 322
Virchow on pathology of cave bears, 187
Viscera, 83

Wainwright, Gerald, 96
Walther, Ph. von, 187
Wear of teeth, 159, 282
Willmore, Dr. J. G., 179, 212, 243, 257, 268
Wormian bones, 158

Lightning Source UK Ltd.
Milton Keynes UK
UKHW021834120419
340955UK00021B/444/P